Architectural Epidemiology

ARCHITECTURAL
Epidemiology

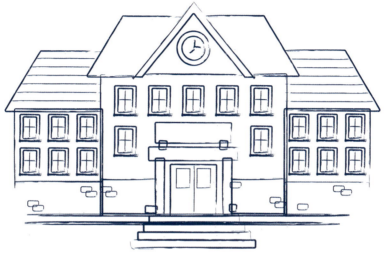

Architecture as a Mechanism for Designing a
Healthier, More **Sustainable**, and **Resilient** World

Adele Houghton
FAIA, DrPH, LEED AP

Carlos Castillo-Salgado
MD, JD, MPH, DrPH

JOHNS HOPKINS UNIVERSITY PRESS
Baltimore

© 2025 Johns Hopkins University Press
All rights reserved. Published 2025
Printed in the United States of America on acid-free paper
9 8 7 6 5 4 3 2 1

Johns Hopkins University Press
2715 North Charles Street
Baltimore, Maryland 21218
www.press.jhu.edu

Library of Congress Cataloging-in-Publication Data

Names: Houghton, Adele, 1977– author. | Castillo-Salgado, Carlos, 1950– author.
Title: Architectural epidemiology : architecture as a mechanism for designing
   a healthier, more sustainable, and resilient world / Adele Houghton and Carlos
   Castillo-Salgado.
Description: Baltimore : Johns Hopkins University Press, [2025] | Includes bibliographical
   references and index.
Identifiers: LCCN 2024021303 | ISBN 9781421450698 (paperback) | ISBN 9781421450704
   (ebook)
Subjects: MESH: Built Environment | Architecture--methods | Epidemiologic Methods
Classification: LCC HC79.E5 | NLM HC 79.E5 | DDC 338.9/27—dc23/eng/20241204
LC record available at https://lccn.loc.gov/2024021303

A catalog record for this book is available from the British Library.

Special discounts are available for bulk purchases of this book. For more information, please contact Special Sales at specialsales@jh.edu.

EU GPSR Authorized Representative
LOGOS EUROPE, 9 rue Nicolas Poussin, 17000, La Rochelle, France
E-mail: Contact@logoseurope.eu

Contents

List of Figures, Diagrams, Boxes, and Tables — vii
Advice for Using This Book — xiii
Online Supplement — xv
Acknowledgments — xvii

Introduction — 1

0.1 Why Do We Need Architectural Epidemiology? — 1
0.2 Our Stories — 2
0.3 How Do We Know the Current System Is Not Working? — 4
0.4 Defining Aspects of Architectural Epidemiology — 4
0.5 How to Use This Book — 16

Chapter 1. An Introduction to Architectural Epidemiology — 19

1.1 Introduction — 19
1.2 A Brief History of Epidemiology's Roots in the Built Environment — 23
1.3 Links between Health and the Built Environment — 24
1.4 Five Myths About Health Data and Design — 28
1.5 The Value Proposition for Architectural Epidemiology — 34
1.6 Why Isn't Architectural Epidemiology Already Standard Practice? — 38
1.7 Summary — 39

Chapter 2. Introduction to Metrics for Built Environment Professionals — 41

2.1 Introduction — 41
2.2 Step 1—Defining the Problem — 43
2.3 Step 2—Measuring the Magnitude of the Problem — 48
2.4 Step 3—Understanding the Key Factors (or Determinants) of Health — 54
2.5 Step 4—Identifying and Developing Evidence-Based Strategies to Prevent and/or Mitigate the Problem — 66
2.6 Step 5—Prioritizing and Recommending the Most Effective Policies and Strategies — 69
2.7 Step 6—Implementing and Evaluating Interventions — 70
2.8 Conclusion — 77

Architectural Epidemiology Toolbox — 79

Introduction — 79
Health Effects of Community Health Conditions — 79
T.1 Toolbox—Community Health Conditions: Cardiovascular Disease — 82
T.2 Toolbox—Community Health Conditions: Respiratory Disease — 89
T.3 Toolbox—Community Health Conditions: Obesity, Diabetes, and Hypertension — 97
T.4 Toolbox—Community Health Conditions: Cancer — 106
T.5 Toolbox—Community Health Conditions: Mental Health — 114
Health Effects of Climate Change — 123
T.6 Toolbox—Health Effects of Climate Change: Extreme Heat — 124
T.7 Toolbox—Health Effects of Climate Change: Flooding — 129
T.8 Toolbox—Health Effects of Climate Change: Air Quality — 141
T.9 Toolbox—Health Effects of Climate Change: Disasters — 148
T.10 Toolbox—Health Effects of Climate Change: Vector-Borne Disease — 157
Toolbox Crosswalk — 167

Chapter 3. Architectural Epidemiology at Each Phase of the Project Delivery Process — 173

3.1 Introduction — 173
3.2 Phase 1—Programming/Visioning — 174
3.3 Phase 2—Schematic Design — 195
3.4 Phase 3—Design Development — 202
3.5 Phase 4—Construction Documents — 206

3.6 Phase 5—Construction Administration	209
3.7 Phase 6—Occupancy	215
3.8 Summary	219

Chapter 4. Applying Architectural Epidemiology to Different Contract and Financing Structures — 221

4.1 Introduction	221
4.2 Architectural Epidemiology and Project Delivery Models	221
4.3 Architectural Epidemiology and Real Estate Investment Models	230
4.4 Scale of Development	255
4.5 Summary	264

Chapter 5. Looking Ahead to the Future of Architectural Epidemiology — 265

5.1 Introduction	265
5.2 What Will It Take to Turn a Ripple into a Wave?	267
5.3 Envisioning a Research Agenda for Architectural Epidemiology	268
5.4 Closing Thoughts	270

Glossary	273
Index	275

Figures, Diagrams, Boxes, and Tables

Figures

5   Figure 0.1. LEED Projects Are Clustered in Low-Risk Neighborhoods and Nearly Absent from High-Risk Neighborhoods

12 Figure 0.2. Harvard Case Study 01—Air Pollution Analysis: Proposed Carbon Offset Program

14 Figure 0.3. Harvard Case Study 02—Air Pollution Analysis: Proposed Gund Hall Renovation

21 Figure 1.1. Architectural Epidemiology Conceptual Diagram

22 Figure 1.2. Green and Healthy Building Approaches Used by Architectural Epidemiology Organized by Spatial Scale and Relevant Project Delivery Phases

25 Figure 1.3. Timeline of Major Trends Linking Public Health and the Built Environment from the 18th Century to the Present

26 Figure 1.4. Baseline Contextual Health Assessment for Bruce Elementary School Houston, Texas, USA

27 Figure 1.5. Health Impact Pyramid

28 Figure 1.6. Hierarchy of Controls: COVID-19 Example

47 Figure 2.1. Potential Health Impacts of the North Houston Highway Improvement Project on Schools Mediated through Mobility, Air Pollution, and Flooding

51 Figure 2.2. Whole Foods Market in Houston Provides Access to Anyone Seeking Free Water and a Cool Place to Sit on Hot Days

53 Figure 2.3. Standard Hierarchy of Census Geographic Entities

64 Figure 2.4. Visual Comparison of the Percentages of Public Schools in Colorado and Florida, USA, Located within 150 m of a Highway, 2010–2011

65 Figure 2.5. Using Buffering, Point Data, and Photographs to Visualize the Connections between the Environment and Malaria Prevalence in Costa Rica

80 Figure T.1. Example of Co-Impact Pathways Linking Selected Building Design and Operations Strategies with COVID-19, Climate Change, and Health Equity Desired Outcomes

84 Toolbox Infographic T.1. Linkages among Cardiovascular Disease, the Built Environment Determinants of Health, Protective Design and Operations Strategies, the Groups Who Are at Highest Risk, and Related Negative Health Outcomes

90 Toolbox Infographic T.2. Linkages among Respiratory Disease, the Built Environment Determinants of Health, Protective Design and Operations Strategies, the Groups Who Are at Highest Risk, and Related Negative Health Outcomes

98 Toolbox Infographic T.3. Linkages among Obesity, Diabetes, and Hypertension; the Built Environment Determinants of Health; Protective Design and Operations Strategies; the Groups Who Are at Highest Risk; and Related Negative Health Outcomes

108 Toolbox Infographic T.4. Linkages among Cancer, the Built Environment Determinants of Health, Protective Design and Operations Strategies, the Groups Who Are at Highest Risk, and Related Negative Health Outcomes

116 Toolbox Infographic T.5. Linkages among Mental Health, the Built Environment Determinants of Health, Protective Design and Operations Strategies, the Groups Who Are at Highest Risk, and Related Negative Health Outcomes

126 Toolbox Infographic T.6. Linkages among Extreme Heat, the Built Environment Determinants of Health, Protective Design and Operations Strategies, the Groups Who Are at Highest Risk, and Related Negative Health Outcomes

130 Toolbox Infographic T.7. Linkages among Flooding, the Built Environment Determinants of Health, Protective Design and Operations Strategies, the Groups Who Are at Highest Risk, and Related Negative Health Outcomes

135 Figure T.2. Historical Climate Trends for Precipitation and Air Temperature in Western Kentucky, USA: Annual and Spring Months

142 Toolbox Infographic T.8. Linkages among Air Quality, the Built Environment Determinants of Health, Protective Design and Operations Strategies, the Groups Who Are at Highest Risk, and Related Negative Health Outcomes

145 Figure T.3. Distance-Decay Gradients of Ultrafine Particulate Matter Near a Busy Expressway in Toronto, Ontario, Canada, Compared with NO_2 and $PM_{2.5}$

150 Toolbox Infographic T.9. Linkages among Disasters, the Built Environment Determinants of Health, Protective Design and Operations Strategies, the Groups Who Are at Highest Risk, and Related Negative Health Outcomes

158 Toolbox Infographic T.10. Linkages among Vector-Borne Disease, the Built Environment Determinants of Health, Protective Design and Operations Strategies, the Groups Who Are at Highest Risk, and Related Negative Health Outcomes

168 Figure T.4. Health-Promoting Green and Healthy Building Strategies Cross-Tabulated by Climate Change and Community Health Categories

179 Figure 3.1. Rendering of the Peninsula Redevelopment, South Bronx, New York City, New York, USA

181 Figure 3.2. Hunts Point Redevelopment Project Map, South Bronx, New York City, New York, USA

182 Figure 3.3. Gillett Square, London, UK

185 Figure 3.4. Diagram of Breathe-Easy Home

187 Figure 3.5. Pocket Park in High Point Neighborhood, Seattle, Washington, USA

188 Figure 3.6. Bon Pastor Redevelopment and SUDS Network, Barcelona, Spain

190 Figure 3.7. New Apartment Buildings and SUDS Installation in Bon Pastor Neighborhood, Barcelona, Spain

196 Figure 3.8. The Family Health Center on Virginia, McKinney, Texas, USA

198 Figure 3.9. Jack London Gateway Senior Housing, West Oakland, California, USA

200 Figure 3.10. Aerotropolis Atlanta, Atlanta, Georgia, USA

203 Figure 3.11. Data Mapping between BIM (ArchiCAD Software) and Energy (Energy Plus Software) Models for the NASA Sustainability Base Project at the Ames Research Center, Moffet Field, California, USA

204 Figure 3.12. Data Flow for Automatic Calculation of LEED Indoor Air Quality—Ventilation Prerequisite and Credit, Bulgari Factory, Valenza, Italy

207 Figure 3.13. Plan of a Classroom Cluster Maximizing Natural Ventilation and Daylighting, St. Antony's School, Gudalur, Tamil Nadu, India

207 Figure 3.14. Perspective View of Classroom Cluster, St. Antony's School, Gudalur, Tamil Nadu, India

210 Figure 3.15. View of Exterior Stairs at Via Verde, South Bronx, New York City, New York, USA

212 Figure 3.16. The Technological and Higher Education Institute Chai Wan Campus, Hong Kong, China, South-Facing Façade Showing Daylighting, Natural Ventilation, and Noise Pollution Design Elements

213 Figure 3.17. Project Rendering of The Technological and Higher Education Institute Chai Wan Campus, Hong Kong, China, and Aerial Photo of the Completed Project

217 Figure 3.18. Erosion in the "Shopping Park" Social Housing Development, Uberlândia, Brazil

229 Figure 4.1. Design Elements Included in Woodson Education Complex, Buckingham County, Virginia, USA, that Promote Physical Activity

232 425 Park Avenue (box 4.2)

234 Santa Monica City Hall East (box 4.3)

236 Harvard Science and Engineering Complex (box 4.4)

238 Heerema Marine Contractors B.V. (HMC) Headquarters (box 4.5)

240 Vancouver Convention Centre West (box 4.6)

242 School of Sustainable Development, Bond University (box 4.7)

246 Health and Wellness District at Frisco Station (under construction) (box 4.8)

248 Genentech Employee Center (box 4.9)

250 JLL Shanghai Office (box 4.10)

252 Floth Headquarters (box 4.11)

258 Dell Children's Hospital (box 4.12)

259 New Karolinska Solna University Hospital (box 4.13)

262 Figure 4.2. Texas Woman's University, Denton, Texas, USA, Master Plan: Health Situation Analysis

Figure A.1. Types of Buffering (online)

Figure A.2. PRISMA Flow Diagram for New Systematic Reviews which Included Searches of Databases and Registers Only (online)

Health Situation Analysis Diagrams

180 HSA 3.1. South Bronx

183 HSA 3.2. Gillett Square

186 HSA 3.3. High Point

189 HSA 3.4. Bon Pastor

197 HSA 3.5. The Family Health Center on Virginia

199 HSA 3.6. Jack London Gateway

201 HSA 3.7. Aerotropolis Atlanta

208 HSA 3.8. St. Antony's School

211 HSA 3.9. Via Verde

214 HSA 3.10. The Technological and Higher Education Institute

218 HSA 3.11. Uberlândia Housing Development

228 HSA 4.1. Buckingham County Primary and Elementary Schools

233 HSA 4.2. 425 Park Avenue

235 HSA 4.3. Santa Monica City Hall East

237 HSA 4.4. Harvard Science and Engineering Complex

239 HSA 4.5. Heerema Marine Contractors B.V. (HMC) Headquarters

241 HSA 4.6. Vancouver Convention Centre West

243 HSA 4.7. School of Sustainable Development, Bond University

247 HSA 4.8. Health and Wellness District at Frisco Station

249 HSA 4.9. Genentech Employee Center

251 HSA 4.10. JLL Shanghai Office

253 HSA 4.11. Floth Headquarters

258 HSA 4.12. Dell Children's Hospital

260 HSA 4.13. New Karolinska Solna University Hospital

Boxes

9 Box 0.1. Architectural Epidemiology in Action—Harvard University Climate Action Plan Test Case, USA

50 Box 2.1. Example—Options for Defining Extreme Heat in the US

50 Box 2.2. Example—Options for Accessing Data on Cardiovascular Disease

50 Box 2.3. Example—Environmental Determinants of Health for Extreme Heat

56 Box 2.4. Example—Health Effects of Climate Change in Rural Kentucky, USA

61 Box 2.5. Example—Health Impact Assessment of an Elementary School in Houston, Texas, USA

62 Box 2.6. Tip—Look for Existing Indices Before Starting from Scratch

64 Box 2.7. Example—Public Schools Near Highways in Colorado and Florida, USA

75 Box 2.8. Example—Comparison of Two Public Elementary Schools in Raleigh, North Carolina, USA

175 Box 3.1. Example—Environmental Exposures Shift from One Neighborhood to the Next in Phoenix, Arizona, USA

176 Box 3.2. Example—Kaiser Permanente Community Health Initiative, USA

176 Box 3.3. Example—Traffic-Related Air Pollution, Hong Kong, China

177 Box 3.4. Example—Green Alley Program, Chicago, Illinois, USA

177 Box 3.5. Example—Sanitation Options for Sustainable Housing Tool, South Africa

179 Box 3.6. Architectural Epidemiology in Action—South Bronx, New York City, New York, USA

182 Box 3.7. Architectural Epidemiology in Action—Gillett Square, London, UK

185 Box 3.8. Architectural Epidemiology in Action—High Point, Seattle, Washington, USA

188 Box 3.9. Architectural Epidemiology in Action—Bon Pastor, Barcelona, Spain

196 Box 3.10. Architectural Epidemiology in Action—The Family Health Center on Virginia, McKinney, Texas, USA

198 Box 3.11. Architectural Epidemiology in Action—Jack London Gateway, West Oakland, California, USA

200 Box 3.12. Architectural Epidemiology in Action—Aerotropolis Atlanta, Atlanta, Georgia, USA

203 Box 3.13. Example—NASA Sustainability Base, Moffet Field, California, USA

204 Box 3.14. Example—Bulgari Manufacturing Plant, Valenza, Italy

207 Box 3.15. Architectural Epidemiology in Action—St. Antony's School, Gudalur, India

210 Box 3.16. Architectural Epidemiology in Action—Via Verde, New York City, New York, USA

212 Box 3.17. Architectural Epidemiology in Action—The Technological and Higher Education Institute Chai Wan Campus, Hong Kong, China

215 Box 3.18. Example—Health Impact Assessment of Bridge Demolition, Cincinnati, Ohio, USA

215 Box 3.19. Example—Construction Air Pollution Study, Montreal, Quebec, Canada

216 Box 3.20. Example—Indoor Air Quality Study, Syracuse, New York, USA

217 Box 3.21. Architectural Epidemiology in Action—Uberlândia, Minas Gerais, Brazil

227 Box 4.1. Architectural Epidemiology in Action—Buckingham County Primary and Elementary Schools, Dillwyn, Virginia, USA

232 Box 4.2. Architectural Epidemiology in Action—425 Park Avenue, New York City, New York, USA

234 Box 4.3. Architectural Epidemiology in Action—Santa Monica City Hall East, Santa Monica, California, USA

236 Box 4.4. Architectural Epidemiology in Action—Harvard Science and Engineering Complex, Boston, Massachusetts, USA

238 Box 4.5. Architectural Epidemiology in Action—Heerema Marine Contractors B.V. Headquarters, Leiden, Netherlands

240 Box 4.6. Architectural Epidemiology in Action—Vancouver Convention Centre West, Vancouver, British Columbia, Canada

242 Box 4.7. Architectural Epidemiology in Action—School of Sustainable Development, Bond University, Robina, Queensland, Australia

246 Box 4.8. Architectural Epidemiology in Action—Health and Wellness District at Frisco Station, Texas, USA

248 Box 4.9. Architectural Epidemiology in Action—Genentech, South San Francisco, California, USA

250 Box 4.10. Architectural Epidemiology in Action—JLL Shanghai Office, Shanghai, China

252 Box 4.11. Architectural Epidemiology in Action—Floth Headquarters, Brisbane, Queensland, Australia

256 Box 4.12. Architectural Epidemiology in Action—Dell Children's Hospital, Austin, Texas, USA

259 Box 4.13. Architectural Epidemiology in Action—New Karolinska Solna University Hospital, Solna, Sweden

261 Box 4.14. Architectural Epidemiology in Action—Texas Woman's University Master Plan, Denton, Texas, USA

Box A.1. Example—Body Mass Index Z-Score Study in Boston, Massachusetts, USA (online)

Box A.2. Example—Study of Health Vulnerabilities in Travis County, Texas, USA (online)

Box A.3. Example—Global Spatial Autocorrelation Analysis of Clustering in Austin, Texas, USA, and Chicago, Illinois, USA (online)

Box A.4. Example—Hot Spot Analysis of the Relationship between Green Building Strategies in Austin, Texas, USA, and Chicago, Illinois, USA, with Extreme Heat and Flooding Vulnerability (online)

Box A.5. Example—Meta-Analysis of Association between Residential Dampness/Mold and Respiratory Disease (online)

Box A.6. Example—HIA of Frogtown Neighborhood in Saint Paul, Minnesota, USA (online)

Tables

7 Table 0.1. Professions Covered by Each Core Competency Category

10 Table 0.2. Harvard Case Study—Architectural Epidemiology Decision-Making Table for Proposed Carbon Offset Program

20 Table 1.1. Aspects of Epidemiology, Environmental Epidemiology, and Social Epidemiology That Are Deployed by Architectural Epidemiology

Page	Table
37	Table 1.2. Stakeholder Analysis of Value Generated Using Architectural Epidemiology
57	Table 2.1. Relative Vulnerability of Green River District Counties to Climate Change by Environmental Public Health Indicator
61	Table 2.2. Air Quality and Extreme Heat Metrics for Bruce Elementary School, Houston, Texas, USA
67	Table 2.3. Sample MeSH Query Terms Searching for Links between the Design and Operation of the Built Environment and Cardiovascular Disease or Air Quality
71	Table 2.4. Factors Influencing Risk Perception, Annotated with Extreme Heat Examples
75	Table 2.5. Results from Social Determinants of Health Post-Occupancy Survey of a Case Elementary School and a Matched Elementary School in the Wake County, North Carolina, USA, Public School System
82	Table T.1. Examples of the Built Environment as a "Cause of Causes" of Cardiovascular Disease, Respiratory Disease, Diabetes, Hypertension, and Obesity
83	Table T.2. Symptoms of Cardiovascular Disease and Stroke
93	Table T.3. Symptoms of Respiratory Disease
101	Table T.4. Symptoms of Obesity, Diabetes, and Hypertension
110	Table T.5. Symptoms of Common Cancers Associated with Environmental Determinants of Health
118	Table T.6. Symptoms of Mental Health Conditions
133	Table T.7. Direct and Indirect Health Effects of Exposure to Floodwaters
144	Table T.8. Air Quality Thresholds: US and World Health Organization (WHO)
145	Table T.9. Direct and Indirect Health Effects of Exposure to Air Pollution
153	Table T.10. Direct and Indirect Health Effects of Exposure to Disasters
161	Table T.11. Vector-Borne Disease: Average Number of Annual Cases, US and Global, Non-US Countries/Regions
163	Table T.12. Direct and Indirect Health Effects of Vector-Borne Diseases
192	Table 3.1. National Health Service England Health Check Scorecard 2018
223	Table 4.1. Role of Architectural Epidemiology (ArchEPI) in the Four Predominant Real Estate Project Delivery Models
	Table A.1. US and International Data Sources and Indicators (online)
	Table A.2. Association between Child and Adolescent Obesity and Characteristics of Neighborhood Walkability (online)
	Table A.3. Extreme Heat and Flooding Environmental Public Health Indicators and Principal Components for Travis County, Texas, USA (online)
	Table A.4. Uses of Spatial Analysis and Associated Methods (online)
	Table A.5. Spatial Autocorrelation (Moran's *I*) Analysis of Green Building Strategy Groupings in Austin, Texas, USA, and Chicago, Illinois, USA (online)
	Table A.6. Local Spatial Autocorrelation (LISA) of Green Building Strategy Groupings in Austin, Texas, USA, and Chicago, Illinois, USA (online)
	Table A.7. Sample EPHIs and Design/Operations Recommendations for a Residence in the Frogtown Neighborhood of Saint Paul, Minnesota, USA (online)

Advice for Using This Book

This book has been designed to fulfill three roles in one.

First, it introduces a new, transdisciplinary field of research and practice to action researchers who are filling gaps in our knowledge about the links between the built environment, social equity, and population health priorities like climate change, chronic disease, and mental health.

Second, it is organized to be easily integrated into discipline-specific courses. Sidebars highlighting discipline-specific core competencies are displayed in the margins and called out in the text with corresponding note numbers; for example, CC1.1 = Core Competency 1.1.

Third, chapter 2, the technical appendices, and the architectural epidemiology toolbox are designed to be used as a field guide for practitioners.

See below for a navigation guide tailored to your user group. (Readers are also advised to read the "How to Use This Book" section in the introduction for additional detail.)

Researchers

1. Read the introduction and chapter 1 to define architectural epidemiology and place it within the larger history linking public health and the built environment. The conceptual model (figure 1.1) in chapter 1 may be particularly helpful in this regard.
2. Read the research agenda in chapter 5 to identify synergies between architectural epidemiology and your primary area of research.
3. Read the remaining chapters that align most closely with your area of research to identify gaps in knowledge that your research could help fill.

Professors

1. Review table 0.1, "Professions Covered by Each Core Competency Category," in the introduction to check whether sections of the book can be used to support accreditation requirements in your department.
2. Search the sidebars and core competency tables in chapters 2–4 to identify the sections of the book that could be added to the curriculum to either add depth to an existing topic covered by the course and/or expand existing material to include topics specific to architectural epidemiology.
3. Use the key messages at the beginning of each chapter to write course learning objectives. Use the discussion questions at the end of each chapter to create assignments and classroom discussion prompts.

Practitioners

1. Read the introduction to learn how public health methods can improve building design and real estate development.
2. Read chapter 1 for the business case underpinning architectural epidemiology.
3. Use chapter 2 and the technical appendices to identify the highest priority environmental health topics in the neighborhood surrounding a building project.
4. Use the toolbox to select the evidence-based design and operations strategies that will bring the greatest co-benefits to both the real estate project and the surrounding neighborhood.
5. Use the case studies in the "Architectural Epidemiology in Action" boxes as models for opportunities to integrate architectural epidemiology into your own work.

Online Supplement

Architectural Epidemiology is supported by an online supplement. It provides expandable versions of some figures, technical appendices, and references. The additional materials for this book can be found by visiting the specific book page on **press.jhu.edu**.

Acknowledgments

The idea behind this book can be traced back to Adele Houghton's tenure with the *Green Guide for Health Care* (GGHC, 2005–2008), where she first realized that the green and healthy building movement suffered from a last mile problem. She would like to thank the GGHC coordinators, Gail Vittori, the late Robin Guenther, Tom Lent, and Walt Vernon, and the entire GGHC Steering Committee for their mentorship and guidance during those crucial years. Adele was inspired by the ingenuity and rigor underlying each individual strategy in best-practice guides like BREEAM, Enterprise Green Communities, the *Green Guide*, Fitwel, Green Star, Just Communities (formerly EcoDistricts), LEED, Living Building Challenge, Passive House, and WELL. But, as time went on, it became more and more apparent that an initial step was missing from the design and development process: how to know which strategies to prioritize for any given project. Best practice guides awarded highest recognition to projects that included the greatest number of strategies in the final building—regardless of whether those strategies met an environmental, community health, or social need amongst occupants or the surrounding neighborhood.

We believe epidemiological methods can be used to fill in that crucial missing step. And most importantly, we believe that using architectural epidemiology to reorient the design and development process has the potential to unleash real estate development as the primary driver of meaningful action on climate change, the United Nations Sustainable Development Goals, and environmental justice. We hope this book will facilitate new collaborative interactions between architects, landscape architects, engineers, community planners, climate change researchers and practitioners, epidemiologists, community-based organizations, environmental and social justice advocates, and local officials in the pursuit of better understanding the role that buildings can play in advancing community and planetary health.

We are indebted to our many colleagues who read early drafts and offered guidance and encouragement. In particular, the many dedicated staff and volunteers at built environment and public health organizations who helped guide our methods and messaging, so that the book can be seamlessly integrated into green and healthy building projects. Special thanks to Seema Bhangar, Kira Gould, Rachel MacCleery, Brendan Owens, Chris Pyke, and Kelly Worden, for sharing their deep knowledge of the green and healthy building industry and acting as thought partners along the way.

Thank you to Liz York for bringing clarity and good humor to editing the book and endlessly cheerleading during the final long months. We are grateful to Xiaolin (Elle) Li whose attention to detail and entrepreneurial spirit were essential to securing image reprint permissions and finalizing numerous figures. We are also grateful to Opus Design for their graphic design support.

Special recognition is due for the support of the Johns Hopkins University Press leadership, the Press Faculty Editorial Board, and, particularly, for Robin Coleman, Adriahna Conway, Kyle Kretzer, and Paul Payson who gave us crucial input and valuable editorial assistance throughout the production of this book.

Most importantly, we wish to acknowledge the sacrifices our families have made over the decade this project has spanned. Many of Adele's childhood memories involve a decade-long book project carried out by her own mother. So, she can relate to her husband Fernando's and children Thomas's and Evelia's experiences over the past 10+ years. While the summer days spent with her mother and sister in a dusty, un-airconditioned attic in the Houston Public Library did not inspire Adele at the time, perhaps watching a book project grow from a conversation about a gap in the historical record into a new archive with thousands of exhibits and spinoff projects gave Adele the staying power she would need when, years later, she recognized a gap that needed to be filled.

Architectural Epidemiology

Introduction

KEY MESSAGES

1 Architectural epidemiology is an emerging transdisciplinary field that analyzes the effects of the built environment[D0.1] on population health. It leverages building design, renovation, and operations to improve health outcomes by reducing exposure to environmental hazards and promoting healthy behavior change.

2 Architectural epidemiology responds to a "last mile" challenge that has made it difficult for community-scale efforts to address climate change and population health conditions (including communicable diseases, non-communicable diseases, and mental health). It does this by influencing building design, renovation, and facilities management decisions made at the parcel level.

> **No man is an Island, entire of itself; every man is a piece of the Continent, a part of the main.**
> —John Donne, *Devotions upon Emergent Occasions* (1624)

0.1 Why Do We Need Architectural Epidemiology?

Imagine a street with three buildings under construction, one next to the other. The local government requires all buildings over a certain size to achieve Leadership in Energy and Environmental Design (LEED) Gold certification. Their idea is that slowly converting the building stock to green buildings will reduce the community's contribution to climate change, improve air quality, and encourage residents to live an active lifestyle.

The first building is an office building that promises future tenants a $0 electric bill. So, the design team specifies high-grade insulation, high-performance windows, and a geothermal heat pump to minimize the electricity needed for climate control. A rooftop solar array and battery are installed to meet tenant electricity needs.

The developer for the second building is concerned about flooding. So, that project raises the ground floor above the 500-year floodplain and installs flood-proof materials and electrical outlets. Outside, the site and the roof are covered with vegetation. An underground cistern is installed to collect stormwater that is not directly absorbed by the landscaping.

The third building is anchored by a wellness center. That design emphasizes active living both indoors and outdoors and focuses on promoting physical and mental health. The wellness center separates its entrance from the busy street and screens outdoor activities from traffic-related noise and air pollution. Interior spaces are designed with views of nature and abundant natural light. The developer recruits a grocery store and a farm-to-table restaurant to occupy the remainder of the ground floor.

All three of these projects meet the community's sustainability requirement of LEED Gold certification. Individually, all three projects also address public health concerns. The first building can continue to function normally during blackouts triggered by heat waves, thereby protecting its occupants from exposure to very hot temperatures. The second building is protected from major flooding events. And the third building is designed to reduce the risk of chronic

DEFINITION 0.1

Built Environment
For the purposes of this text, "built environment" is defined as structures, sites, landscapes, streetscapes, zoning, transportation options, food access and other physical attributes designed, constructed, and maintained by humans for human activity including living, working, and recreation day to day.

disease by encouraging an active lifestyle and increasing access to fresh and healthy food, while also promoting safety, enhancing mood, and reducing exposure to traffic-related noise and air pollution.

The problem arises when we take a step back and consider whether, collectively, these developments are meeting the community's needs. When the city council reviews local trends in urban heat island, flood risk, obesity, and air pollution over time, they see that there is no difference before and after the sustainability regulations were put in place more than a decade earlier. How could that be?

In this book, we propose that the current approach to green and healthy building design has not resulted in community-scale environmental and health benefits, because it is blind to the unique needs and context of a given project site. In short, there is a disconnect between what happens inside and outside the project boundary.

The three building projects in our example were focused entirely on the developer and future occupants' needs within the project boundary. The city council was focused on the community as a whole. And the tools designed to link community goals with project-specific goals (e.g., building codes and zoning) do not currently incentivize projects to look for opportunities to catalyze positive healthy change in the surrounding neighborhood.

Yet, in reality, individual projects both influence and are influenced by their surroundings. They change the microenvironment on and around their site. And they contribute to the economic and social composition of a neighborhood, which, in turn, can improve the social and economic value of the project itself.

The COVID-19 pandemic brought into high relief the influence of design and operations decisions on population health and social equity. The odds of contracting airborne viruses like SARS-CoV-2 (the virus that causes COVID-19) are orders of magnitude higher in indoor spaces compared with outdoor gatherings.[1] As a result, design guides like the American Institute of Architects Re-occupancy Assessment Tool,[2] the Fitwel Viral Response Module,[3] and the WELL Building Health-Safety Rating[4] all encourage designers and facility operators to increase outdoor air supply, use high-efficiency filters, and introduce natural ventilation where possible—to dilute and filter out as many viral particles as possible. However, as Dr. Howard Frumkin's commentary "COVID-19, the Built Environment, and Health"[5] points out, the geographic disparities in COVID infection and death rates cannot be explained by architectural or land use design alone. They reflect the spatial clustering of low income and minority communities, who are both more likely to live in crowded and poorly ventilated homes (which increases risk of transmission) and more likely to be employed in service industry jobs that expose them to large numbers of people every day.

We developed architectural epidemiology to help real estate[D0.2] teams, local government, and community groups bridge the property boundary, so that each individual project considers design within its social context. Our goal is to enable projects to touch off a positive ripple effect on their surroundings that results in tangible benefits, at the site level and beyond.

0.2 Our Stories

During her time at university, Adele Houghton was drawn to architecture because the profession presented itself as both reflecting and helping shape the ideals of the society it represents. Environmental sustainability appeared to be her generation's vehicle for making societal change. So, Adele trained in passive design,

---

DEFINITION 0.2

Real Estate
The term "real estate" is defined in this book to be inclusive of the entire sector that creates, finances, develops, designs, builds and maintains buildings, sites, landscapes, streetscapes, infrastructure and other elements of the built environment. It includes developers, architects, engineers, public health professionals, environmental consultants, contractors, program managers, property managers, maintenance engineers, code officials, and zoning boards, as well as officials and others who govern and influence the built environment.

energy efficiency, and non-toxic materials selection. After working as a sustainability consultant at a commercial architecture firm for a few years, she ran the *Green Guide for Health Care* (*Green Guide*), the first green building best practices toolkit in the US to identify health as a primary driver for environmental sustainability. As hospitals using the *Green Guide* began to see health and wellness benefits on campus, they became increasingly frustrated that recovering patients were returning to their communities and facing unhealthy surroundings. Responding to hospital requests, Adele began to research the aspects of the built environment outside of healthcare campuses that contributed to disease. The more she learned about these environmental determinants of health, the more she began to question whether the one-size-fits-all approach common to green building systems—including the *Green Guide*—was generating the environmental and health benefits their founders envisioned. Industry metrics tended to focus on process: the number and square footage of certified buildings, for example, rather than on the actual effects of the strategies. Adele realized she needed to learn a new skillset to understand the pathway linking building design and operations with health outcomes. She returned to school to pursue a Master of Public Health (MPH) at the Johns Hopkins Bloomberg School of Public Health. There, she met Professor Carlos Castillo-Salgado, a professor of epidemiology and spatial statistics, who helped her explore the ways environmental and social drivers operate differently in various local contexts.

After earning her MPH, Adele was given the opportunity to convene a multidisciplinary group of architects, developers, urban planners, public health officials, and academics in Saint Paul, Minnesota, USA, to explore how to tailor green building design to the immediate environmental and human health needs of three sites along a four-mile stretch of land straddling the twin cities. Even though all three projects involved affordable housing, the way traffic patterns, access to green space, and demographics changed from one neighborhood to the next resulted in three different sets of design recommendations. Perhaps even more striking, the conversation in the workshop between disciplines who had never worked together before offered Adele a glimpse into a future where cross-sectoral collaboration could lead to meaningful environmental and health benefits for building occupants, their neighbors, and the larger community. This book attempts to bring that successful engagement to scale.

Carlos Castillo-Salgado came to this subject from a slightly different perspective. Carlos is an epidemiologist, medical doctor, and lawyer. As he sees it, the needs of society have changed during the 21st Century—demanding major overhauls to traditional scientific paradigms. Massive amounts of knowledge and data have been generated. But they have accumulated inside of disciplinary silos rather than being translated into problem-solving methods that could enhance the quality of life of billions of individuals and social groups.

To address "wicked" challenges like climate change and chronic disease, researchers and practitioners will need to engage in truly transdisciplinary collaborations across previously siloed areas of research and practice. Architectural epidemiology—the new, transdisciplinary subfield proposed by this book—is one example of this approach. Architecture, the art and science of shaping the human environment, is unavoidably connected to the public health field of epidemiology. Building safe and livable neighborhoods and cities requires accurate and accessible epidemiological information. People, time, and place, the three key characteristics of epidemiology, are also important factors to consider in the design process for buildings. Basic epidemiological methods can be used as part of the design process to better understand the effects of people, time, and place on a proposed project. For example, they can help design teams measure and address environmental health challenges like climate change, ecological diversity, clean air, clean water, access to healthy food, and opportunities for physical activity. In this way, epidemiological methods offer a new tool for designers and developers as they strive to build better buildings that support healthy individuals and populations and advance a more equitable society.

0.3 How Do We Know the Current System Is Not Working?

Around 2005, Adele worked with the Central Texas chapter of the US Green Building Council to designate bonus points for LEED credits that addressed neighborhood environmental priorities. Called "regional priority credits" or RPCs, the idea was that offering a bonus point for some credits would prompt green building projects to address environmental problems requiring collective effort: such as air pollution, urban heat islands, and flood risk.

Influence of LEED Regional Priority Credits in Austin, Texas, USA, and Chicago, Illinois, USA

In 2012, Adele and Carlos set out to discover whether the RPC program was achieving its desired results. We analyzed the LEED credits awarded to 74 LEED-certified projects in Austin, Texas, USA, and 393 LEED-certified projects in Chicago, Illinois, USA, from 2001–2012 (figure 0.1). Our goal was to understand whether LEED was being used as a tool by the real estate sector as a whole to enhance resilience to the two major climate-related hazards in both communities: extreme heat and flooding. We found the opposite was true. The real estate sector seemed to be acting agnostically without regard to health risk for these hazards. Not only were the LEED projects that were awarded climate-protective RPCs not clustered in neighborhoods at high risk of heat and/or flooding, but LEED projects overall were more heavily clustered in low-risk neighborhoods that, arguably, were less in need of the intervention. A detailed description of the study has been published elsewhere.[6]

What forces are at play here? In 2020 and 2021, Adele interviewed 24 real estate developers from across the US, representing all building types and both the for-profit and non-profit sectors. To a person, they all confirmed that the current financial and regulatory system governing the real estate market strongly incentivizes them to focus on the needs of the individual project over and above all other considerations. Projects that have prioritized community health needs have done so either quietly—without the knowledge of their financial backers—or loudly challenging regulations that stand in the way of community benefit design.

Chapter 1 proposes a value proposition for using architectural epidemiology as an analysis-based tool enabling developers to overcome the "last mile" and "wrong pocket" barriers that prevent so many of them from capitalizing on "community benefit" to generate new value streams for their projects.

0.4 Defining Aspects of Architectural Epidemiology

By definition, transdisciplinary[7] fields like architectural epidemiology are practiced differently by different members of its community. This section describes three sets of benefits that naturally arise as a result: collaboration, scalability, and flexibility.

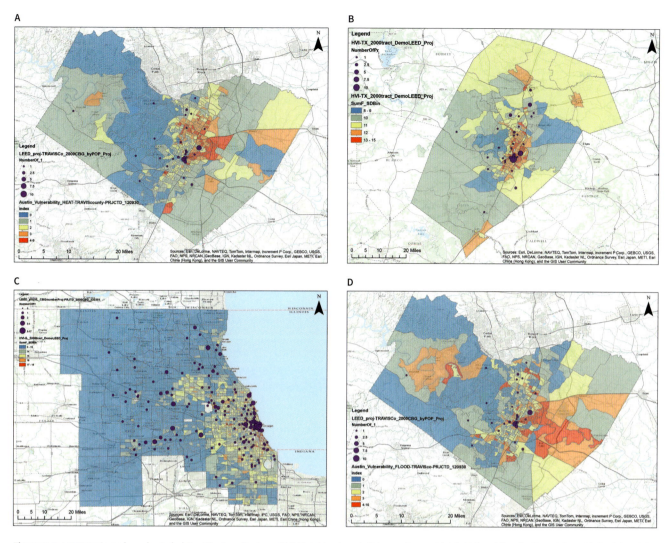

Figure 0.1. LEED Projects (*purple circles*) Are Clustered in Low-Risk Neighborhoods (*blue and green highlights*) and Nearly Absent from High-Risk Neighborhoods (*orange and red highlights*). Numbers of LEED-Certified Projects Overlaid on Vulnerability Indices in Austin, Texas, USA, and Chicago, Illinois, USA: (A) Austin Cumulative Heat Vulnerability Index in Travis County, Texas; (B) Austin Heat Vulnerability Index; (C) Chicago Cumulative Heat Vulnerability Index; (D) Austin Flood Vulnerability Index. *Source:* Houghton and Castillo-Salgado 2020[6]

1. Architectural Epidemiology Fosters Collaboration

Multi-disciplinary collaboration is not new to either the real estate sector or public health.

The real estate development process requires input from 5–10 design trades, technical consultants, a general contractor overseeing at least as many subcontractors, financial backers, legal advisors, and regulatory oversight (which could involve a number of municipal departments).

Similarly, public health agencies partner with area health centers, laboratories, and hospitals to track disease and to alert the community about timely public health threats. They work with the office of emergency management, which is itself a collection of many local departments, to plan for and respond to natural and man-made disasters. And they are increasingly consulted by sister agencies overseeing the built environment (such as zoning, public works, and watershed protection) who are interested in maximizing the health co-benefits of their work and avoiding or minimizing its co-harms.

This book is a first step in expanding both groups' sizable network of professional colleagues to include each other. Chapter 1 includes a brief overview of the history connecting these two fields, which overlapped a great deal in the 19th century. In fact, many of the professions who will collaborate on architectural epidemiology projects today worked together in the 19th century to improve sanitation and fire safety in the overcrowded neighborhoods of industrialized cities like London and New York.

The idea that built environment and public health practitioners should work more closely together is also not new. In 2017, eight membership organizations representing over 450,000 professionals in the US signed a Joint Call to Action to Promote Healthy Communities[8] calling on their members to work together to promote population health and health equity. The call to action reflects a groundswell of support within the real estate, public health, and allied industries to start designing, modifying, and operating the built environment to support health and wellness, particularly among vulnerable groups.

This book will be particularly useful to projects pursuing one of the corollaries to the conversations that led to the Joint Call to Action: health impact assessment credits in best practice guides like LEED, Enterprise Green Communities, and WELL. Architectural epidemiology makes use of many of the tools that are necessary to perform cross-sectoral collaborations and to measure the effectiveness of interventions over time. Many of the metrics used in architectural epidemiology are similarly multi-disciplinary, such as the UN Sustainable Development Goals, the US Healthy People 2030 goals, and the Paris Climate Agreement, among others.

In the spirit of supporting the Joint Call to Action's prompt for more transdisciplinary collaboration on real estate development projects, we include core competency tables throughout this book to help clarify the roles and responsibilities of each discipline engaged in delivering an architectural epidemiology project. Table 0.1 provides an overview of the specific disciplines covered by each of the five categories in the core competencies tables: epidemiology, real estate development, design and construction, sustainability, and philanthropy. The guidance in later core competency tables is drawn directly from these disciplines' core competency requirements for academic accreditation or professional licensure. In this way, they guide you through the responsibilities of each profession and the roles they play at different points in the process. See the "How to Use this Book" section below for a more detailed explanation of ways to use the core competency tables in practice or as a pedagogical tool.

Finally, to support collaboration across the many stakeholders who will participate in an architectural epidemiology project, we have annotated chapters 2–4 with callout boxes highlighting opportunities for three primary stakeholder groups—the real estate team, the local government, and community groups—to contribute to the project's success. See table 1.2 ("Stakeholder Analysis of Value Generated Using Architectural Epidemiology") in chapter 1 for a more in-depth review of the factors that motivate these three groups to support a real estate development process that generates community benefit.

2. Architectural Epidemiology is Scalable

Architectural epidemiology starts from the premise that robust structures for developing health-promoting strategies already exist within the real estate project delivery process on the one hand and the community planning process on the other. The challenge has been finding a way to bridge across the project

TABLE 0.1.

Professions Covered by Each Core Competency Category

Core Competency	Professions
Epidemiology[9]	• Applied epidemiologists • Public health officers • Schools of public health
Real estate development[10]	• Real estate developers • Capital finance providers • Corporate service providers • Public-private partnerships
Facility design, construction, operations[11–15]	• Architects • Landscape architects • Interior designers • Professional engineers • Community planners • General contractors • Program managers
Sustainability[16–18]	• Green building consultants • Healthy building consultants • Climate change consultants/officers • Building certification systems • Adaptation/resilience consultants
Philanthropy[19]	• Strategic planners • Grant officers

boundary, so that individual real estate projects begin to use neighborhood-level metrics to inform their environmental and health design priorities.

Because the essence of the methodology is communication transfer between and among multiple disciplines, architectural epidemiology can be applied at any scale—from an interior design renovation to a campus master plan and beyond. The key is to use the method to identify leverage points that will set off a health-promoting ripple effect in surrounding areas.

Case studies embedded throughout this book demonstrate how individual building projects have applied population-level data to inform design decisions, how those strategies have improved daily life for occupants and the surrounding neighborhood, and how they advance community goals related to climate change and chronic disease. Additionally, many of the methodologies presented in the book could be applied at larger scales. Several case studies demonstrate how architectural epidemiology could be applied at the neighborhood and community scale to ramp up implementation of local climate, health, and equity plans in underserved neighborhoods.

3. Architectural Epidemiology is Flexible

Architectural epidemiology practitioners develop location-specific metrics that translate across scales to facilitate multi-disciplinary collaboration. Given the field's transdisciplinary nature, its methods need to be flexible enough that a wide range of built environment, public sector, and community stakeholders can deploy them for multiple end uses.

The Harvard University Climate Action Plan test case in box 0.1 offers one example of how flexible the architectural epidemiology method can be. It applies the approach laid out in chapter 2 of this book to two very different questions of practice:

1. What selection criteria could help Harvard invest in carbon offset projects that maximize both cost efficiency of carbon sequestration and co-benefits of social and population health?
2. What metrics would help Harvard project teams assess the environmental and population health implications of a building project, so that new buildings, renovations, and facility operations maximize co-benefits for carbon reduction and human health?

As the Harvard case demonstrates, the architectural epidemiology approach remains constant, but its output adjusts to meet the needs of the project, its context, and the goals of each stakeholder group.

Finally, the output from an architectural epidemiology analysis is flexible enough both to inform the design of an individual building and to add built environment metrics to local public health tracking programs on topics like climate change, environmental health, air pollution, and chronic and infectious diseases. It does this by establishing a link between building attributes and two data streams that are routinely included in tracking platforms: environmental exposures and population health needs.

Using the Harvard case study as an example, the rooftop solar microgrid project in the Mission Hill neighborhood links an individual building attribute (i.e., carbon emissions per square foot) with numerous metrics in the City of Boston Climate Action Plan,[20] that is, reduction in carbon emissions, increased megawatts of solar capacity, and reduction in criteria air pollutants. It also contributes to metrics in the Climate Ready Boston[21] plan (i.e., district-level energy solutions) and the Boston Community Health Implementation[22] plan and Health Equity Now[23] plan (i.e., increase economic security in low-income neighborhoods and reduce resident displacement). Architectural epidemiology provides a framework for tracking all of these issues in relation to each other, so that city policies, neighborhood strategic plans, and, ultimately, individual building design can address them in a coordinated fashion.

BOX 0.1.

Architectural Epidemiology in Action
Harvard University Climate Action Plan Test Case, USA

The Harvard University Climate Action Plan has set the ambitious dual goal of achieving carbon neutrality by 2026 and becoming fossil fuel free by 2050.[24] The *2016–2017 Harvard University Climate Change Task Force Report* acknowledges the human health effects of climate change, particularly related to air pollution that is generated through fossil fuel combustion.[24] The plan explicitly calls for human health to factor into the selection of carbon offset projects and allows other projects to prioritize interventions based, in part, on the extent to which they benefit human health—particularly in vulnerable and underserved communities. This case study considers two ways architectural epidemiology could be used to implement the Harvard University Climate Action Plan.

The first approach ranks three possible carbon offset projects according to total sequestered carbon and the social and population health benefits of the project within the surrounding community, on campus at Harvard, in the Boston area, and in the larger region.

In order to decide between the three options, it is necessary to consider the demographics, socioeconomic status, and health status of the populations living around each offset project site (figure 0.2). All three project communities demonstrate need.

1. *Option 1:* Protect an Old Growth Forest in Western Massachusetts. This project benefits three small towns in western Massachusetts. The median income in all three towns is lower than the median of the Commonwealth of Massachusetts. Holyoke, in particular, has a disproportionately large Hispanic population, a lower level of educational attainment, a lower median income, and a higher poverty rate than both Massachusetts and the US as a whole. Holyoke residents also report high rates of asthma, heart disease, and overall poor physical health.
2. *Option 2:* Invest in a Landfill Methane Gas-to-Electricity Plant in a Suburb of Boston. This project benefits the health of New Bedford, Massachusetts, residents both by reducing air pollution from the local landfill and by generating job opportunities. New Bedford is a town that would benefit from this kind of investment, because it reports a low median income, high poverty rate, and high asthma rates.
3. *Option 3:* Invest in a Solar Microgrid in the Mission Hill Neighborhood of Boston. This project would arguably be the best option for Harvard from a community relations point of view, as long as it was not perceived as a mechanism to speed up the displacement of low-income residents that appears to be underway. On the one hand, the neighborhood is more ethnically diverse than both Boston

and Massachusetts. It also boasts a very high percentage of college graduates. On the other hand, its median income is quite low, and its poverty rate is four times the average in Massachusetts and the US.

Table 0.2 and figure 0.2 present a decision-making framework that could be used to weigh cost considerations against greenhouse gas (GHG) emission offsets, social impact, and the value of engaging with communities surrounding the Harvard campus.

The second approach zooms into the building level. It demonstrates how architectural epidemiology can be used to help project teams assess the environmental and population health implications of a new construction, addition, or renovation project. Used well, the framework could lead to building designs, renovations, and facility policies that maximize benefit for both carbon reduction and human health. This approach starts from the hypothetical premise that the home of the Harvard Graduate School of Design, Gund Hall, has been slated for renovation. After considering the health concerns of Harvard students, faculty, and staff regarding air quality, as well as those of the surrounding community, the analysis considers air pollution source (both indoors and outdoors) and exposure pathways (figure 0.3).

The analysis returned a slate of possible interventions. Indoor interventions included restricting emissions-producing activities to designated rooms, exhausting air directly to the exterior, and verifying that these rooms are already negatively pressurized. Ventilation and filtration recommendations might include upgrading the air filters in the mechanical system, moving outdoor air intakes to the alley behind the building (away from the busy streets on both sides), and only allowing operable windows on the alley side. In this way, the building could act as a wall protecting occupants from exposure to the worst of the traffic-related air pollution (TRAP). The most extreme outdoor intervention would be to move the building to a new location or farther away from the street. The existing bike lanes on the side of the street next to the Graduate School of Design is an example of a more feasible strategy. These lanes both calm traffic (thereby reducing overall emissions) and push the traffic a few feet farther away from the building. The next step in traffic design might suggest building a roundabout at the corner, which would reduce localized TRAP by largely eliminating traffic congestion. The school could institute a no idling rule in the loading dock to minimize the quantity of exhaust that enters the building every time a delivery truck arrives. And the plantings between the sidewalk and the street could be designed to block and filter out particulate matter.

BOX 0.1. (cont.)

TABLE 0.2.

Harvard Case Study—Architectural Epidemiology Decision-Making Table for Proposed Carbon Offset Program

	Option 1: Forest Preservation	Option 2: Landfill Gas Capture and Electricity Production	Option 3: Rooftop Solar Microgrid in Mission Hill
Project cost	$–$$$	$$$$	$$$
Annual GHG offset (tons CO₂e)	163,492.66	130,000	117,500
GHG impact/cost	+++	++	+
Social impact/cost	+	++	++
Harvard community engagement value/cost	+	++	+++
Population health and sociodemographic profile on and surrounding the project site	Urban parks that benefit the local community Low income High minority population High asthma rates High cardiovascular disease rates Poor health	Low income High asthma rates	Gentrifying neighborhood Low income High minority population
Project benefits for underlying social determinants of health in the surrounding community	Helps sustain tourism economy, which reduces the risk of poverty	Creates employment opportunities for the neighborhood, which reduces the risk of poverty	↑ Energy security, which reduces the financial strain of utilities on low-income residents
Project Air-Quality Benefits			
Surrounding Community	↓ NOx, ↓ SOx, ↓ VOCs, ↓ PM, ↓ Ozone precursors	↓ NH₄, ↓ CO₂	N/A
Harvard	N/A	N/A	N/A
Boston	N/A	↓ NH₄, ↓ CO₂	N/A
Region	↓ NOx, ↓ SOx, ↓ VOCs, ↓ PM, ↓ Ozone precursors	↓ NH₄, ↓ CO₂	↓ NOx, ↓ SOx, ↓ VOCs, ↓ PM, ↓ Ozone precursors

TABLE 0.2. (*cont.*)

	Option 1: Forest Preservation	Option 2: Landfill Gas Capture and Electricity Production	Option 3: Rooftop Solar Microgrid in Mission Hill
Project Benefits for Health			
Surrounding Community	↓ Risk of respiratory and cardiovascular disease from air pollution	↓ Risk of respiratory and cardiovascular disease from air pollution	↑ Energy connectivity, leading to ↓ health risk from electricity blackouts (medical device; climatic exposure)
Harvard	Indirect through region	N/A; small installation	Reflected community health benefit
Boston	Indirect through region	N/A; small installation	↓ Risk of heat- or cold-related injuries from brownouts, blackouts
Region	↓ Risk of respiratory and cardiovascular disease from air pollution	N/A; small installation	↓ Risk of heat- or cold-related injuries from brownouts, blackouts
Project Advancement of Local Climate Action and/or Public Health Goals			
Surrounding Community	Helps advance carbon neutrality and air quality goals	Helps advance air quality goals in an environmental justice community	Helps reduce population vulnerability to extreme heat and extreme cold events (may not be directly correlated with a specific policy)
Harvard	Helps achieve carbon neutrality goals	Helps achieve carbon neutrality and health equity goals	Helps achieve carbon neutrality and health equity goals (demonstrates shared value from an anchor institution)
Boston	N/A	Helps advance carbon neutrality, air quality, and health equity goals	Helps advance carbon neutrality, emergency preparedness, and health equity goals
Region	Helps advance carbon neutrality and air quality goals	Helps advance carbon neutrality, air quality, and health equity goals	Helps advance carbon neutrality, air quality, and health equity goals

Note: GHG = greenhouse gases; NOx = nitrogen oxides; SOx = sulfur oxides; PM = particulate matter; VOCs = volatile organic compounds.

BOX 0.1. (cont.)

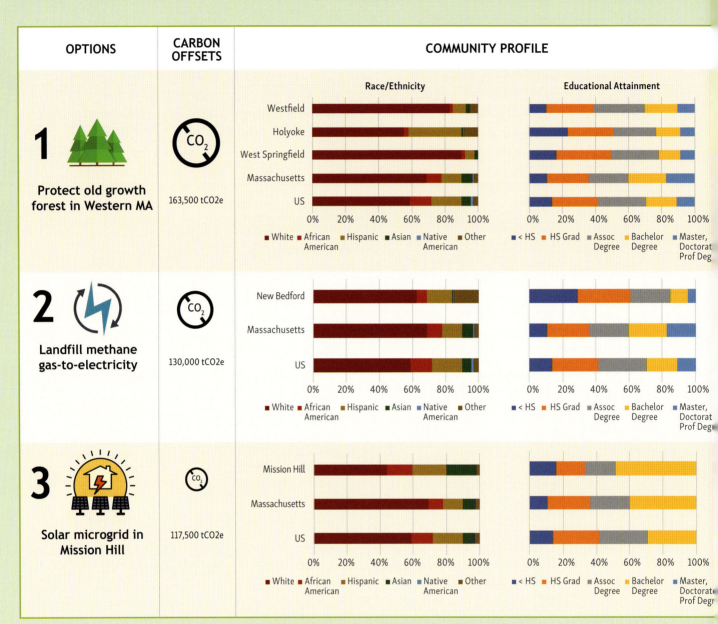

Figure 0.2. Harvard Case Study 01—Air Pollution Analysis: Proposed Carbon Offset Program. *Source:* Adele Houghton

12 ARCHITECTURAL EPIDEMIOLOGY

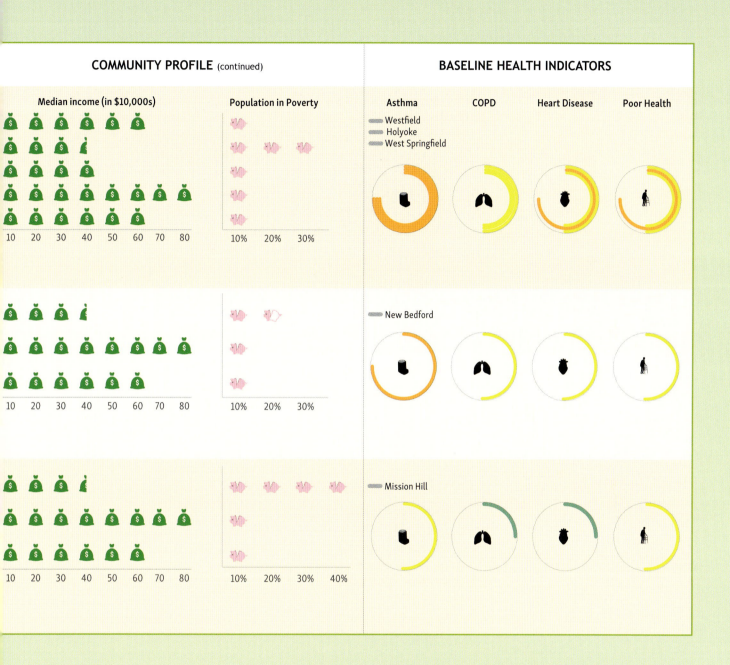

INTRODUCTION 13

BOX 0.1. (cont.)

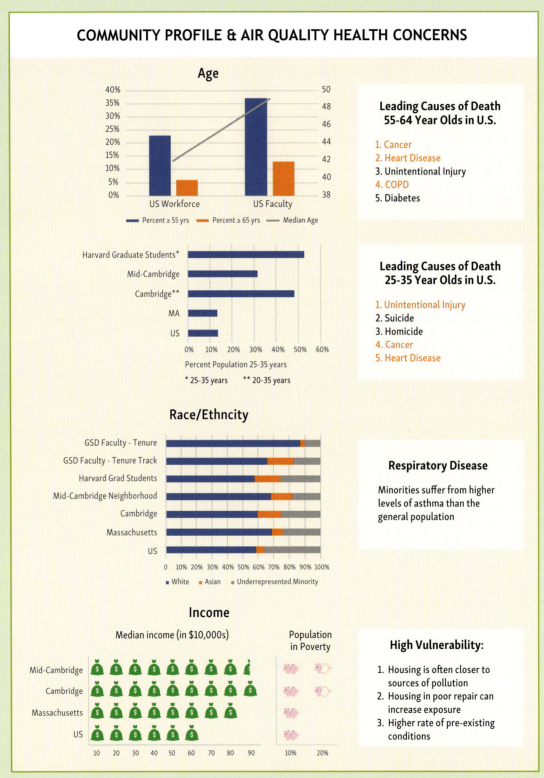

Figure 0.3. Harvard Case Study 02—Air Pollution Analysis: Proposed Gund Hall Renovation. *Source:* Adele Houghton

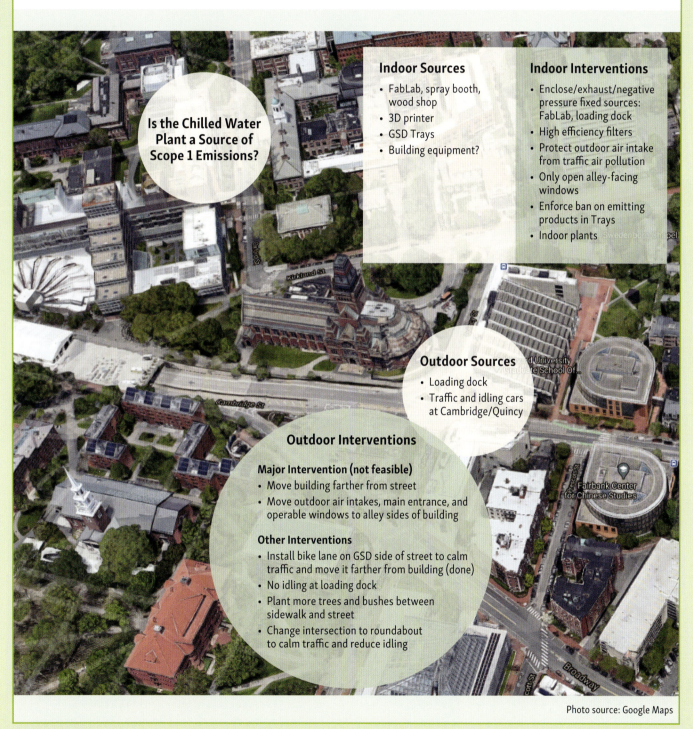

Figure 0.3. (cont.)

0.5 How to Use This Book

This book has been designed to fulfill three roles in one.

First, it proposes a new, transdisciplinary field of research and practice called architectural epidemiology. Approached from that perspective, the book may be read cover to cover. It places architectural epidemiology within the history and current context of the two fields it straddles: real estate development and public health (chapter 1). It presents a methodology for applying architectural epidemiology in the field (chapter 2). It identifies opportunities for adding value to each phase of the real estate project delivery process (chapter 3). And it envisions different roles for architectural epidemiology, depending on who is developing the project, who will occupy the project, and how the construction contract is organized (chapter 4). The appendices go into greater detail about how to perform the more technical pieces of the problem-solving framework. Additionally, the toolbox lays out the current state of the evidence linking architecture and epidemiology in 10 factsheets. These visual aids orient you to the relationship between building design and 10 health topics (5 related to climate change and 5 related to chronic disease and mental health). They identify groups who are particularly vulnerable to poor health outcomes in each topic. And they list the green building and operations strategies that have been shown in scientific studies to reduce the risk of poor health outcomes related to the topic of interest. In the conclusion, we identify gaps in research and propose a research agenda that will help quantify the relative benefit of certain strategies in one setting versus another. For example, it is not immediately obvious which green building strategies would maximize health co-benefits and minimize co-harms for a school that aims to reach net zero energy use, reduce the risk of airborne disease transmission, is located next to a busy road, and includes outdoor playgrounds and practice fields as part of the program. Additional research may be required to quantify the relative health benefits associated with strategies that reduce exposure to heat and outdoor air pollution, coupled with indoor strategies that both increase filtered outdoor air supply and meet high energy efficiency requirements.

Second, the book was designed to be integrated into academic degrees and executive education courses about sustainability, climate change, and public health. Chapter 2 and the technical appendices are organized into discrete sections that could be included in spatial analysis and statistics courses as vertical, in-depth technical topics. The problem-solving framework in chapter 2 could also be taught as a horizontal topic, integrating epidemiological methods into the design process. Real estate courses could combine the value proposition in chapter 1 with the discussion of real estate investment models and contract frameworks in chapter 4 to demonstrate how architectural epidemiology could be used to generate new value streams. As noted above in the "Defining Aspects of Architectural Epidemiology" section, the material presented in chapters 1–4 is punctuated with tables referencing core competency requirements for degree programs in epidemiology, real estate development, design and construction, sustainability, and philanthropy. This information, as well as the discussion questions at the end of chapters 1–4, are designed to facilitate the integration of architectural epidemiology concepts and methods into a range of academic and professional development syllabi. The core competency tables in particular can be used during the accreditation process to document how a transdisciplinary course on architectural epidemiology supports core competencies in all relevant disciplines.

Third, chapter 2, the technical appendices, and the toolbox are designed to be used in concert as a field guide for practitioners. Concepts that are described using broad brush strokes in the text are fleshed out as detailed guidance in the technical appendices. Practitioners can follow the problem-solving framework in chapter 2 and supporting technical appendices to identify the top one to three priority health topics of concern for their project. They can then turn to the infographics in the toolbox, which share talking points that help teams communicate the significance of priority health topics to clients and stakeholders. The infographics also list evidence-based design and operations strategies that can be used on the project to protect occupants and the surrounding community from negative environmental exposures. Architectural epidemiology practitioners can use the environmental exposure, population health, and design and operations metrics they develop with this two-step process as a common language when real estate developers, local government, and neighborhood groups begin conversations about ways the project can generate value for all stakeholders. Finally, the core competency tables interspersed throughout the book can support practitioners in outlining desired qualities and attributes when hiring team members or defining performance specifications within their scopes of work.

We now move to chapter 1, where we introduce architectural epidemiology, its historical roots, and the value it can generate for real estate developers, community members, and local governments alike.

CHAPTER 1
An Introduction to Architectural Epidemiology

KEY MESSAGES

1. The built environment influences population[D1.1] exposure to elements of the environment[D1.2] that could promote or harm their health and wellbeing.

2. The relationship between building design/operations and population health is best understood through the dual lens of the health impact pyramid and the hierarchy of controls framework.

3. Architectural epidemiology analyzes baseline environmental health conditions of a building project site, identifies exposure pathways that can be effectively influenced using building design and operations interventions, considers the impact of mediating factors, and estimates the results on population health outcomes.

4. Architectural epidemiology uses neighborhood metrics as a common language to generate new value streams for real estate developers, local government, and community members.

1.1 Introduction

This book introduces a new, transdisciplinary[1] field of action research and practice called architectural epidemiology. As its name suggests, architectural epidemiology engages scientists and practitioners from the public health, real estate, government, and community sectors in a shared conceptual framework that describes the unique combination of environmental exposures and human health needs in and around a building project site. Each member of the coalition contributes knowledge and expertise to identifying the top health priorities for the site and the set of evidence-based design and operations strategies that will most effectively address those priorities.

This transdisciplinary framework is populated with environmental, demographic, socioeconomic, and health metrics at the neighborhood scale, which act as a bridge between the real estate project team, local government, and community groups. At its best, architectural epidemiology fosters collaboration among these three stakeholder groups and generates financial and health benefits for all three.

1.1.a Defining the Epidemiology Half of Architectural Epidemiology

According to *A Dictionary of Epidemiology*, **epidemiology** is defined as "[t]he study of the occurrence and distribution of health-related events, states, and processes in specified populations, including the study of the determinants influencing such processes, and the application of this knowledge to control relevant health problems."[2(p95)] It is a large field of research, encompassing a number of sub-fields, including environmental and social epidemiology. **Environmental epidemiology** includes the study and application of interventions to control "the health effects on populations

> **DEFINITION 1.1**
>
> **Population**
> In public health, population refers to a group of people in a particular area, ethnic group, or other defining characteristic. It could also mean an entire population for a region, city, etc.

> **DEFINITION 1.2**
>
> **Environment**
> In public health, environment can have at least two meanings. In this case, it means the localized physical environment such as you would find within the building, area, or region of a particular location. Environmental supports include anything in the localized physical environment that guides or supports behaviors or creates conditions that lead to healthier outcomes. Environment can also mean the larger ecosystem primarily of the natural features of the world. Environmental health is concerned with both the natural and man-made physical surroundings that have an effect on health.

> **DEFINITION 1.3**
>
> Environmental Determinants of Health
> The elements in the built and natural environment that influence population health outcomes

> **DEFINITION 1.4**
>
> Social Determinants of Health
> The underlying demographic, political, social, and economic factors that influence population health outcomes

of physical, chemical, and biological processes and agents external to the human body."[2(p93),D1.3] **Social epidemiology** "studies the role of social structures, processes, and factors in the production of health and disease in populations. It uses epidemiological knowledge, reasoning, and methods to study why and how the frequency and distribution of a health state is influenced by factors such as ethnicity, socioeconomic status and position, social class, or environmental and housing conditions."[2(p264),D1.4]

Architectural epidemiology draws from both environmental and social epidemiology to study how the social forces underlying real estate development practices and land use regulation shape the architectural design process, which ultimately changes the pathways of environmental exposures for future building occupants and the surrounding community (table 1.1). In short, architectural epidemiology provides a framework for using building design and operations as a social mechanism for addressing environmental hazards.

Like other sub-disciplines of epidemiology, architectural epidemiology identifies factors that can benefit population health. It does not delineate a direct causal pathway between architectural design and an individual's health outcomes. Instead, it identifies the attributable factors in building design and operations that could lead to positive or negative health outcomes among the building occupant population and the population in the surrounding community.

Figure 1.1 presents architectural epidemiology in the form of a conceptual diagram illustrating the way that environmental and social epidemiological forces converge around building projects. Every parcel of land is exposed to a range of environmental hazards, such as heat, air pollution, flooding, and biological pathogens. The mechanisms of exposure are called built environment determinants of health. Social epidemiology tells us that socioeconomic and political forces create disparities in differential exposure. In other words, the built and natural environment are designed to expose some neighborhoods to negative determinants of health and other neighborhoods to positive determinants of health. The combination of environmental exposures and social determinants of health varies widely in the US, leading to disparities in health outcomes. Taking an extreme example, the combination of built environment and social determinants of health have created a patchwork of life expectancy in US cities. In some cities, the disparities are so stark that life expectancy varies more than 20 years

TABLE 1.1.

Aspects of Epidemiology, Environmental Epidemiology, and Social Epidemiology That Are Deployed by Architectural Epidemiology

	Aspects
Epidemiology	• Addresses population health risk distributions, not the health outcome of any single individual • Maps exposure pathways of environmental and social determinants of health that are mediated by building design and operations
Environmental epidemiology	• Traces the pathways linking environmental hazards with population exposures through the built and natural environment and related health outcomes
Social epidemiology	• Uses architecture and allied disciplines in the real estate industry as the mechanism for epidemiological interventions

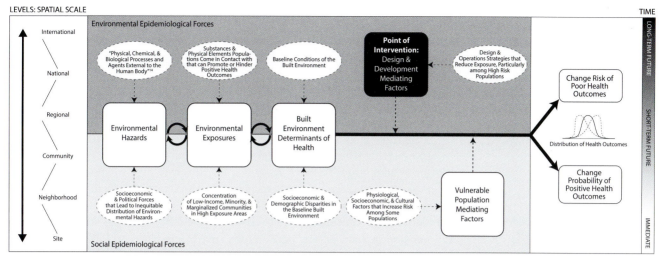

Figure 1.1. Architectural Epidemiology Conceptual Diagram. *Sources:* Adapted from Birn et al. 2017;[4] Krieger 2008;[5] Schulz and Northridge 2004;[6] and World Health Organization 2007[7]

from one neighborhood (i.e., census tract) to the next.[3] Architectural epidemiology's innovation is to use design and operations strategies to reduce exposure to environmental hazards, particularly in neighborhoods with high concentrations of people who are at heightened risk of a poor health outcome. The result is a development that reduces the risk of poor health outcomes and increases the probability of positive health outcomes both among people who use the site and in the surrounding neighborhood.

At its core, architectural epidemiology is a problem-solving discipline. It analyzes the baseline environmental health situation, identifies the exposure pathways that can be most effectively influenced using building design and operations interventions, considers the impact of mediating factors, and estimates the result on population health outcomes.

1.1.b The Role of Space and Time in Architectural Epidemiology

Architectural epidemiology aims to link conversations and design decisions at the building and interiors scale to the needs of the building occupancy, the neighborhood, and the community. The range of health topics that can be influenced by building design operations is broad and varied. A project guided by architectural epidemiology might lead to both short-term and long-term impacts on population health. As a result, architectural epidemiology necessarily operates at multiple scales—in terms of both time and place.

Figure 1.2 displays how commonly practiced approaches to green and healthy building design[CC1.1] fit into an architectural epidemiology framework across spatial scales and at each point in the project delivery process. For example, green and healthy building approaches to community planning are often actively considered as part of very early decisions—such as a site selection. But they can have an outsized impact over important topics like economic development long after completion of construction. Meanwhile, decisions about the interior of the building often start as a general concept during the design development phase and are continually refined as the project delivery process proceeds into construction documents (e.g., materials specification) and construction administration (e.g., conversations about construction sequencing). Finally, material performance is dependent on approaches to cleaning and maintenance during the occupancy

CORE COMPETENCY 1.1

Sustainability
Integrative Strategies

phase. See chapter 3 for more details about the appropriate use of architectural epidemiology during each phase of the project delivery process.

Refer back to this graphic as you read the case studies in chapters 3 and 4 to pinpoint the spatial and project delivery milestones that are influenced by the health-promoting strategies in each project. Over the course of the book, you will begin to recognize patterns, as a convergence of neighborhood conditions, building type, and design and operations strategies lead to strategic interventions that are designed to bring the most co-benefits to climate, health, and equity.

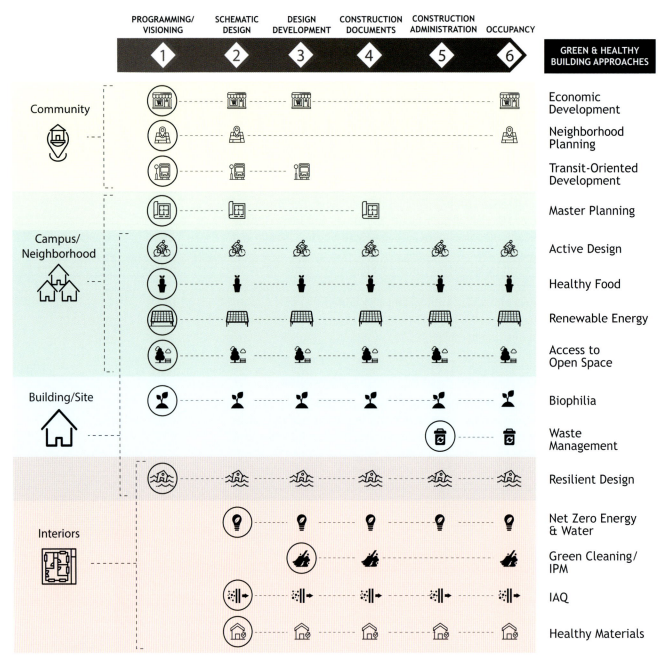

Figure 1.2. Green and Healthy Building Approaches Used by Architectural Epidemiology Organized by Spatial Scale and Relevant Project Delivery Phases. *Note:* The numbered diamonds across the top of the figure refer to the phases of the project delivery process: (1) programming/visioning, (2) schematic design (3) design development, (4) construction documents, (5) construction administration, and (6) occupancy.

1.1.c Why Focus on Climate Change and Chronic Disease?

In theory, architectural epidemiology could be used to address any number of environmental health hazards. In practice, building design is most likely to influence two major categories of hazard: climate change and community health conditions (including communicable diseases, non-communicable diseases, and mental health).

Buildings account for nearly 40% of global greenhouse gas emissions[8] and up to 20% of preventable deaths from chronic disease.[9] While the green and healthy building industries have made great strides over the past 20 years, resulting in over 15.5 billion square feet of construction,[10,11] they have had limited success shifting the trend lines for greenhouse gas emissions and chronic disease. Over the past decade, global building related emissions increased almost 10%,[12] the percentage of US adults suffering from heart disease hovered around 10%,[13] and the percentage of obesity among US adults rose from 27%–30%.[14]

The good news is that the commitments to address climate change made by local government and private companies are so significant that they could bring the world into alignment with achieving the 2°C limit in the Paris Climate Agreement on their own.[15] In order to do this, they will need to convince *all* property owners to work towards the common good—not just the highest and best use of their individual asset. The private real estate sector has the potential to rapidly propel local government in the direction of meeting their goals, because up to 70% of greenhouse gas emissions reduction in the building sector will take place on private property.[16]

Architectural epidemiology presents a methodology and an incentive for the real estate sector (including building design, construction, and operations), local government, and community groups to design projects with the goal of triggering a ripple effect on greenhouse gas emissions, community resilience, and prevalence of community health conditions like chronic disease and mental health.

1.2 A Brief History of Epidemiology's Roots in the Built Environment

The modern practice of epidemiology traces its origins to a debate in 1840s London over water sanitation.[17] But the connection with the built environment began a century earlier. In the 18th century, technological innovations in agriculture and industry in Great Britain resulted in a large-scale migration of rural families to cities. Agricultural innovations increased food supply, which, in turn, facilitated the reduction of the childhood mortality rate. When it became clear that the agrarian economy could not support larger families, workers began to move in large numbers to London, where automation in the textile sector had sparked a rapid economic expansion.[18] Industrialists built living and working quarters as quickly and densely as possible to accommodate the newcomers. Manufacturing hubs like London densified so quickly that the British government found itself incapable of setting or enforcing building safety and sanitation regulations—both because of the overwhelming volume of construction and because of the political power wielded by industrialists. The government's ineffective oversight extended to the water system, which was supplied by a patchwork of largely unregulated private companies, some of whom did not filter the water before pumping it to customers.[19,20]

The two seminal pieces of epidemiological research coming out of this period are the *Report on the Sanitary Condition of the Labouring Population of Great Britain*

(1843)[59] by Edwin Chadwick, which traced a cholera outbreak to dirty water supplied by a private water company, and *On the Mode of Communication of Cholera* (1855) by Dr. John Snow, which traced a cholera outbreak in 1854 to a public water pump in Broad Street, Soho, London.[17] The public outcry accompanying the revelations that private water companies delivering contaminated drinking water had caused cholera outbreaks led to the passage of the UK Public Health Act in 1848, the first of its kind.[17]

During the second half of the 19th century, cities in the UK, the US, and elsewhere around the world responded to the lessons of those first epidemiological studies by installing separate potable water and sanitary sewer systems to service their populations. They also strengthened building regulations to protect occupants from risk of fire and structural collapse.[17]

The modern system of building codes and regulations reflects a similar public health social contract between private landowners and the state. Each society has codified a minimum threshold of "health, safety, and welfare" to which new buildings are held accountable. In most industrialized societies, those codes address, at a minimum, structural integrity, sanitation (i.e., water, sewage, and trash), access to daylight and clean air, and access to electricity and/or gas. In 2009, the International Code Council began the process of adding environmental stewardship to that social contract through the development of the International Green Construction Code (IgCC).[21] The IgCC highlights the public health priorities that have overtaken communicable disease in the 21st century: chronic disease and climate change, both of which are strongly linked to the rise of car culture during the second half of the 20th century.[22] The COVID-19 pandemic that began in 2020 reminded the world that buildings should continue to be designed to reduce the risk of communicable disease transmission. The growing evidence that COVID-19 patients exposed to climatic events like extreme heat[23] or suffering from preexisting chronic disease conditions[24] are at increased risk of poor outcomes reinforces the need to retool the built environment so that it promotes human and environmental health.

Figure 1.3 displays these key historical events in relation to each other on a timeline.

1.3 Links between Health and the Built Environment

The built environment is often described as setting the context for population health.[CC1.2] In practice, that means that the way we design our communities and our buildings influences population exposure to elements of the environment that could promote or harm their health and wellbeing. For example, land use decisions place some neighborhoods adjacent to freeways and others at a distance. The neighborhoods next to and downwind from the freeway are exposed to higher concentrations of traffic-related air pollution—and associated health concerns—than neighborhoods that are farther away—not to mention increased risk of bike/pedestrian collisions with fast-moving vehicles. (The air pollution fact sheet in the toolbox explains the links between the built environment, air pollution, and human health in more detail.) At the building scale, architects and developers working in the neighborhood next to the freeway must adapt their design to protect building occupants as much as possible from exposure to the air and noise pollution and fast-moving vehicles coming off the freeway.

CORE COMPETENCY 1.2

Epidemiology
Assessment and Analysis

Real Estate Development
Location Analysis

Facility Design, Construction, Operations
Contextual Analysis

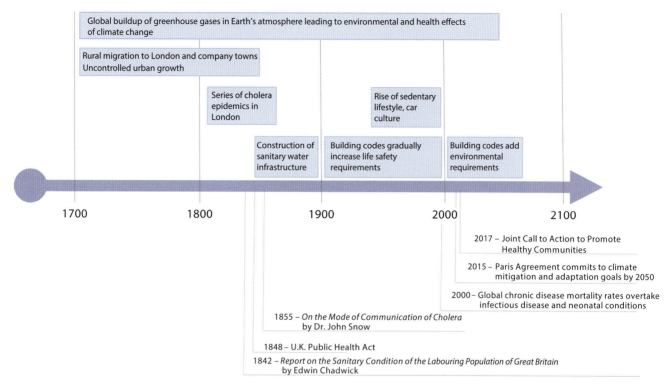

Figure 1.3. Timeline of Major Trends Linking Public Health and the Built Environment from the 18th Century to the Present. *Sources:* American Institute of Architects et al. 2017;[56] Chadwick 1843;[59] Dannenberg et al. 2011;[22] Institute of Medicine 1988;[17] Snow 1855;[30] U.N. Framework Convention on Climate Change 2015;[60] and World Health Organization 2020[58]

A health impact assessment (HIA)* of a proposed freeway expansion in Houston, Texas, USA, carried out by author Adele Houghton and colleagues at Air Alliance Houston illustrates this connection. Bruce Elementary, a school located across the street from a freeway, reports higher asthma rates and lower test scores than the school district average (figure 1.4). Given the school's proximity to the freeway and the unfeasibility of building a new building in a different location, HIA design recommendations[CC1.3] for protecting students and staff after the freeway expansion focused on improving air filtration within the building, minimizing additional sources of air pollution associated with school operations (such as turning the campus into a no-idle zone), and using vegetation to screen the school from at least some of the particulate matter blowing off of the freeway. See box 2.5 in chapter 2 for a more detailed description of the HIA design recommendations.

The design recommendations for Bruce Elementary describe its relationship with an environmental exposure[CC1.4]—air pollution—in two ways. First, they consider the relationship between the school and its surrounding community—both in terms of the physical campus and by addressing where the students live and how they travel to and from school each day. Second, the recommendations consider how the school building and campus could be used to protect students and the neighborhood behind the school from the traffic-related air pollution generated by the freeway. These two approaches correspond to two frameworks: the health impact pyramid and the hierarchy of controls.

CORE COMPETENCY 1.3

Sustainability
Integrative Strategies; Strategic Execution

CORE COMPETENCY 1.4

Epidemiology
Community Dimensions of Practice;
Cultural Competency

Facility Design, Construction, Operations
Programming and Analysis

Sustainability
Integrative Strategies; Strategic Execution

---

*See chapter 2 for more information about this tool.

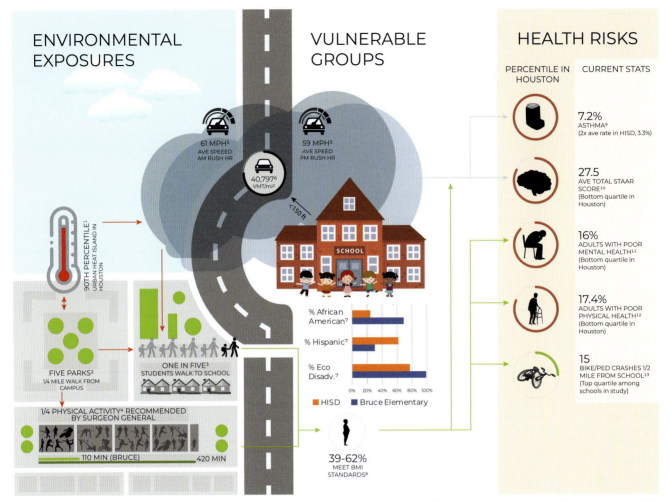

Figure 1.4. Baseline Contextual Health Assessment for Bruce Elementary School Houston, Texas, USA. *Source:* Adapted from Air Alliance Houston NHHIP Health Impact Assessment

1.3.a Health Impact Pyramid

The health impact pyramid is a public health framework that was popularized by former director of the US Centers for Disease Control and Prevention Dr. Thomas Frieden (figure 1.5).[25] It organizes major categories of public health intervention into a pyramid, with actions that will impact the largest number of people at the bottom progressing up to more and more individualized interventions towards the top.

Land use planning, real estate development, and building design and construction sit in the second tier from the bottom: changing the context to make individuals' default decisions healthy. This position means that the building industries have a large-scale impact on the health of both building occupants and the surrounding community. Additionally, the fact that the building sector sits one slot above the bottom tier—socioeconomic factors—indicates that design and operations have the potential to lead to even greater health benefits if they address the social determinants of health unique to the neighborhood where they are situated.

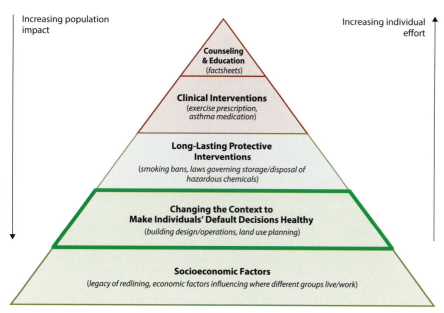

Figure 1.5. Health Impact Pyramid. *Source:* Adapted from Frieden 2010[25]

1.3.b Hierarchy of Controls

The hierarchy of controls (HOC) framework approaches buildings and land use from the perspective of protecting occupants from exposure to something that could harm their health. Figure 1.6 uses COVID-19 as an example of how the HOC works. Similar to the health impact pyramid, interventions that sit in the widest tiers of the pyramid benefit the greatest number of people with the least amount of individual responsibility for making a behavior change.

In the case of the COVID-19 pandemic, the safest way to stay virus-free when case counts were high would be to eliminate exposure to the virus in a workplace or other public setting by working from home. If it is not possible to work from home, then the next most effective approach would be to substitute exposure to the virus SARS-CoV-2 with exposure to the vaccine (in healthy individuals) or medication (in infected individuals). The building sector is not directly involved in those first two tiers of the pyramid. Our sweet spot is the third tier, engineering controls. Design elements (like programmed outdoor spaces) and building systems (like HVAC equipment fitted out with high efficiency MERV 13 filters) can protect building occupants from exposure and reduce the risk of disease transmission. Facility managers are more active than designers in the next tier, administrative controls. However, architects and engineers are often tasked with designing and specifying the building monitoring systems that facility managers then use to implement administrative controls. Finally, at the tip of the pyramid sits personal protective equipment (PPE), which in the case of the COVID-19 pandemic was symbolized by the face mask.

Architectural epidemiology applies these two frameworks to the design and operations process by combining the complementary skillsets of the design fields and epidemiology. Epidemiology helps uncover (1) the role architecture plays in exposure to health promoting or health inhibiting forces and (2) the relationship between the building design and operations and social determinants of health. The design fields take that information and translate it into a building project that is tailored to maximize its contribution to the health co-benefits of its location and community and minimize its co-harms.

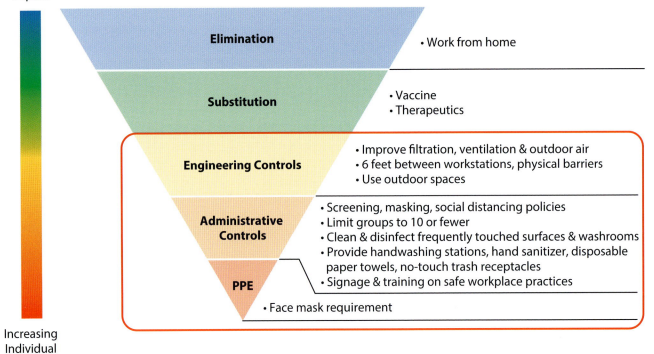

Figure 1.6. Hierarchy of Controls: COVID-19 Example. *Source:* Adapted from US Centers for Disease Control and Prevention[26]

As we discuss in the next sections, the act of defining and quantifying those co-benefits can generate new value streams for real estate developers, local government, and the neighborhood where the project is located.

1.4 Five Myths About Health Data and Design

The World Health Organization identifies the physical environment as one of three factors fundamental to human health. The other two factors, or determinants of health, are the social and economic environment, and individual characteristics and behaviors.[27] Over 90% of health-related expenditures in the US are targeted to individuals—such as offering medical services and encouraging individual behavior changes.[28] However, even limited changes to the physical environment removing barriers to health and promoting healthy choices can benefit a larger proportion of the population than interventions that are targeted to individuals.[29] This is the take-home message depicted in the Health Impact Pyramid above.

If the physical environment is fundamental to a healthy community and if changing it to promote health is more effective than focusing exclusively on individual care, then why are health data not *already* considered as fundamental to the design process as topography, access to public utilities, and the local building code? While the architecture and green building communities are showing growing interest in promoting health through design, the following five myths have kept health at the margins of standard practice.

28 ARCHITECTURAL EPIDEMIOLOGY

1.4.a Myth 1: Not Enough Evidence Supports a Direct Link between Design and Health

While it is true that scientific research exploring the links between health and the built environment cannot be conducted in a laboratory environment, an abundance of evidence points to strong correlations between specific land use configurations and population health status. These studies can be analyzed to identify which design strategies are likely to be the most beneficial or the most detrimental to health and wellness. The toolbox synthesizes the current state of the evidence for 10 health topics to facilitate their application to design projects in the field.

One famous example of a change to the built environment that had direct and immediate health benefits was John Snow's epidemiological research mapping the cholera outbreak in August 1849. (See section 1.2 above.) After tracing the source of the outbreak to a communal water pump on Broad Street in the Golden Square neighborhood of London, Snow persuaded the authorities to remove the handle until the well was decontaminated.[30] Another example is Florence Nightingale's book *Notes on Hospitals* (1863), which lays out specific design considerations to increase ventilation, sanitation, and other physical characteristics that can speed the healing process. While Nightingale openly admits that data are lacking to fully support her argument, she publishes the data that are available. And she devotes a chapter in the third edition to proposing an improved method for gathering hospital statistics, so that her theories of improved hospital design can be tested after pilot projects have been constructed.[31] A more recent example of applying population health evidence to influence design is the suite of regulations in California that require school and child-care facilities to consider the proximity of mobile sources of air pollution in the siting process. Specifically, these facilities may not be sited within 500 feet of busy roadways or within 1,000 feet of other mobile sources of air pollution (such as distribution centers, diesel truck idling stations, rail yards, and ports).[32]

1.4.b Myth 2: Population Health Considerations Do Not Generate Profit

This myth traces its origin to the fee-for-service business model practiced by most health systems in the US. Under this model, health care providers benefit financially from treating illness. The financial benefits of wellness are considered savings (not profits) and are shared by: healthy individuals; their health insurance companies who bring in more premiums than they pay out to reimburse medical care; and the public sector, which benefits from a reduction in demand for safety net services such as ambulances and indigent care.

Real estate developers could leverage the evidence published in public health literature and open-source health and vulnerability data (as outlined in the toolbox) to predict future savings associated with their design. They could be reimbursed prospectively (through public sector concessions such as expedited plan review, increases in square footage allowances, etc.) or after occupancy (by sharing in the savings associated with reduced medical services). Potential partners for a shared savings model might include the Centers for Medicare and Medicaid Services, private health insurance companies, integrated health systems (that provide both insurance and health care services), large employers, and/or private investors participating in health impact bonds. For example, Fresno, California, USA, pilot tested a health impact bond designed to reduce local childhood asthma rates. The program combines clinical care with changes to the home environment that have been shown through scientific research to reduce asthma triggers. The resulting reduction in medical reimbursements will be shared by participating insurance companies and program investors.[33] The Affordable Care Act increases the value of the shared savings model in the US by tying Medicare and Medicaid reimbursements to health outcomes associated with a handful of chronic diseases that are expensive to treat. By incorporating the environmental determinants underlying these diseases into the community health assessments that are developed every few years by local health departments and non-profit health systems, changes to the built environment could be factored into future reimbursement schema.

Unfortunately, when a new building or development leads to reduced medical expenditures, neither developers, property owners, nor their design and construction teams currently receive a share of those savings.

Instead, other opportunities have begun to appear that leverage population health benefits to generate reasonable profit for real estate projects.[CC1.5]

CORE COMPETENCY 1.5
Real Estate Development
Market Research Analysis

1.4.b.i Opportunity 1: Increase Operational Revenue

Building projects can leverage research showing a correlation between healthy indoor environments and worker productivity, which increases a green and healthy building's value to corporate tenants. For example, a study of 10 office buildings in five US cities from 2015–2016 found that cognitive test scores among office workers at LEED-certified buildings were 26.4% higher compared with working in non-certified buildings. The same study found that workers in LEED-certified buildings self-reported 6.4% higher sleep quality scores and 30% fewer sick building syndrome symptoms than their counterparts at non-certified buildings.[34] A 2022 study of 60 properties in Canada and the US conducted by the Center for Active Design converted evidence-based design and operations strategies like the ones in the cognitive function study into quantifiable value by linking higher Fitwel scores (a green and healthy building rating system) with higher net promoter scores (i.e., the likelihood that an occupant would recommend the building to peers)—indicating that occupants value green and healthy building strategies even if they are not aware that the building was designed to promote health and wellbeing.[35] Some companies have translated employee satisfaction into savings tied to human resources and productivity. For example, after Cundall, an engineering services firm in London, UK, moved into an office space that was certified at the Gold level under the WELL building certification system, they measured a 27% reduction in staff turnover and a 50% reduction in absenteeism over the following year, resulting in £122,000 and £90,000 in savings, respectively.[36]

The commercial real estate market has also begun to translate occupant health benefits into predicted value streams on the operational pro forma. For example, a study of over 22,000 leasing transactions conducted by commercial real estate services firm CBRE found that office buildings that certified under green and healthy rating systems in Europe from 2015–2020 were leased more quickly, experienced lower vacancy rates, and commanded 21% higher rents on average than non-certified buildings.[37] A triple bottom line tool called Autocase translates green and healthy building performance metrics into a predicted return on investment for design strategies that exceed minimum code requirements. For example, the tool predicted that achieving LEED Gold Certification for the 236,000 ft² (22,000 m²) Howard County, Georgia, USA Circuit Courthouse project would increase capital expenditures by 2.5% over code minimum. But the $1.10/square foot ($0.10/square meter) predicted reduction in operations costs per year associated with those additional capital expenditures would result in $40.1 million in lifetime savings for the owner ($2.6 million), building occupants ($15.4 million), and the community ($22.1 million), primarily in the form of enhanced productivity and reduced health care costs associated with indoor air quality.[38]

1.4.b.ii Opportunity 2: Reduce the Cost of Capital

Government tax-credit and loan programs offer a second pathway for green and health-promoting real estate projects to capitalize on the value they create for occupants and the community. One example is the Healthy Housing Rewards program managed by Fannie Mae, which offers a 15-basis point reduction in the construction or renovation loan and covers certification costs for affordable housing projects (e.g., properties serving households earning 80% or less of Area Median Income) that achieve a minimum two-star certification under Fitwel. One example of this approach, Edgewood Court Apartments in Atlanta, Georgia, USA, combined Fannie Mae's Healthy Housing Rewards program with their Green Rewards program (which underwrites 75% of energy and water upgrades), and their mortgage-backed securities as tax-exempt bond collateral program (another mechanism to reduce loan interest rates). The resulting project preserved 204 very low-income affordable housing units in a neighborhood that was experiencing rapid escalation of rental rates. Additionally, the budget was able to accommodate a 4,500 ft² (418 m²) community center, community gardens, outdoor play areas, indoor fitness facilities, safe paths for pedestrians and cyclists, and enhanced indoor air quality.[39,40]

1.4.b.iii Opportunity 3: Attract New Sources of Capital

The Healthy Neighborhoods Equity Fund (HNEF), a $50 million private equity fund[CC1.6] managed by the Conservation Law Foundation, exclusively invests in real estate development projects that show potential to improve neighborhood social and environmental determinants of health. For example, HNEF funded almost 16% ($2.9 million out of an $18 million total development cost) of the Bartlett Station redevelopment (2019) in the Nubian Square (previously Dudley Square) neighborhood of Boston, Massachusetts, USA. This project converted a brownfield that had been used as a bus yard into a mixed-income, green, walkable, and health-promoting development with retail space on the ground floor and rental units above. HNEF's goal in funding the project was to support changes to the built environment that would help address the shocking disparities in life expectancy in the Nubian Square neighborhood (58.9 years) compared with the average in Massachusetts (80.5 years).[41]

CORE COMPETENCY 1.6

Philanthropy
Collaboration/Partnership

1.4.b.iv Opportunity 4: Future-Proof the Property

Population health and vulnerability data can also be used to reduce capital expenditures and future-proof the long-term value of real estate investments. For long-term owners and building occupants, this value can be enhanced over time by measuring the behavioral and health outcomes associated with the building after it is occupied. At the federal level, the Federal Emergency Management Agency has recognized the need to fund projects enhancing local resilience by launching the Pre-Disaster Mitigation Grant Program. New York City carried this idea to the local scale in the PlaNYC report following the devastation caused by Superstorm Sandy in 2012: *A Stronger, More Resilient New York*. The report reviewed climate-related vulnerabilities in five neighborhoods and outlined specific resiliency measures that could be applied at the building level to reduce vulnerability to future events. A chapter was also devoted to funding opportunities targeted at increasing the resilience of the built environment.[42]

1.4.c Myth 3: Population Health Data Are Not Site-Specific

This myth may be the most baseless barrier to applying population health data to the design process. The Enterprise Foundation and the National Center for Healthy Housing overcame this concern by collecting site-specific data for a demonstration project in Worthington, Minnesota, USA. The project assessed the health outcomes associated with using a combination of green building and healthy housing principles to renovate an affordable housing development. The research team trained residents on how to operate their home according to healthy housing principles; asked residents to fill out a baseline health questionnaire before the renovation and again 12 and 18 months after its completion; performed breathing tests and height and weight measurements on residents diagnosed with asthma; performed visual examinations of the building before and after renovation; and measured building performance characteristics, such as energy use and ventilation rates, before and after the renovation. The study results found improvements in health indicators, improved operational efficiency in the complex as a whole, reduced numbers of pest infestations, and reduced instances of graffiti one year after completion of the renovation.[43]

Collecting new data is often time- and cost-prohibitive for new construction projects. And while it is true that, in the past, population health data available from federal agencies such as the US Centers for Disease Control and Prevention (CDC) was often not coded to a geographic area smaller than the county level, geospatially coded health and vulnerability data sets are becoming increasingly available at smaller spatial scales, such as the census tract (i.e., neighborhood scale). Executive Order 13642: Making Open and Machine Readable the New Default for Government Information,[44] issued in 2013, resulted in a barrage of open data being made available by public entities at all levels of government. Much of that data is now available at the census tract level and can contribute to the site assessment process for real estate development projects. See chapter 2 for detailed guidance on how to find and use neighborhood-scale data sets to support design decisions.

For the South Lincoln redevelopment master plan in Denver, Colorado, USA,[45] the Denver Housing Authority developed an HIA using data sets from federal agencies (such as the US Census and the CDC), local sources (such as the Tri-County Health Department and the Colorado Asthma Program), and project-specific resident surveys. The resulting recommendations include specific design strategies for public spaces (such as neighborhood streets and parks). They also include building strategies that would reduce exposure to poor air quality, promote physical activity, and increase public safety. A few examples of the HIA's recommendations include

- providing amenities (e.g., benches, game tables, barbeque pits, public art, etc.) that would encourage residents to spend more time in streetscapes and parks
- designing schools to accommodate community activities during off-hours
- designing stairwells to encourage their use and discourage use of elevators[45]

1.4.d Myth 4: Community Health is Not "Our" Responsibility

Licensed architects and engineers are held to professional codes of conduct to protect the "health, safety, and welfare" (HSW) of the public.[46,47] The scope of this professional obligation is often interpreted as limited to the building structure and fire safety. As a result, the health of community members beyond the building's walls is sometimes overlooked or considered irrelevant to the design process.

However, a number of organizations have started to expand the definition of HSW in interesting ways. In 2010, New York City released the *Active Design Guidelines*,[48] a set of design strategies at both the building and urban scales that promote health and wellbeing through increased physical activity. In 2012, the American Institute of Architects launched an advocacy initiative called "The Decade of Design"[49] that begins to expand the definition of HSW beyond the design of a single building to the urban context. In 2013, the US Green Building Council published a report, *Health is a Human Right. Green Building Can Help.*, which seeks to redefine green building as actively supportive of health and wellbeing.[50] And, in 2016 the CDC launched Fitwel,[51] a healthy building certification system that compiles hundreds of public health studies into actionable strategies for designers and owners to implement in new construction and existing buildings to improve the health-promoting aspects of their facilities. All of these initiatives point to a growing realization in the design industry that community health *IS* our responsibility—at least, in part.

Finally, every $1 of expenditure on natural disaster emergency preparedness is estimated to avoid $15 (net present value) of future damages.[52] Therefore, if a building or development is located in an area whose population is particularly vulnerable to disease, injury, or death from climate-related events, it may be in the property owner's financial interest to prioritize design strategies that either reduce exposure (such as planting trees in urban heat islands) and/or support the community's ability to shelter in place during and after the event. Furthermore, to the extent that community health influences property values, it is in an owner's best interest to design, construct, and operate properties that support positive health outcomes. Investing in design and programmatic strategies that promote health benefits everyone.

1.4.e Myth 5: Analyzing Health Data Will Slow Down the Project

It is true that, on the whole, public health research has traditionally followed a lengthier schedule than a typical real estate development project. If the goal of the research is to influence a particular building's design, it is not helpful if the results of the data analysis are released after completion of construction. While this was a real concern in the past, the confluence of increased availability of data, new technologies, and streamlined assessment tools has radically shortened the minimum timeframe required to develop credible recommendations.

As discussed in chapter 2 of this book, population health and vulnerability data are becoming increasingly available at spatial scales that can be used to inform design decisions. Design tools such as building information management (BIM) systems can use this newly available information to inform design decisions. Chapter 2 will also present public health methodologies like Health Situation Analysis and HIAs, which can be used to develop recommendations that are tailored to a specific design project. Comprehensive, or in-depth, HIAs often take six months or longer to complete. On the other hand, health situation analysis and less intensive "rapid" and "desktop" HIAs can often be completed in days to weeks.[53]

1.5 The Value Proposition for Architectural Epidemiology

Architectural epidemiology starts from the premise that the real estate industry is a complex adaptive system in capitalist economies like the US and Europe. This means that, while it is governed by a set of generic regulations, the forces that lead real estate development teams to prioritize one set of design strategies over another are largely determined by individual interactions between competing properties within the marketplace. One way to visualize a complex adaptive system is to imagine a flock of birds. There is no single, organizing leader. But one bird influencing its immediate neighbors can swiftly touch off a rapid shift in direction for the entire flock.

The real estate sector could be described in a similar manner. Building projects are bought and sold as discrete financial assets—disconnected from their surroundings. For example, a chain reaction of green or healthy building certifications among class A office buildings in a certain market, each of which is seeking to create competitive advantage for an individual project, could quickly cause a distortion in that portion of the building market, similar to the flock of birds.

Crucially, the way real estate projects interact with each other is divorced from their environmental and social context. Instead, comparisons are made based on building use, size, age, and rental rates. Meanwhile, the health impact pyramid and the hierarchy of controls frameworks tell us that buildings influence occupant and community health and wellbeing regardless of whether or not they are designed or operated with that reality in mind. Seen through a business lens, this state of affairs is a market failure. Both the real estate developer and the local government stand to lose value if buildings continue to be developed as though they stood separate and apart from their context.

Architectural epidemiology proposes a method for touching off a context-adaptive chain of events by addressing two unintended consequences of the current system: the last mile problem and the wrong pocket syndrome.

1.5.a The Last Mile

The idea of a "last mile" originated in the 19th century with the telegraph industry. It referred to the last step in a telegraph's journey. After traveling quickly and efficiently through a network of cables, it was transcribed at a local office and delivered by hand to its final destination. Today, "the last mile problem" is used in the real estate industry to call out land use planning that invests in centralized public transit infrastructure but does not upgrade the surrounding streets to safely accommodate pedestrians and cyclists charting unique paths from the bus or train stop to their ultimate destination. The definition has also expanded beyond its original reference to distance. It is used in many industries to refer to the gap between a generic strategy that applies to all situations and the personalization that is required to put the strategy into action. As the book *The Last Mile* by Dilip Soman chronicles across a wide swath of economic sectors, the last mile can determine the success or failure of any number of efforts—from employee decisions regarding health insurance coverage to COVID vaccination rates.[54]

In this book, the last mile refers to the gap between large-scale societal and economic interests on the one hand and the project-specific interests of real estate teams on the other.

1.5.a.i Large-Scale Interests

Societal interests are codified in the built environment through local policies and regulations like building codes, zoning requirements, and climate action plans. Local governments use these instruments to signal to the market the importance that real estate developers should place on life safety, carbon emissions, protection from infectious disease, and the social and economic character of the community. In contrast, economic interests in real estate are dominated by lending institutions and private equity firms whose key performance indicators are influenced by market forces that are larger than any single community. Neither set of interests are easily tailored to the specific needs of a building project surrounded by a unique combination of environmental exposures and population health characteristics.

1.5.a.ii Project-Specific Interests

Most real estate teams limit their focus to inside the boundaries of the project site. The developer tasks the design team with producing a project that balances programmatic needs with the budgetary constraints set by financial backers. The building program and decisions about the quality of construction are determined by financial comparisons with similar projects nearby. Sustainability and health criteria are the only aspects of the project that are not responsive to neighborhood characteristics—such as traffic-related air pollution, urban heat island effects, or lack of access to grocery stores. Projects often minimize communication with community members and local regulators out of concern that additional contact might lead to expensive requests or unwarranted oversight. They only interface with elements outside the property boundaries to connect with utilities, sidewalks, and other public infrastructure.

1.5.b The Wrong Pocket

The other major misalignment preventing building teams from prioritizing community health in their designs, the wrong pocket syndrome, refers to the gap between who pays for the project (i.e., the developer) versus who reaps its health benefits over time (i.e., building occupants, medical insurance companies, and local government). This conundrum is called the wrong pocket syndrome because the party who takes on the financial risk of developing the project is not the same party who "pockets" the proceeds in the form of lower medical bills and improved health.[SR1.1]

In the building sector, the wrong pocket syndrome is exacerbated by time delays between the completion of construction and eventual benefits to health outcomes. In the case of design strategies that protect future occupants from climate-related hazards, the original investment might not reap any monetized health benefits for years or even decades after completion of construction.

1.5.c Using Architectural Epidemiology to Create New Value Streams

The way to overcome the last mile and wrong pocket conundrums is to demonstrate to real estate developers, local government, and community groups who might initially oppose the project or overlook the possibilities for improving population health outcomes that they are leaving value on the table by not coordinating more closely with each other. Architectural epidemiology can be used by all three groups to identify and quantify opportunities for value creation by tailoring

STAKEHOLDER ROLES 1.1

  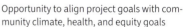

Opportunity to align project goals with community climate, health, and equity goals

STAKEHOLDER ROLES 1.2

Opportunity for local regulators to tailor requirements and incentive programs to address neighborhood needs

STAKEHOLDER ROLES 1.3

ArchEPI increases the visibility of community voices, particularly in relation to climate, health, and equity goals.

building design and operations to advance improvements in neighborhood environmental health conditions (table 1.2).

Value generation begins with the real estate team performing a health situation analysis of the building site and surrounding neighborhood (usually defined as its census block group or census tract). Chapter 2 describes in detail how to prioritize the top one to three health issues of importance to the neighborhood, both in terms of environmental exposure and population health needs.[SR1.2] A set of 10 health infographics in the toolbox are designed to help project teams deploy evidence-based strategies tailored to address their stated priorities. Chapter 2 also explains how to link project metrics with local goals related to climate change and chronic disease.

Local government has a number of levers at its disposal to generate value for the real estate development team. Actions that shorten the length of the construction loan are particularly of interest to developers, because construction loan rates often fluctuate on a monthly basis and have higher interest rates than fixed-rate loans. Table 1.2 lists both monetary and non-monetary opportunities for a range of governmental departments to generate value for the developer, including zoning, permitting, code enforcement, engineering and public works, sustainability and climate change, and public health. It is important to note that interdepartmental exchange of information and pooling of resources can be a challenge in local government. However, if an administration is able to break down siloes between departments, a great deal of value can be created. In many communities, the permitting department would act as the main point of contact with the real estate development team. They would funnel climate mitigation, resilience, and chronic disease metrics to the departments that are tasked with tracking progress on those topics. And they would funnel incentives in the other direction from their sister departments to the development team.

Community groups are an often-overlooked source of value creation for both the development team and the local government. The architectural epidemiology method starts by gathering data from reports and data portals. By including the community early in the process, the project team can ground-truth their preliminary assumptions about which environmental exposures and health concerns should be prioritized and how recommended design and operations strategies could coordinate with other elements in the neighborhood to create a ripple effect promoting community and planetary health.[SR1.3]

Community groups can act as partners and intermediaries as the project seeks to establish relationships and cooperative agreements with other landowners in the neighborhood. And they can be particularly powerful as advocates on behalf of families who are exposed to environmental toxins, economically disadvantaged populations, and neighborhoods that have suffered the environmental and health effects of racist policies like redlining. Engaging these groups as equal partners in the negotiation about value generation can result in a wide range of social and economic benefits to neighborhood residents and the community as a whole that otherwise would not have been considered. Understanding a wide range of perspectives during the project development process can create a win–win–win for the community, the municipality, and the project team.

Author Adele Houghton conducted a proof-of-concept of this approach from 2022–2023 with three real estate projects in three different communities across the country. At the end of the pilot, 43 participants (89.6% response rate) representing all three stakeholder groups (community, design/development team, and local government) reported that the approach presented in this section successfully expanded the cost–benefit conversation beyond the property line. In other words, all three stakeholder groups reported feeling that both their own group

TABLE 1.2.

Stakeholder Analysis of Value Generated Using Architectural Epidemiology

Stakeholder	Motivation	Timeframe	What Value Can Be Created?	Who Benefits?	What Is the Role of Architectural Epidemiology?
Developer	Pay off construction loan as quickly as possible	Development process (usually two to five years)	• Health-promoting strategies tailored to neighborhood needs • Baseline neighborhood environmental health metrics aligned with community metrics	Local government and community groups	• Methodology to prioritize climate-related and chronic disease health outcomes and link them to protective green building and operations strategies • Create a conceptual framework for each priority health concern and designate metrics (and identify existing data sets) for each component of the framework
Local government	Reduce expenses from social services	Long-term	• *Zoning Department*: Increase floor area ratio; approve expanded use; trade automobile parking requirements for bicycle racks or transit improvements • *Permitting Department*: expedite approvals; lower real estate taxes • *Code Enforcement Department*: expedite code review • *Engineering/Public Works Department*: pay for infrastructure improvements • *Climate Change/Sustainability/Public Health*: make a portion of grant funding available for real estate projects that demonstrate targeted benefit for resilience, reduced health effects of climatic events, and/or chronic disease	Developer	• Makes it possible for the project team to generate something of value that can be exchanged for monetary and non-monetary concessions from the local government
Community groups	Reduce chronic disease, health effects from exposure to climatic events; improve quality of life, economic opportunities; protect affordability	Long-term	• Share local knowledge and a coordinated vision for how to advance their population's health • Help the project establish relationships and cooperative agreements with other landowners in the neighborhood	Developer and local government	• Methodology encourages broad, multi-disciplinary collaboration • Methodology makes it possible to identify the priority environmental health concerns specific to the neighborhood—with input from community members

and other stakeholder groups received more benefit from the aligned vision for the project than they would have received through the conventional real estate development process.[55]

In summary, architectural epidemiology makes it possible to create new value streams by using neighborhood metrics as a common language. Community members use metrics to communicate the unique conditions in their neighborhood that would benefit from a design or operations intervention. Real estate development teams use metrics to demonstrate that their project will make a substantive contribution to local efforts to address climate change and/or chronic disease. And local government uses metrics to justify the kind and quantity of concessions made to the development project based on its contribution to local priorities.

Look for callout boxes in chapters 2–4 highlighting leverage points where one or more of the stakeholder groups engaged in the architectural epidemiology process are particularly well positioned to generate value for themselves and the project as a whole.

1.6 Why Isn't Architectural Epidemiology Already Standard Practice?

Given how much value can be created by aligning building project priorities with local government priorities around climate change and chronic disease, the question naturally arises: why don't all real estate projects tap into this opportunity? The last mile problem and wrong pocket syndrome are part of the reason. But there are also legal, technical, and process objections that must be overcome before architectural epidemiology can be widely adopted across the real estate industry.

1.6.a Legal Objections

The traditional legal position of real estate and design firms regarding health outcomes is too narrow to allow for health considerations to be integral to the decision-making process. Legal advice has steered firms away from making population-level health claims out of concern that they may be held liable if an individual occupant is harmed or does not attain the benefits outlined in the claim. There is also concern that the evidence base linking design decisions with health outcomes is not robust enough to warrant any claims of reduced health risk or potential improvements to health outcomes.

All of these objections were rebutted by a Joint Call to Action to Promote Healthy Communities that was released in 2017 by eight US built environment and public health membership organizations representing 450,000 members.[56] Since that time, interest in using design and operations to promote health and wellbeing has grown across the real estate sector. As practitioners have become more knowledgeable about the health effects of building and land use decisions, concerns about an individual suing an organization for making a claim about reductions in population health risks have begun to subside. Chapter 2 speaks specifically to the question of how to distinguish between causation and correlation or association in health claims. The health factsheets in the appendices demonstrate the growing body of knowledge validating the movement towards raising up health promotion as a primary goal of every real estate project.

1.6.b Technical Objection

The technical objection argues that post-secondary education in the design, real estate development, and public health fields does not teach students the analytical skills and underlying, cross-disciplinary concepts required to integrate neighborhood-level environmental health information into the design process.

This objection is largely true at the present time. Author Adele Houghton's research of US and global institutions of higher learning shows that only a handful of public health courses are available to university design and engineering students; most design students do not receive any education on statistical methods; and only a handful of built environment courses are available to public health students.[57] This book was designed to fill that gap in several ways. It can be used as a textbook for a standalone course teaching architectural epidemiology. Portions of it can be integrated into courses focused on specific design, health, or climate topics. As a practical tool, it can be used as a reference book by individuals working in real estate, design, government, and community advocacy.

1.6.c Project Delivery Process Objection

Two assumptions about how health data might disrupt the project delivery process also stand in the way of using it to help guide decision-making for design and operations. First, many people assume it is not available at a small enough scale to be relevant to real estate projects. Second, even if it is available, the concern is that analyzing it would slow down the design process too much to make it a practical addition to other contextual information such as topography, soil composition, and connections to public utilities.

Chapter 2 and the technical appendices share the enormous progress that has been made over the past decade increasing access to neighborhood scale datasets. While health data is still difficult to obtain at small spatial scales due to privacy concerns, many health outcomes and proxies are available down to the census tract level and sometimes further. In terms of the time cost of the analysis, experienced design teams can gather and analyze health data within a similar timeframe as other existing conditions for the project site.

1.7 Summary

This chapter places architectural epidemiology within the field of epidemiology and within its historical context. Real estate development, building regulations, and public infrastructure have profoundly influenced public health practice since its inception in 1840s London. However, societal recognition of the intertwined nature of these two fields waned in the late 19th century. The rise of bacteriology led to a shift in public health policy and investment away from large-scale capital works (like municipal water systems) and towards research into vaccines and therapeutics to combat infectious diseases like malaria, tuberculosis, and smallpox.[17] It was not until annual deaths from chronic diseases surpassed deaths from infectious diseases around the turn of the 21st century[58] that public health's origins in land use and building design rose again to prominence. As the factsheets in the toolbox explain in detail, mounting evidence suggests that tailoring land use and building design to promote positive health outcomes will be critical to successfully reversing the upward trend in chronic disease and climate-related death rates around the world.

The remainder of the book will present the architectural epidemiology method in detail (chapter 2) and recommend ways to use it effectively at each phase of the real estate project delivery process (chapter 3) and within different contract and financing structures (chapter 4).

Summary of Core Competencies Relevant to Architectural Epidemiology

Field	Core Competencies
Epidemiology	• Assessment and analysis • Community dimensions of practice • Cultural competency
Real estate development	• Location analysis • Market research analysis
Facility design, construction, operations	• Practice management • Programming and analysis • Contextual analysis
Sustainability	• Integrative strategies • Strategic execution
Philanthropy	• Collaboration/partnership

DISCUSSION QUESTIONS

1. Explain the historical connection between public health and the real estate sector including design and construction activities.
2. Describe what is meant by the concept of the last mile and give an example.
3. Compare and contrast two tiers within the Health Impact Pyramid and describe where buildings and sites would fit within the pyramid.
4. How has the question of the building sector's responsibility to protect the health of building occupants and/or the surrounding community evolved over time?
5. Describe three issues that impede Architectural Epidemiology from widespread adoption across the real estate industry.

CHAPTER 2

Introduction to Metrics for Built Environment Professionals

KEY MESSAGES

1. Architectural epidemiology (ArchEPI) assessments provide site-specific environmental public health indicators (EPHIs) that define the environmental exposure and population health context of a site, the drivers behind positive and negative health outcomes for site occupants and the community, and opportunities for design and operations to reduce negative exposures and amplify positive exposures.

2. ArchEPI assessments follow the six-step Guyer Problem-Solving Framework in order to strike a balance between scientific rigor and the fast pace of building design and facility operations projects.

3. Meaningful EPHIs will measure the environmental hazard of interest, the severity of exposure, the prevalence of vulnerable populations, the availability of building and operational strategies that can reduce exposure, and negative human health outcomes. An ArchEPI assessment identifies and develops site-specific EPHIs and provides recommendations focused on identifying and promoting the mediating factors that are most likely to benefit the health of building occupants and the surrounding neighborhood.

4. Developing site-specific EPHIs involves defining each indicator, deciding which geographic unit to use for the data set, taking measures to protect privacy, prioritizing the most relevant environmental public health hazards for the project, and performing spatial analysis to determine the extent to which negative health outcomes are occurring in a localized cluster.

2.1 Introduction

At its core, architectural epidemiology is a problem-solving discipline. It helps developers, designers, and facility managers understand the environmental public health context of a site, the drivers behind positive and negative health outcomes, and opportunities for design and operations to reduce negative exposures and amplify positive exposures.

As cross-disciplinary endeavors, architectural epidemiology (ArchEPI) assessments should be designed to meet two sets of requirements that can be in tension with each other. They must both meet the level of scientific rigor expected by epidemiologists and also respond to the fast pace of building design and facility operations projects.

Happily, the Guyer Problem-Solving Framework[1]—a clear, six-step approach to problem-solving in public health—meets both of these requirements:

1. Defining the problem
2. Measuring the magnitude
3. Understanding its key factors (or determinants)
4. Identifying and developing strategies to prevent and/or mitigate the problem
5. Prioritizing and recommending the most effective policies and strategies
6. Implementing and evaluating interventions

It lays out an evidence-based approach to addressing public health challenges. However, it allows for flexibility in the design of the assessment. And it emphasizes implementation and evaluation as integral components of the overall process.

This chapter uses the Guyer Problem-Solving Framework to introduce a set of tools drawn from the field of public health that can be used to decide which environmental health concerns should be prioritized by a design or facility operations project, which design/operations strategies should be implemented to address the problem, and how to measure success. While the chapter has been written with built environment professionals in mind, public health professionals may gain additional insight into the role of public health approaches within the built environment by reviewing this discussion of epidemiological inquiry within a design process framework.

You may find it valuable to reference the architectural epidemiology conceptual framework in chapter 1 (figure 1.1) as you explore the methods in chapter 2 that activate that diagram. The goal is to turn the architectural epidemiology conceptual framework into a powerful tool for decision-making, stakeholder alignment, and value creation.

2.1.a The Value of Understanding the Relationship (i.e., Correlation) between Environmental Exposures and Health Outcomes

If you have spent any time reviewing public health literature, you have been exposed to the difference between correlation and causation. Just because an outcome occurs when a variable is present does not mean that the variable causes the outcome. It merely means that the two phenomena are present simultaneously. The fact that statistical results fall short of estimating a causal connection between a variable and the outcome of interest is not a reason to ignore the variable. Instead, the fact that the two phenomena are correlated may indicate opportunities to reduce negative outcomes. It is important to note that almost all of the methodologies outlined in this chapter identify relationships (association/correlation) without quantifying the extent to which an environmental exposure or intervention is predicted to result in a certain health outcome (causation).

Causality is notoriously difficult to prove for environmental public health topics, because there are so many variables involved. Also, unlike randomized controlled trials, it is usually not ethical to randomize who lives in a certain neighborhood or who is exposed to traffic-related air pollution at their school.

While it is important to keep the distinction between correlation and causation front of mind during ArchEPI assessments, project teams should not be disheartened by the lack of causal predictability between building design strategies (e.g., building weatherization) and positive health outcomes (e.g., fewer occupants in weatherized buildings are diagnosed with heat stroke). It would be difficult to estimate a cause–effect health metric for such a small scale with any accuracy, because so few people would be included in the study design and analysis. The value of performing a site-specific correlation analysis stems instead from its ability to place the project within its context. By understanding the strength of association between the project's environmental assets and liabilities and the corresponding assets and liabilities of its surroundings, the project team can develop design strategies that maximize health and climate resilience benefits for the entire neighborhood, not just building occupants.[SR2.1] What ArchEPI practitioners are doing, in effect, is determining the population risk of a particular health outcome for the factors identified. They are not determining exactly how many people will be affected. Instead, they are identifying a risk for populations similar to the one in a specific project area.

> **STAKEHOLDER ROLES 2.1**
>
>
>
> Opportunity for alignment among developers, local government, and community groups

Using correlated data helps us understand the big picture and could arguably be more effective at addressing large-scale health epidemics like chronic disease and climate change than the current, high-level approach to developing public policy. It also opens the door to collaboration between the project team, communities, and public sector authorities who are working to address the same problems across cities, regions, and even globally.[SR2.2] See chapter 1 (table 1.2) for more detail about how to leverage the valuable information generated by ArchEPI assessments into a mutually beneficial relationship with policymakers.

STAKEHOLDER ROLES 2.2

Opportunity for alignment among developers, local government, and community groups

2.2 Step 1—Defining the Problem

Arguably the most significant step in the problem-solving framework—and the step that is most often lacking in current built environment practice—is the first one: defining the environmental health problem that could be improved through changes to the built and natural environment.

All design and facility operations projects confront a barrage of competing priorities from the very outset, ranging from financing to regulatory constraints to concerns about marketability. Assuming that health promotion is one of the project's central goals, the first and most important question confronting the project team is: Which health concerns should we target? (See chapter 1 for additional information about the business case in support of prioritizing health in the building sector.)

"Health" is a broad topic that is influenced by location (e.g., is the building located in an urban heat island?), demographics (e.g., will the building serve the young, the elderly, or both?), social equity (e.g., could the project make progress towards dismantling the legacy of racist policies like redlining?), socioeconomic status (e.g., could the project fill a gap for underserved populations?), and time or season (e.g., is there a seasonal threat of natural disasters like hurricanes or wildfire?).

In order to perform the first step in the problem-solving framework—define the problem—the team will need to perform a health situation analysis to assess the environmental and human health assets and liabilities associated with the project site and its surroundings and identify stakeholder groups.[CC2.1]

2.2.a Health Situation Analysis

A *health situation analysis (HSA)* is defined in A Dictionary of Epidemiology as the *"[s]tudy of a situation that may require improvement. This begins with a definition of the problem and an assessment or measurement of its extent, severity, causes, and impacts upon the community; it is followed by appraisal of interactions between the system and its environment and evaluations of performance."*[2(p262)] Context is fundamental to the concept of a situation analysis. The purpose of the analysis is to identify aspects of a building project's context that need to be improved and to rank those needs by severity, so that decision-makers can base their decisions to prioritize some actions over others on a review of the evidence.

An HSA could be seen as ArchEPI's contribution to the site assessment process that occurs at the inception of all real estate projects. Site assessment often includes mapping the site's topography, sunlight, and wind patterns; identifying the location of city utilities serving the site; performing preliminary code review; and analyzing the real estate market surrounding the site. Its purpose is to establish the regulatory, fiscal, and environmental assets and constraints of the site that, together, will form a framework within which the project will be designed.

CORE COMPETENCY 2.1

Epidemiology
Assessment and Analysis

Facility Design, Construction, Operations
Programming and Analysis

STAKEHOLDER ROLES 2.3

Opportunity for alignment among developers, local government, and community groups

CORE COMPETENCY 2.2

Epidemiology
Cultural Competency

Facility Design, Construction, Operations
Contextual Analysis

Sustainability
Project Surroundings and Public Outreach

STAKEHOLDER ROLES 2.4

Opportunity for community to revise and add richness to analyses based on secondary data sets

DEFINITION 2.1

Community-Based Participatory Research
Scientific enquiries in which scientific and community researchers collaborate on all aspects of the study, including defining the research question, establishing methods, data collection, data analysis, forming conclusions, and implementing actions based on the study results

CORE COMPETENCY 2.3

Epidemiology
Basic Public Health Services

STAKEHOLDER ROLES 2.5

Opportunity for local government to tailor open-source data sets to support design decisions

CORE COMPETENCY 2.4

Real Estate Development
Location Analysis

Sustainability
Location and Transportation

By performing a health situation analysis alongside traditional site assessment topics, the ArchEPI team will ensure that the most pressing environmental public health challenges facing building occupants and the surrounding neighborhood have been defined and articulated before design begins.[SR2.3]

2.2.a.i What Are the Primary Health Concerns of Stakeholders Such as the Building Occupants, Surrounding Neighborhood, and Community?

As you begin to develop the HSA, build a list of the environmental health concerns that are priorities for the community where the project is located[CC2.2] and may turn out to be of particular significance on-site. This information can be gathered directly from community members[SR2.4] by adding an environmental health topic to community meetings and stakeholder events. It could also be gathered using community-based participatory and action research methods[D2.1] in partnership with local universities, non-profits, and/or the public health departments. See appendix A for resources on how to conduct community-based participatory and action research.

Public health agencies[CC2.3] routinely gather information about the incidence, prevalence, and precursors (i.e., risk factors) of disease based on geography, demographics, and socioeconomic status.[SR2.5] Sometimes these data are publicly available down to the zip code or neighborhood level (e.g., census tract or census block group). Data sets may also be accessible to researchers down to the address or block level after removing information that would allow identification of a specific individual. Section 2.3.e goes into more detail about how health data is aggregated to protect personal privacy. By simply searching for published environmental, demographic, and community health data and public health resources related to the project site, you can improve the site assessment's ability to identify high priority environmental health opportunities for the site and surrounding neighborhood. Compare neighborhood-scale data with larger spatial scales (such as community, state, and country) to develop a short list of potential environmental health goals for the project.

See appendix B for resources on how to research local environmental public health priorities. Examples of publicly available data sets that can be used to develop environmental public health indicators include Healthy People 2030 (https://health.gov/healthypeople) and the National Center for Health Statistics (https://www.cdc.gov/nchs/index.htm) in the US. The Global Observatory (https://www.who.int/data/gho) at the World Health Organization (WHO) and the United Nations Sustainable Development Goals (SDGs) (https://unstats.un.org/sdgs/indicators/database/) are commonly used global data sets.

2.2.a.ii What Are the Environmental Conditions Surrounding the Project Site that Promote or Act as Barriers to Optimal Health Outcomes?

After identifying a short list of potential environmental health concerns for prioritization, project teams need to identify built environment strategies for reducing the severity or incidence of those health concerns.[CC2.4]

For example, if air pollution and mental health are identified as neighborhood health priorities, the project design could respond by including

- vegetative barriers that separate occupants from off-site sources of air pollution,
- outdoor rooms which increase occupants' direct access to nature,
- renewable energy installations and battery storage to reduce on-site sources of air pollution,

- enhanced ventilation and filtration in the heating, refrigeration, and air conditioning (HVAC) system,
- low emitting and non-toxic finish materials, and
- access to daylight and views of nature.

These features can reduce exposure to toxins and create a context supportive of health-promoting behaviors.

The toolbox is designed to help project teams connect the dots between priority environmental health conditions and evidence-based strategies that can reduce the risk of negative health outcomes and/or promote positive health outcomes.[CC2.5] In addition to accessing national databases, it can be helpful to research local "open data" portals and local reports on the same topics. A variety of public agencies and non-governmental organizations collect information about environmental conditions—often at very granular geographic scales.

CORE COMPETENCY 2.5

Sustainability
Integrative Services

2.2.b Existing Public Health Definitions

In many cases, data are already being gathered at the local, state, national, and/or international level about the health concerns that will emerge as priorities for the project team through the HSA.

Appendix C shares an example of existing data definitions related to extreme heat. In the US, many definitions are drawn from the Healthy People program managed by the US Centers for Disease Control and Prevention (CDC) (https://www.cdc.gov/nchs/healthy_people/index.htm). Internationally, definitions are often drawn from the World Health Organization's Global Health Observatory (https://www.who.int/data/gho) and the U.N. Sustainable Development Goals (https://unstats.un.org/sdgs/indicators/database/). Understanding the concepts and definitions can facilitate cross-disciplinary discussion and collaboration.

Crafting site-specific environmental health priorities using existing data definitions benefits the project in three ways:

1. It makes it possible for the project to use existing data sets, rather than gathering data specific to the project population. Gathering health data can be slow, labor intensive, and expensive. Using existing data sets is often free and easy to accomplish.
2. Using an existing data set allows the project to make comparisons with other locations, which can be helpful both for benchmarking and for measuring the long-term success of interventions.
3. Using data definitions that have been adopted by the local climate action plan, the neighborhood strategic plan, the community health implementation plan, and other local policies allows the project to quantify its response to specific needs identified by the surrounding neighborhood and community. That approach opens the door to conversations about how the neighborhood and community could support the project in achieving the metrics laid out in its design concept.[SR2.6]

STAKEHOLDER ROLES 2.6

Opportunity for the development team to demonstrate how the design supports community goals

The downsides, of course, are that the existing data definition may not exactly reflect the health concern of highest priority to the project team. And data may not be available at a small enough geographic unit to reflect the specific conditions within a neighborhood.

Whether or not the team decides to make use of existing public health definitions or craft their own definitions and gather data from future occupants and the surrounding community to establish baseline conditions, the next step in the ArchEPI assessment is to draft operational definitions for the short list of health challenges faced by the population affected by the project.

STAKEHOLDER ROLES 2.7

Opportunity for alignment among developers, local government, and community groups

CORE COMPETENCY 2.6

Real Estate Development
Market Analysis

Sustainability
Strategy Planning

Philanthropy
Vision Setting

2.2.c Develop a Conceptual Framework for the Health Concern

Conceptual frameworks are used in social science disciplines like public health to diagram the major relationships linking concepts that, together, can help explain a complex health problem.[3] They are useful within the context of environmental public health, because the relationships between environmental hazards, design interventions, and health outcomes are often influenced (i.e., mediated) by other factors, such as demographics, socioeconomic status, and behavioral choices.[4,SR2.7]

Conceptual frameworks lay out the major variables (also called indicators) that help explain how natural hazards (like climate change) and characteristics of the built environment (like poorly maintained buildings located in an urban heat island and/or flood plain) can contribute to the vulnerability of at-risk populations (such as the elderly) to related health concerns (like heat exhaustion and cardiovascular disease). These conceptual frameworks help visually describe the system that is acting on or creating the conditions associated with specific health outcomes of interest.

A strong conceptual framework is

- simple,
- easy to read from left to right, and
- contains all of the variables that will be measured by the ArchEPI project.

See the architectural epidemiology conceptual framework in chapter 1 (figure 1.1) for a generic example. Figure 2.1 demonstrates how a conceptual model can be used to uncover the relationship between environmental exposures and health outcomes. The figure displays three conceptual frameworks developed by author Adele Houghton and colleagues at Air Alliance Houston for a health impact assessment (HIA) that considered potential co-harms to the health of students and staff in elementary schools adjacent to a proposed freeway expansion in Houston, Texas, USA. By mapping out the relationship between the freeway expansion and three environmental health exposures (air pollution, flooding, and mobility), the team was able to identify opportunities for a single design strategy or set of strategies to reduce exposure to more than one environmental hazard.[CC2.6]

2.2.d Core Competencies

Defining the Problem: Core Competencies

Field	Core Competencies
Epidemiology	• Assessment and analysis • Basic public health services • Cultural competency
Real estate development	• Location analysis • Market research analysis
Facility design, construction, operations	• Programming and analysis • Contextual analysis
Sustainability	• Integrative Services • Location and transportation • Project surroundings and public outreach • Strategic planning
Philanthropy	• Vision setting

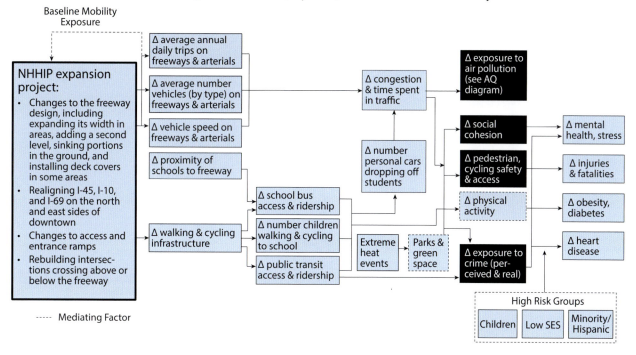

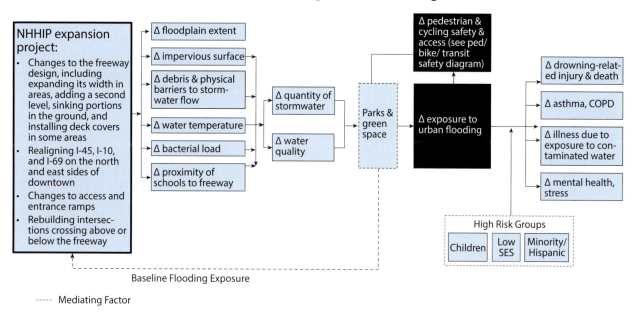

Figure 2.1. Potential Health Impacts of the North Houston Highway Improvement Project on Schools Mediated through Mobility, Air Pollution, and Flooding. *Source:* Air Alliance Houston NHHIP Health Impact Assessment

Potential Health Impacts of the NHHIP Project on Schools Mediated through Air Quality

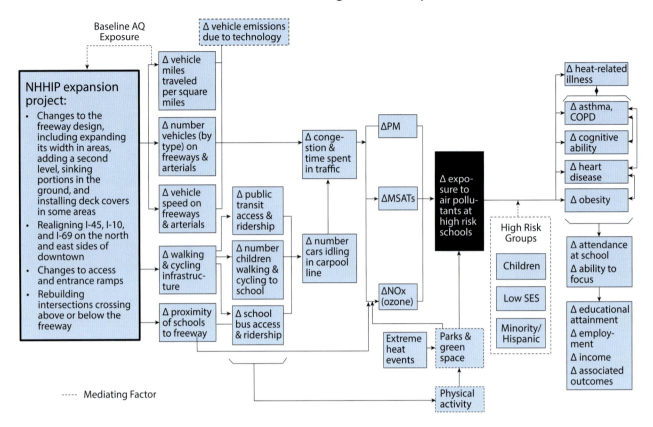

Figure 2.1. (cont.)

DEFINITION 2.2

Environmental Public Health Indicators
Data that provide "information about a population's health status with respect to environmental factors"

U.S. CDC, National Environmental Public Health Tracking, 2022. https://ephtracking.cdc.gov/indicatorPages

CORE COMPETENCY 2.7

Epidemiology
Basic Public Health Services

STAKEHOLDER ROLES 2.8

Opportunity for local government to tailor open-source data sets to support design decisions

2.3 Step 2—Measuring the Magnitude of the Problem

2.3.a Introduction to EPHIs

It is often difficult or impossible to establish a direct causal link between exposure to an environmental hazard and a health outcome among a defined group of people in a specific location. EPHIs[D2.2] help overcome that hurdle by measuring factors—both direct and indirect—that link human health with environmental hazards.[5]

EPHIs are often used by local, state, and federal public health officials to track a population's health status in relation to an environmental hazard.[CC2.7] For example, a state or local health department might use a set of EPHIs to understand whether or not neighborhoods with a high percentage of impervious surface, elderly residents, families living in poverty, racial and ethnic minorities, and/or homes lacking central air conditioning have experienced a higher rate of hospital visits and/or death during heat waves.[SR2.8]

After setting a baseline, EPHIs can be used to evaluate over time whether certain interventions—such as weatherization programs, air conditioning giveaway programs, low-income electricity protection programs, and tree planting programs—help bring residents living in high-risk neighborhoods closer to the health profile of low-risk neighborhoods.

48 ARCHITECHTURAL EPIDEMIOLOGY

2.3.b Developing Indicators Linking the Built Environment to Health Outcomes

Most EPHIs touch on at least three topics: environmental hazard, environmental exposure, and human health outcomes resulting from exposure.[5] In this book, we add two mediating factors—vulnerable populations and design/operational interventions. These two mediating factors can either increase or decrease the risk of a bad health outcome after exposure to the environmental hazard in question.[SR2.9]

An ArchEPI assessment prioritizes site-specific EPHIs (e.g., percent impervious surface and homes without central air conditioning, etc.) and built environment recommendations (e.g., tree planting and weatherization programs) that promote the mediating factors that are most likely to benefit the health of building occupants and the surrounding neighborhood.[CC2.8] When developing the final set of indicators that will be used by the project to set its architectural epidemiology goals and track progress, it is important to integrate community input and questions of social equity, so the project's vision translates into tangible benefit for the surrounding community after completion of construction.

Note: You may find it useful to keep the architectural epidemiology conceptual framework in chapter 1 (figure 1.1) at hand as a visual guide while reading the following sub-sections. The infographics at the end of each health topic in the toolbox provide specific examples for each step. And figure T.4 in the toolbox shares a crosswalk of climate change and community health co-benefits associated with common design and operations strategies.

2.3.b.i Environmental Public Health Hazard

It is important to include a recognized definition of each environmental public health hazard[D2.3] under consideration for the project.[CC2.9] For example, the definition of extreme heat changes in response to location and context. It is defined differently in Seattle, Washington; Houston, Texas; and Phoenix, Arizona, USA. As the project team moves from conversations about generic health topics to the specific concerns of future occupants and the surrounding neighborhood, it may become necessary to consider a range of possible definitions and selecting the option that is most relevant to the project.[SR2.10]

2.3.b.ii Environmental Exposure

Environmental exposure indicators[CC2.10] measure conditions that increase or decrease the risk of building occupants and others coming in contact with the environmental public health hazard (see section 2.3.b.i). The conceptual frameworks in the toolbox divide environmental exposure into two categories: natural environment determinants of health and built environment determinants of health. The indicators measuring natural environment determinants of health refer to the specific environmental processes with which the population could come in contact as a result of the environmental public health hazard. The built environment determinants of health, on the other hand, measure the extent to which the built environment acts as a conduit for or protection from exposure to the environmental hazard.

STAKEHOLDER ROLES 2.9

Opportunity for alignment among developers, local government, and community groups

CORE COMPETENCY 2.8

Epidemiology
Cultural Competency

Facility Design, Construction, Operations
Research, Technical and Analytical

Philanthropy
Planning; Vision Setting

DEFINITION 2.3

Environmental Public Health Hazard
An environmental situation or agent that is capable of causing harm to a population's health

CORE COMPETENCY 2.9

Epidemiology
Basic Public Health Services

STAKEHOLDER ROLES 2.10

Local agencies often set local definitions for environmental public health hazards like heat events.

CORE COMPETENCY 2.10

Real Estate Development
Location Analysis

Facility Design, Construction, Operations
Site Inventory; Physical Analysis

Sustainability
Site Assessment

BOX 2.1.

Example—Options for Defining Extreme Heat in the US

The CDC Environmental Public Health Tracking Network (EPHTN) offers several options for defining an extreme heat event in the US. Depending on local priorities, an extreme heat day could be defined using absolute temperature, heat index (i.e., temperature plus humidity), or percentile thresholds. Similarly, an extreme heat event could be defined as meeting the desired threshold over two or more days or over three or more days.[6] This level of flexibility is particularly important for heat events, because the same sets of conditions might trigger concerns about heat-related illness in some locations but not in others. For example, researchers in Seattle, Washington, USA, have found that negative health outcomes from heat begin to rise at 78.6°F (25.9°C).[7] In comparison, researchers in Miami, Florida, USA, use 100°F (37.8°C) as the threshold for defining an extreme heat day.[8] See the extreme heat section of the toolbox for more information.

BOX 2.2.

Example—Options for Accessing Data on Cardiovascular Disease

Cardiovascular disease is the leading cause of death both in the US and worldwide.[9,10] In the US, the CDC PLACES (formerly 500 Cities)[11] data portal provides estimates of average adult coronary heart disease prevalence at the census tract level. Measures of current disease can indicate how widespread it is in the population, but they may not provide information about severity. The EPHTN (see box 2.1) tracks three additional indicators that can shed light on the severity of cases and how well the disease is managed in the community: heart attack mortality, hospitalizations for heart attack, and ischemic heart disease mortality. But these data sets are only available down to the county level.[6] Twenty-six states have developed state and local tracking programs, which may include data on cardiovascular disease mortality at the census tract or block group level. But, in states without a tracking program, it may be necessary to request data from the local health department or regional health systems to calculate the rate of cardiovascular disease mortality in a particular neighborhood or community. The WHO and SDGs data portals lump four chronic diseases into a single definition: "mortality rate attributed to cardiovascular disease, cancer, diabetes, or chronic respiratory disease."[12,13] As discussed in the toolbox, the mechanisms linking the built environment to health outcomes are quite different for cardiovascular disease compared with cancer and respiratory disease. So projects located in regions that follow WHO or SDG tracking programs may face barriers to accessing cardiovascular disease data isolated from other chronic diseases. See the toolbox section on cardiovascular disease for more information.

BOX 2.3.

Example—Environmental Determinants of Health for Extreme Heat

Continuing with the example of extreme heat, the infographic in the toolbox lists increased average temperatures and an increase in the number, frequency, duration, and severity of heat waves as natural environment determinants of health attributable to climate change. The built environment determinants of health for extreme heat include the urban heat island, access to outdoor activities, stress on plant and animal life, food insecurity, water quantity and quality, habitat availability for disease-carrying vectors, sources of air pollution, building materials and ventilation contributors to indoor air quality, and level of electricity grid stability.

2.3.b.iii Population Vulnerability

Physiological, social, and economic differences can at least partially explain why some individuals are at higher risk than others of negative health outcomes after exposure to a specific environmental public health hazard. It is important for design and facility operations projects to understand the potential vulnerabilities of building occupants and the surrounding community.[CC2.11] Sometimes, the populations touched by a project may exhibit low vulnerability to the priority environmental public health concerns in the neighborhood. But in other cases (e.g., projects serving children, the elderly, the immunocompromised, or low-income groups), the project team may find that significant portions of the population within their sphere of influence are vulnerable to one or more priority hazard. In that case, the team may decide to emphasize evidence-based design strategies that are particularly effective with the priority hazard and de-emphasize some other potential design choices.

CORE COMPETENCY 2.11

Epidemiology
Assessment and Analysis

2.3.b.iv Design and Development Mediating Factors

Design and development mediating factors refer to changes to the building, site, public right-of-way, and facility operations that could either reduce exposure to the environmental public health hazard in question or increase population resilience to the hazard.[CC2.12] For example, adding trees along sidewalks or including an onsite park with shade and water to reduce the heat island effect of the hard surfaces on the property would be a design and development mediating factor for the hazard of extreme heat. Design can also increase equitable access to a property. For example, the Montrose Whole Foods Market in Houston, Texas, USA, includes an indoor–outdoor seating area with freely available cups and a water dispenser (figure 2.2). Anyone is free to enter the seating area without entering the store. As a result, people walking down the street can use the air-conditioned seating area as an informal cooling center and source of water regardless of whether they plan to purchase groceries.

CORE COMPETENCY 2.12

Facility Design, Construction, Operations
Project Planning and Design

Sustainability
Integrative Services; Location and Transportation

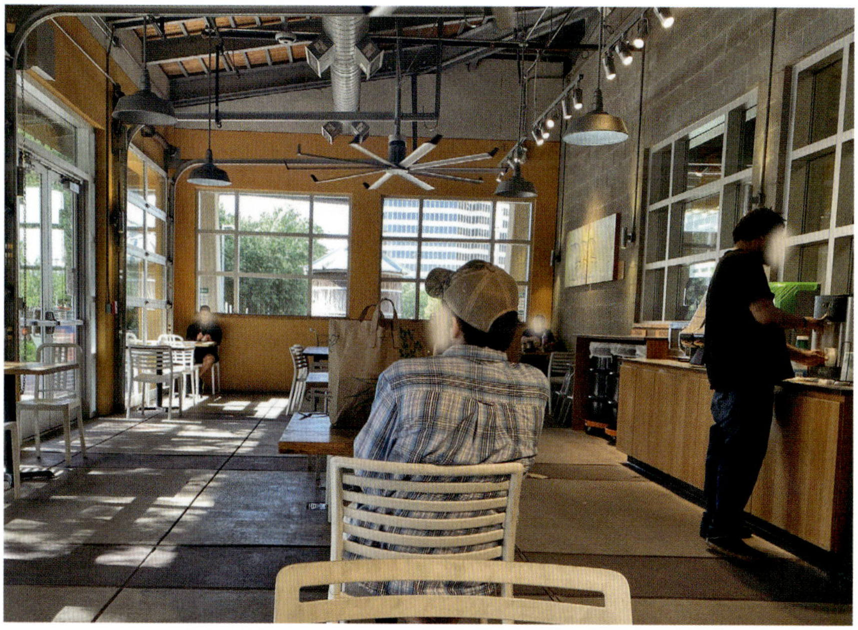

Figure 2.2. Whole Foods Market in Houston Provides Access to Anyone Seeking Free Water and a Cool Place to Sit on Hot Days. *Photo credit:* Adele Houghton

The goal of performing an ArchEPI assessment on a design or facility operations project is to develop recommendations highlighting the design and behavioral mediating factors that will have the greatest positive impact on the health of the project's population of interest. A well-performed assessment will also highlight the synergies between interventions that are recommended for health reasons and the ways in which they benefit other priorities of the project, such as marketability, reduced risk from natural disasters, social equity, and sustainability goals. Building on our previous example, a well-designed onsite park would demonstrate how it mediates extreme heat health concerns while also sustainably managing stormwater on the site, expanding access to open space, reducing habitat for disease-carrying vectors, and providing a marketable amenity for the project.[CC2.13]

2.3.b.v Health Outcomes

Depending on which environmental public health hazards are short-listed for prioritization, project teams may focus exclusively on direct health outcomes (such as heat-related injury and death in the extreme heat example) or both direct and indirect health outcomes.[CC2.14] Indirect health outcomes associated with extreme heat include exacerbated heart disease, respiratory disease, and diabetes; increased risk of infectious disease; and deterioration in mental health.[SR2.11]

2.3.c Geographic Hierarchy

All indicators include a geographic description as part of their definition. However, until recently, the three standard geographic scales for many public health indicators—national, state, and county—were much too large to be useful for real estate developments.

Figure 2.3 shows the relationships between geographic scales captured by the US Census. For an ArchEPI assessment of a single site, obtaining data at the smallest spatial scale—census block—would be the ideal scenario. The smaller the spatial scale, the more insight can be gained about similarities and differences between the ArchEPI project and its surroundings. However, small spatial scales may return too few results, which can both compromise the integrity of a statistical analysis and raise concerns about protecting privacy.

Many demographic, socioeconomic, and population health data sets are now available at the census tract level, which corresponds roughly to the size of a neighborhood. Environmental data, on the other hand, is often mapped as points or grids rather than according to census boundaries. For example, urban impervious surfaces in the US National Land Cover Database have been mapped onto a 30 square meter (323 square foot) grid.[14]

If environmental data is available at a granular geographic scale but other data sets are only available at larger scales, projects can use the environmental data at the site or census block scale to inform their understanding of which neighborhood characteristics related to demographics, socioeconomic status, and population health status are most relevant to the project site and its eventual occupants. See section 2.4 ("Understanding the Key Factors of Health") below for more detail.

CORE COMPETENCY 2.13

Real Estate Developer
Market Research Analysis

CORE COMPETENCY 2.14

Epidemiology
Assessment and Analysis

STAKEHOLDER ROLES 2.11

Opportunity for local public health department to advise the project whether to track direct or indirect health outcomes

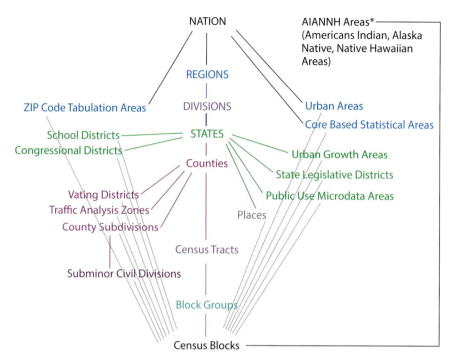

Figure 2.3. Standard Hierarchy of Census Geographic Entities. *Source:* Rossiter, Katy. Understanding Geographic Relationships: Counties, Places, Tracts and More. *Random Samplings* Blog. U.S. Census Bureau, 2014. https://www.census.gov/newsroom/blogs/random-samplings/2014/07/understanding-geographic-relationships-counties-places-tracts-and-more.html (public domain)

2.3.d Where to Obtain Data

Data are becoming increasingly accessible both within the US and internationally. Over 90 countries have made national statistics freely available, and many countries have made a wide array of government data sets free and easily downloadable by the public.[15] The US federal government has made a wide array of data sets openly available, ranging from census data to building efficiency data to health data. Every state in the US[16] and more than 100 municipalities[17] have also made local data available to anyone who would like to download it. At the international level, major organizations like the United Nations,[13] the World Health Organization,[12] and the World Bank[18] have made country-level data sets available for indicators measuring a wide array of environmental, governance, and health topics.[SR2.12]

Data sets that are "open access" (i.e., within the public domain) are preferable for ArchEPI projects. Being free and easily accessible, they will not affect the project budget or timeline. It is essential that comparison statistics use the same definition. So, pre-existing data sets are also used to illustrate where a neighborhood stands in relation to the rest of its community, the state or region, and the national average. While existing data sets may not measure the exact metric desired by the project team, it is often possible to approximate the desired relationship using related data sets—called "proxies." For example, if measurements of increased ambient temperature are not available to measure the urban heat island effect, a reliable substitute (or proxy) could be the percentage of impervious surface, because impervious surfaces have been found to increase nearby ambient temperature in comparison with vegetated spaces.

See appendix C for examples of data sources that could be used as EPHIs for extreme heat.

STAKEHOLDER ROLES 2.12

Opportunity for local government to tailor open-source data sets to support design decisions

2.3.e Protecting Privacy

Design and facility operations projects often avoid making use of building occupant behavioral and health data to protect occupant anonymity. While these concerns touch on the extremely important question of protecting an individual's right to privacy, legal parameters have been established in many countries that set boundaries for using data sets in a responsible manner.

Appendix D lays out the questions project teams should consider before beginning to work with potentially sensitive data.

2.3.f Core Competencies

Measuring the Magnitude of the Problem: Core Competencies

Field	Core Competencies
Epidemiology	• Assessment and analysis • Basic public health services • Cultural competency
Real estate development	• Location analysis • Market research analysis
Facility design, construction, operations	• Site inventory • Physical analysis • Project planning and design • Research, technical and analytical
Sustainability	• Integrative services • Location and transportation • Site assessment
Philanthropy	• Planning • Vision setting

CORE COMPETENCY 2.15

Epidemiology
Assessment and Analysis

STAKEHOLDER ROLES 2.13

Opportunity for developers, local government, and community to align project goals with community climate, health, and equity goals

---

CORE COMPETENCY 2.16

Epidemiology
Assessment and Analysis; Basic Public Health Services; Cultural Competency

Facility Design, Construction, Operations
Research, Technical and Analytical

2.4 Step 3—Understanding the Key Factors (or Determinants) of Health

Often, project teams discover that a large array of potentially useful data is available. But they are not sure how to identify priority indicators or compare one indicator with another. An experienced public health professional, epidemiologist, or data scientist can help organize and analyze environmental health data for the team to discuss and prioritize together.[CC2.15] This section will address the question of how to select a short list of priority indicators once a preliminary collection has been assembled.[SR2.13]

2.4.a Align Indicator Definitions with Data Sets Compiled by Trusted Sources[CC2.16]

The first step in prioritizing indicator development often requires looking to local, regional, and national health outcome experts or institutions for advice.

- Which health outcomes have been designated as high priority by local and regional health departments, health systems, or community-based organizations? Are priorities available for individual neighborhoods or sections of the community? Are the community's priorities the same or different from priorities in the project's neighborhood? What is different about land use, environmental assets and hazards, population demographics, and economic development in the neighborhood surrounding the project site compared with the rest of the community?

    Primary reference document(s): Community health needs assessment and/or HIA, which are often developed by the local health department and/or local hospital system.

- Which climate change hazards are prioritized for the community or region? Why? Are there aspects of the project site, surrounding land use, building occupants, and neighbors in the surrounding community that might increase or decrease the project's vulnerability to certain high-risk climate hazards?

    Primary reference document(s): National climate assessment; National, regional, state, and local climate vulnerability, action, and resilience plans.

- Which environmental, health, economic, social justice, and climate change topics have groups active in the project's neighborhood identified as high priority? Whose voice is missing from the current community conversation on these topics? How could their concerns be folded into the larger ArchEPI conversation between the development team, the community, and local government?

    Primary reference document(s): Neighborhood master plan, results from citizen-science and community-based participatory research projects.

If any indicators are drawn from expert reports, the project team should try to use the same data definition at the project scale. This approach will increase the validity of the ArchEPI investigation. And it will allow the team to compare the site-specific indicator with a reference data point, as will be explained more fully in the next section.

2.4.b Compare Baseline Indicators with Reference Data Sets and Health Standards

Comparing the site's value for each indicator with local, regional, national, and international data sets is an effective way to understand where the project site stands prior to the planned design or operations intervention.[CC2.17]

It can be helpful to use indicator definitions that are available at larger geographic scales for historical data, model projections (such as climate models), and aspirational goals for changes to environmental or health outcomes. For example, the Healthy People 2030[19] program through the US Department of Health and Human Services offers both historical data and aspirational goals for a number of indicators on individual behavior and health outcomes associated with chronic diseases like cardiovascular (i.e., heart) disease. Healthy People 2030 has set two general goals for improving overall cardiovascular health in adults by 2030: (1) improving the mean cardiovascular health score from 3.2 to 3.5 out of a scale of 7.0 and (2) reducing the rate of coronary heart disease deaths from 90.9 per 100,000 population to 71.1 per 100,000. The first indicator is drawn from the National Health and Nutrition Examination Survey, which is a nationally representative survey. As such, it is not easy to downscale. The second indicator, on the other hand, is more readily available down to the county level. But it may not have enough data points to be useful at the neighborhood level.

CORE COMPETENCY 2.17

Epidemiology
Assessment and Analysis

Facility Design, Construction, Operations
Research, Technical and Analytical

In that case, a project team may decide to use the CDC PLACES[20] indicator, percent coronary heart disease among adults, as a proxy, because it uses the same definition for the health condition as Healthy People 2030 and provides estimates at the census tract level.

Similarly, the SDGs[21] track both historical indicators for each participating country and an aspirational goal for each indicator. For example, SDG 3.4.1 sets a goal of reducing by 30% the probability of dying from non-communicable diseases like cardiovascular disease. Many jurisdictions around the world have begun to collect data on the SDGs that are highest priority in their region, so that SDGs have quickly become indicators that are available at a range of geographic scales.

Comparing site-level indicators with larger scale data sets can be divided into two general categories: direct comparison and ranked importance.

2.4.b.i Direct Comparison

Compare the smallest geographic scale available for an indicator with data using the same definition at as many larger geographic scales as would be relevant to project decision-makers: surrounding neighborhoods, community, regional political boundary (such as a county), state/province/autonomy, country, continent, and world. Develop a color-coded schema to display which project-level baseline indicators are equivalent to or better than indicators at larger scales and which indicators fall short. Use aspirational indicators to demonstrate where the site and other geographic units fall in comparison with local, regional, national, and international goals.

BOX 2.4.

Example—Health Effects of Climate Change in Rural Kentucky, USA

Author Adele Houghton led an assessment of the health effects of climate change in seven rural counties in Kentucky, USA, which ranked environmental exposure, human health outcomes, population vulnerability, and environmental vulnerability according to how well the county performed in comparison with the other six counties in the study, the rest of Kentucky, and the United States as a whole (table 2.1).

TABLE 2.1.

Relative Vulnerability of Green River District Counties to Climate Change by Environmental Public Health Indicator

Vulnerability	Daviess	Hancock	Henderson	McLean	Ohio	Union	Webster
Environmental Exposure							
High				• Exposure to heat waves • Exposure to drought • Exposure to air pollution • Exposure to heavy precipitation events			
Moderate							
Low							
Human Health Outcome[a]							
High	• Flooding-related morbidity		• Heat-related morbidity	• Heat-related morbidity	• Flooding-related morbidity	• Heat-related morbidity	• Heat-related morbidity
Moderate	• Heat-related morbidity		• Flooding-related morbidity		• Heat-related morbidity	• Flooding-related morbidity	• Flooding-related morbidity
Low	• Heat-related mortality • Flooding-related mortality	• Heat-related morbidity & mortality • Flooding-related morbidity & mortality	• Heat-related mortality	• Heat-related mortality • Flooding-related morbidity & mortality	• Heat-related mortality • Flooding-related mortality	• Heat-related mortality • Flooding-related mortality	• Heat-related mortality • Flooding-related mortality

(cont.)

TABLE 2.1. (cont.)

Population Vulnerability

Vulnerability	Daviess	Hancock	Henderson	McLean	Ohio	Union	Webster
High	• Children • Elderly • Homeless • Mental health • Long-term care	• Children • Elderly • Outdoor workers • Diabetes • Heart disease • CLRD[b] • Long-term care	• Children • Elderly • Diabetes • CLRD • Asthma • Cerebrovascular disease	• Children • Elderly • Outdoor workers • Diabetes • Heart disease • Cerebrovascular disease • Long-term care	• Children • Elderly • Poverty • Outdoor workers • Diabetes • Heart disease • Long-term care	• Elderly • Outdoor workers • Obesity • Heart disease • Cerebrovascular disease	• Elderly • Outdoor workers • Obesity • Diabetes • Heart disease • CLRD • Asthma • Cerebrovascular disease
Moderate	• Poverty • Heart disease • CLRD • Cerebrovascular disease	• Obesity • Cerebrovascular disease • Mental health	• Poverty • Outdoor workers • Obesity • Heart disease • Mental health • Long-term care	• Poverty • CLRD • Asthma • Mental health	• Homeless • Obesity • CLRD • Cerebrovascular disease • Mental health	• Poverty • Non-Hispanic Blacks • CLRD • Mental health	• Children • Poverty • Mental health • Long-term care
Low	• Non-Hispanic Blacks • Outdoor workers • Limited English proficiency • Obesity • Diabetes • Asthma • Ambulatory difficulty	• Poverty • Non-Hispanic Blacks • Limited English proficiency • Ambulatory difficulty	• Non-Hispanic Blacks • Homeless • Limited English proficiency • Ambulatory difficulty	• Non-Hispanic Blacks • Limited English proficiency • Obesity • Ambulatory difficulty	• Non-Hispanic Blacks • Limited English proficiency • Asthma • Ambulatory difficulty	• Children • Limited English proficiency • Diabetes • Asthma • Ambulatory difficulty • Long-term care	• Non-Hispanic Blacks • Limited English proficiency • Ambulatory difficulty

TABLE 2.1. (cont.)

Vulnerability	Daviess	Hancock	Henderson	McLean	Ohio	Union	Webster
Environmental Vulnerability							
High	• FEMA floodplain	• FEMA floodplain	• FEMA floodplain • Stressed housing	• FEMA floodplain	• FEMA floodplain	• FEMA floodplain	
Moderate							
Low	• Stressed housing	• Stressed housing		• Stressed housing	• Stressed housing	• Stressed housing	• FEMA floodplain • Stressed housing

Source: Green River District Health Department 2016.[22] Reproduced with permission.

Note: High = falls short of both Kentucky and US indicators, or, if no larger scale data is available, in comparison with other Green River District (GRD) counties; moderate = falls short of either Kentucky or US indicators or in comparison with other GRD counties; low = improvement over Kentucky and US indicators or in comparison with other GRD counties.

[a] Drought reportable human health outcomes to be determined.
[b] CLRD = chronic lower respiratory disease.

2.4.b.ii Ranked Importance

A more involved approach for comparing baseline indicators would rank the site's baseline value against all of the other values within the community or surrounding region. This type of comparison often divides up the results into four or five non-parametric categories: quartiles and quintiles. It can be useful both because it compares the site's baseline status objectively with other neighborhoods in the community and because it can demonstrate where the community as a whole stands in comparison with aspirational goals set by reference institutions like the national CDC or the UN SDGs. For example, if the project neighborhood's value falls within the bottom quartile for its community but even the bottom quartile meets or exceeds the aspirational goal for that indicator, then the project may not need to prioritize design strategies that address that particular environmental public health issue. If, on the other hand, the project falls within the top quartile within a community that, as a whole, does not meet the aspirational goal for the indicator, then the project may want to double down on efforts to prioritize that indicator in order to support neighborhood efforts to move their population across the goalpost for a chronic condition like asthma or a climate change vulnerability like urban heat island.

See appendix E for step-by-step instructions on how to classify the variables mapped using this approach.

2.4.c Develop a Composite Index to Set Priorities

Statistical analysis offers a more sophisticated and scientifically sound way to select a short list of EPHIs that are particularly critical for the project site's baseline conditions.[CC2.18] It moves one step beyond a visual comparison with reference indicators by estimating the strength of correlation between an environmental exposure, mediating factors, and related health outcomes.

See appendix F for a more detailed explanation of why it might be beneficial to a project to employ biostatistical methods, that is statistical modeling related to questions associated with human health.

Two statistical methods—z-score indices and principal component analysis—have been found to be particularly useful for environmental public health assessments. They allow teams to identify a group of variables that, as a group, explain the majority of the correlation between an environmental hazard and specific health outcomes.

Visit appendix G and appendix H for detailed instructions on how to use these two statistical methods to prioritize EPHIs.

2.4.d Perform Spatial Analysis

Spatial analysis can be a useful tool for understanding the spatial distribution of high priority EPHIs on the project property and in surrounding areas.[CC2.19] At a minimum, visualizing the index created in section 2.4.c on a map will help communicate its most salient points to project decision-makers. More complex forms of spatial analysis can estimate the extent to which project indicators are influenced by location.

Visit appendix I for an introduction to geographic information system (GIS) spatial analysis.

CORE COMPETENCY 2.18

Epidemiology
Assessment and Analysis

Facility Design, Construction, Operations
Research, Technical and Analytical

CORE COMPETENCY 2.19

Epidemiology
Assessment and Analysis

Facility Design, Construction, Operations
Research, Technical and Analytical

BOX 2.5.

Example—Health Impact Assessment of an Elementary School in Houston, Texas, USA

Author Adele Houghton led an HIA in Houston, Texas, USA, which used the quartile approach to demonstrate the ways in which schools located less than 50 m (150 feet) from an existing freeway would likely be impacted by a proposed expansion project. Table 2.2 shares air quality and extreme heat data on one such school: Bruce Elementary. Data have been provided for natural and built environment determinants of health, health behaviors, and health outcomes for extreme heat and air quality. Cells under the Bruce Elementary column were highlighted in red if the campus value fell within the worst quartile for that indicator in comparison with its reference geography.

TABLE 2.2.
Air Quality and Extreme Heat Metrics for Bruce Elementary School, Houston, Texas, USA

Metrics	Bruce	Reference Data Set
Natural Environment Determinants of Health		
Number of days the Heat Index was ≥ 108°F in a given Census Tract, 2010–2016[a]	321	217.5 (COH PLACES average)
Number of days ozone concentrations were ≥ 70 ppb in a given Census Tract, 2010–2016 (June–September)[a]	32	36.7 (COH PLACES average)
Number of days ozone concentrations ≥ 70 ppb and the Heat Index was ≥ 108°F in a given Census Tract, 2010–2016[a]	11	10.7 (COH PLACES average)
Built Environment Determinants of Health		
Vehicle miles traveled per square mile[b]	40,797	10,124 (AISD/HISD average)
Number of parks within 400 m of campus[c]	2	1.2 (AISD/HISD average)
Acreage of parks within 400 m of campus[c]	2.9	11.4 (AISD/HISD average)
Number of places to get cool and designated cooling centers within 400 m of campus[d]	1	Total COH PLACES: 225 Average per census tract: 0.4
Location of places to get cool and designated cooling centers within 400 m of campus[d]	Swiney Park Community Center	
Health Behaviors and Health Outcomes		
Outdoor activity per week[e]	110 min (26.2% of recommendation)	
Percentage of students diagnosed with asthma[e]	7.2%	3.3% (HISD average)
School limits outdoor exercise on extreme heat days or ozone action days[e] (yes/no)	Yes	No district-wide rule
Average STAAR score[f]	27.5	44.9 (HISD average)

[a]Data received directly from National Center of Atmospheric Research.
[b]Texas Department of Transportation, 2016. Roadway Inventory (https://www.txdot.gov/inside-txdot/division/transportation-planning/roadway-inventory.html).
[c]Trust for Public Land, ParkServe® Parks (https://parkserve.tpl.org/).
[d]City of Houston Department of Health (2014).
[e]Communication received directly from schools.
[f]Texas Education Agency, State of Texas Assessment of Academic Readiness (STAAR) Resources, 2017–2018 (https://tea.texas.gov/student.assessment/staar/staar-resources).

Notes: Published with permission from Air Alliance Houston. Red highlight indicates the census block group is located in the highest quartile in the City of Houston or above the local average. COH PLACES = City of Houston geographic extent as defined by the US CDC's PLACES project (previously 500 Cities; https://www.cdc.gov/places/); AISD = Aldine Independent School District; HISD = Houston Independent School District.

(cont.)

BOX 2.5. (*cont.*)

To mitigate exposure to extreme heat and traffic-related air pollution, the health impact assessment made the following design and operations recommendations.

Building and Operations
1. Install MERV 13 filters throughout the school to reduce exposure to outdoor air pollution inside the building.
2. Ban idling around campus (carpool line, school buses, deliveries, etc.).
3. If an outside air intake, door, or operable window is adjacent to a pollution source, move one or the other.
4. Schedule most recess in the morning to avoid the higher pollution and traffic in the afternoon.
5. Introduce activities into indoor recess using services like Go Noodle. https://www.youtube.com/user/GoNoodleGames
6. Introduce walking school bus to increase student safety walking to and from school.

Campus
1. Plant drought-resistant trees around play areas to screen children from particulates and traffic noise and to increase access to nature.
2. Plant drought-resistant plants outside school room windows to give students a view of nature, which can help improve concentration, mental health, etc.
3. Plant drought-resistant shade trees along the sidewalks to reduce urban heat island for pedestrians.
4. Install bike rack for cyclists, if there isn't one already.
5. Convert the two campus detention ponds into playing fields to increase access to athletics.

Pedestrian/bike/bus infrastructure
1. Build a direct hike/bike link from Bruce Elementary to the Buffalo Bayou hike and bike trail.
2. Expand the width of sidewalks, fill in gaps along walking routes, and plant shade trees along walking routes to and from school.
3. Paint cycling paths along the main walking routes. Add physical barrier on Jensen Drive to protect cyclists.
4. Change the Jensen Drive exit so that cars slow down before they reach the school.
5. Increase the safety of the intersection of Jensen Drive under I-10 and reopen the pedestrian/bike access to the east side of I-69.

Larger Scale, Time, and Money Recommendations
1. Model the changes to air quality resulting from depressing the freeway.
2. Consider moving the school to the Bayou East development, building a gym and playing fields, and funding a physical education department.
3. Link streets in the Bruce neighborhood with downtown to increase access into downtown.

BOX 2.6.

Tip—Look for Existing Indices Before Starting from Scratch

Before developing a project-specific index, check with the local health department, local research institutions, local non-governmental organizations, and the scientific literature to verify that an index has not already been created in the project's community. The best-case scenario for an ArchEPI project is to use existing chronic disease, climate change, and environmental public health and justice indices to support project decision-making, rather than re-inventing the wheel.

2.4.d.i Data Exploration and Summary

The first step in any data analysis is to become familiar with the data set. This often involves running summary statistics to understand the frequency and distributions of the data, whether the data follows a normal distribution (also known as a bell curve), and whether there are any outliers in the data. With geospatially coded data, it is also important to decide how the data will be classified (e.g., by quartile, standard deviation, or other classifications schemes) and what colors will be used on chloropleth maps to designate larger and smaller values.

Exploratory spatial analysis is used to quantify the extent to which data depart from complete spatial randomness. It is often used to form a hypothesis about spatial autocorrelation that is then tested using spatial clustering analysis techniques. See section 2.4.d.iv and appendix L for more information about how to perform these techniques.

To protect anonymity, it can be preferable to aggregate point data into the smallest political boundary that is comparable across indicators. These aggregated data can then be categorized into quartiles or quintiles, so that spatial variations can been seen both among the original indicators and among the indices developed in section 2.4.c. See section 2.3.e and appendix D for a more detailed review of how to protect privacy—an important topic, even when teams use openly available data sets.

2.4.d.ii Visualization

Visualization refers to displaying maps of different indicators next to each other to allow for inferences based on visual comparison between two or more maps. Examples of spatial visualization methods include rate maps, dot maps, SMR maps, kernel density maps, and case count maps.

Many openly available data sets are accessible online using viewer plug-ins that facilitate this type of data utilization. On the positive side, these viewers make data much more accessible and easily understood than was previously the case. On the negative side, some online portals do not allow users to manipulate the data, so it is not possible to measure the strength or weakness of associations between different variables in the data set.

Visit appendix J for guidance on GIS tools used to perform visualization in spatial analysis.

2.4.d.iii Buffering

Buffering refers to drawing a zone around a map feature measured in units of distance or time. It is used to perform proximity analysis. For example, a project interested in proposing a neighborhood solar rooftop microgrid might use buffering to count the number of existing rooftop solar arrays already installed within a certain distance of the building site. Similarly, a project considering the idea of installing the necessary equipment to convert a portion of the building into a cooling center during power outages might use buffering to count the number of households within a quarter-mile radius without access to central air conditioning. A park project might use buffering to count the number of households within a quarter-mile walking distance.

BOX 2.7.

Example—Public Schools Near Highways in Colorado and Florida, USA

Using the US National Environmental Public Health Tracking Data Portal, it is possible to generate a visual comparison at the county level of the percentage of public schools located within 150 m of a highway in different US states. For example, figure 2.4 compares Colorado, USA, and Florida, USA. Schools located within 150 m of heavily trafficked roads are more likely to be exposed to traffic-related air pollution. (See the air quality section of the toolbox for additional information.)

From this visual comparison, it is easy to see that many more schools are located near busy roads in Florida than in Colorado.

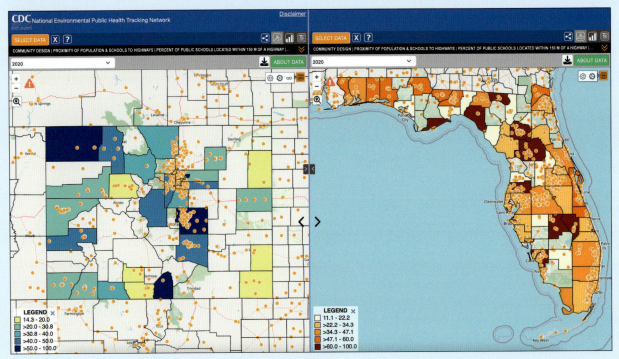

Figure 2.4. Visual Comparison of the Percentages of Public Schools in Colorado and Florida, USA, Located within 150 m of a Highway, 2010–2011. *Source:* US Centers for Disease Control and Prevention Environmental Public Health Tracking Network. https://ephtracking.cdc.gov (public domain)

In addition to measuring and counting environmental exposures and existing assets surrounding a site, buffering can be a powerful visualization tool. For example, figure 2.5 shows how the buffer tool in ArcGIS can be used to overlay *Anopheles* mosquito breeding sites (the primary vector species for malaria) and the distance the mosquito might typically travel on top of the location of malaria-positive residents in a town in Costa Rica. This kind of data visualization coupled with photographs of the breeding sites and the architectural features of the homes with positive cases creates a compelling case for prioritizing design interventions that will reduce breeding sites and keep mosquitoes out of homes. See the vector-borne disease section of the toolbox for additional information.

Visit appendix K for guidance on GIS tools used to perform buffering in spatial analysis.

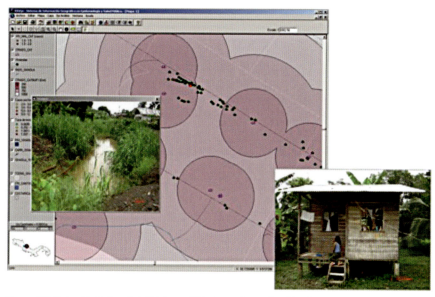

Figure 2.5. Using Buffering, Point Data, and Photographs to Visualize the Connections between the Environment and Malaria Prevalence in Costa Rica. *Source:* Carlos Castillo-Salgado

2.4.d.iv Spatial Clustering Analysis

Spatial clustering analysis is used to estimate the strength of association between spatial distribution and the health outcome of interest. This is a more advanced spatial analysis technique, which can be useful for identifying gaps that do not become apparent through visualization.

For example, spatial clustering can help identify areas of town that would benefit from a grocery store, more pocket parks, or an increase in weatherization incentives.

See appendix L for technical instructions on how to perform the three most commonly used geospatial autocorrelation techniques: global spatial autocorrelation, local spatial autocorrelation, and hot and cold spot analysis.

2.4.e Select Two to Four EPHIs for Further Development

Pausing a moment to review, the first three steps in the ArchEPI methodology move the project from a general understanding of which environmental public health concerns are most pressing in the project's region and community to a more precise understanding of the unique interplay of environmental hazards, vulnerable populations, and mediating factors at the project site level.[SR2.14]

This section will help the ArchEPI project develop a partial conceptual framework and a set of EPHIs for two to four priority environmental public health topics. The conceptual framework should include indicators defining the natural and built environment determinants of health, vulnerable population mediating factors, and direct and indirect health impacts associated with each environmental public health topic.[CC2.20]

When selecting EPHIs to prioritize, the team should consider

- the level of risk from the environmental hazard,
- the level of vulnerability among occupants on-site and in the surrounding neighborhood (present and future), and
- the extent to which the project can plug into existing public health or healthy community policies and funding sources.[SR2.15]

STAKEHOLDER ROLES 2.14

Opportunity for the development team to demonstrate leadership in community benefit design

CORE COMPETENCY 2.20

Real Estate Development
Location Analysis; Market Research Analysis

Facility Design, Construction, Operations
Contextual Analysis; Societal Impact; Sustainability and Environmental Impact

Sustainability
Integrative Services; Site Assessment; Project Surroundings and Public Outreach

Philanthropy
Planning

STAKEHOLDER ROLES 2.15

Opportunity for community to revise and add richness to analyses based on secondary data sets

Using science-based methods to identify site-specific health issues that should be prioritized by an architectural or facilities operations project is a distinguishing feature of architectural epidemiology. Step 3 in the Guyer Framework—described in this section—marks the end of that process. The following three steps (sections 2.5–2.7) use well-known public health methods to translate the priority EPHIs into project-specific design and operations recommendations and evaluation criteria.

2.4.f Core Competencies

Understanding Key Factors (or Determinants) of the Problem: Core Competencies

Field	Core Competencies
Epidemiology	• Assessment and analysis • Basic public health services • Cultural competency
Real estate development	• Location analysis • Market research analysis
Facility design, construction, operations	• Contextual analysis • Societal impact • Sustainability and environmental impact • Research, technical and analytical
Sustainability	• Integrative services • Site assessment • Project surroundings and public outreach
Philanthropy	• Planning

2.5 Step 4—Identifying and Developing Evidence-Based Strategies to Prevent and/or Mitigate the Problem

CORE COMPETENCY 2.21

Epidemiology
Assessment and Analysis

Facility Design, Construction, Operations
Research, Technical and Analytical

Sustainability
Integrative Services

STAKEHOLDER ROLES 2.16

Opportunity for local public health practitioners to perform this task, coach others, and/or provide quality control

After developing a short list of priority EPHIs for the design or facility operations project and validating it through a participatory community engagement process, the next step in the ArchEPI process is to develop an evidence-based list of relevant design and operations strategies that are protective of human health.[CC2.21]

The short list of priority EPHIs that were selected at the end of step 3 of the Guyer framework (section 2.4) are not design or operations strategies in and of themselves. However, they are metrics that have been measured and studied by social scientists and epidemiologists. They can therefore be used to search scientific databases for promising, evidence-based interventions.[SR2.16]

This book shares the results of this exercise for 10 environmental health topics—five related to climate change and five related to chronic disease and mental health. Two sections in each toolbox topic share the results of that effort ("How Does the Built Environment Increase the Risk of [topic]?" and "How Can Design Help?"). Certification programs like LEED (https://www.usgbc.org/about/priorities/human-health), Fitwel (https://www.fitwel.org/fitwel-solutions), and WELL (https://www.wellcertified.com/research) have also conducted extensive narrative literature reviews, ranked the evidence on the strength of the interventions, and prioritized building-level interventions for a range of health hazards and outcomes.

While most people who will read this book will rely on the infographics in the toolbox to link the priority health topics identified in step 3 of the Guyer framework (section 2.4) with relevant evidence-based strategies, we include the following information to support teams who are searching for specific evidence-based strategies (such as design strategies that are culturally appropriate for certain groups, such as Indigenous communities) or are investigating a health topic that is not included in the toolbox.

To search the scientific literature for evidence of building design, landscape design, civil engineering practices, land use and transportation practices, and operational policies and procedures that have been found to be protective of human health within the framework of a specific EPHI, it can be helpful to craft queries that align with existing keywords in the database of interest. For example, table 2.3 converts the natural and built environment determinants of health, vulnerable population mediating factors, and direct and indirect health impact indicators for cardiovascular disease and air quality in the toolbox into query terms using MeSH (US National Library of Medicine medical subject headings) keywords.

There are three primary approaches to conducting a literature review. The least quantitative option, narrative literature review, is presented below. The more advanced methods required to perform a systematic literature review and meta-analysis are detailed in appendix M.

Of the more advanced methods covered in the appendices, systematic literature reviews can be particularly useful, because they help correct for blind spots arising from team composition. Meta-analyses can add value to projects that want to take a deep dive into a specific area of inquiry that has benefited from a great deal of quantitative research. Unfortunately, many aspects of the

TABLE 2.3.

Sample MeSH Query Terms Searching for Links between the Design and Operation of the Built Environment and Cardiovascular Disease or Air Quality

Search	Example Queries
Cardiovascular disease	"Cardiovascular diseases" [C14] AND "built environment" [N06.230.145.500] OR "sustainable development" [N06.230.080.900] OR "urban health" [N01.400.548.875] OR "cities" [N06.230.069] OR "urbanization" [I01.880.853.400.726]]
Air quality	"Air pollution" [N06.850.460.100] AND "climate change" [G16.500.175.374] AND "built environment" [N06.230.145.500] OR "sustainable development" [N06.230.080.900] OR "urban health" [N01.400.548.875] OR "cities" [N06.230.069] OR "urbanization" [I01.880.853.400.726]]
	"Air pollution" [N06.850.460.100] AND "climate change" [G16.500.175.374] AND "extreme heat" [N06.230.300.100.725.232.500] AND "Built Environment" [N06.230.145.500] OR "sustainable development" [N06.230.080.900] OR "urban health" [N01.400.548.875] OR "cities" [N06.230.069] OR "urbanization" [I01.880.853.400.726]]

Note: See the cardiovascular disease and air quality sections of the toolbox and appendix B for more detail.

built environment have not been rigorously studied to quantify the co-benefits and co-harms to human health of one design or operating strategy compared with another. So, most architectural epidemiology assessments will likely rely on narrative and systematic literature reviews rather than meta-analysis.

2.5.a Narrative Literature Review

Narrative literature reviews summarize the results of a handful of relevant studies (generally less than 10). Within the context of an ArchEPI project, they may be used to provide an overview of the role the built environment plays in protecting people (particularly at risk groups) from environmental exposures and in setting a context that promotes healthy behaviors.[SR2.17]

Their primary advantage is the speed at which they can be produced—assuming the team has access to a subject-matter expert who is familiar enough with the material to feel comfortable summarizing the scientific evidence on the basis of a few key studies.

On the other hand, limiting the scope of the review to a handful of studies that have been subjectively selected and interpreted by a small number of researchers may contribute to what is known in epidemiology as "unconscious bias." In other words, the author of the review will naturally feel a tendency towards focusing on the topics with which he or she is most familiar. The resulting summary may provide an incomplete picture of the current state of the evidence. An even more insidious bias is "publication bias," which refers to the studies that were never selected for publication because they did not return positive results or because their topics were outside the mainstream. For that reason, narrative literature reviews should be limited to summarizing the environmental public health context for a health topic. They are not recommended as a tool for identifying design and operations interventions.

See appendix M for a detailed explanation of how to conduct a systematic literature review to summarize the state of the science specific to individual strategies.

2.5.b Core Competencies

Identifying and Developing Strategies to Prevent and/or Mitigate the Problem: Core Competencies

Field	Core Competencies
Epidemiology	• Assessment and analysis
Real estate development	• Not applicable
Facility design, construction, operations	• Research, technical and analytical
Sustainability	• Integrative services
Philanthropy	• Not applicable

STAKEHOLDER ROLES 2.17

Opportunity for community to revise and add richness to analyses based on secondary data sets

2.6 Step 5—Prioritizing and Recommending the Most Effective Policies and Strategies

At this point in the ArchEPI assessment,

- the team has developed a complete conceptual diagram and set of EPHIs for two to four environmental public health topics, and
- the literature review has generated a set of design and operations strategies that are supported by scientific evidence as having the potential to protect building occupants and the surrounding neighborhood from at least some of the negative health consequences of the prioritized health concerns.

The next step is to consider each of the evidence-based strategies in turn and decide which ones to incorporate in the project design.[CC2.22] There are many ways to prioritize strategies using various rubrics or evaluation methods that weight the information based on the project site, surrounding populations, or current events. One empirical way to do this analysis is by conducting an HIA,[D2.4,CC2.23] which is a public health tool that has been used for many years in the public sector to develop evidence-based recommendations on a range of policy-related topics.[23,SR2.18]

The HIA methodology, which is flexible and emphasizes objectivity, is particularly well adapted to addressing the health effects of the built environment. Over the past two decades, it has gained traction in the US, particularly among community planners.[24] For example, according to the American Planning Association, one-third of the more than 350 HIAs performed in the US from 2004–2014 focused on built environment topics.[25] HIAs are often used in the policy realm to justify a policymaking approach called Health in All Policies (HiAP). The HiAP approach requires policies to integrate accountability around health equity into their performance criteria.[26] In a sense, architectural epidemiology applies the HiAP approach to building design and operations, perhaps changing the acronym to HiARE (Health in all Real Estate)

Traditional HIAs generally include a discussion of socioeconomic and racial equity as part of a focus on at-risk populations. However, for projects located in environmental justice communities or in neighborhoods undergoing rapid population displacement due to gentrification, social equity may be such an urgent topic that it should be overlaid on top of the traditional HIA framework. This method is commonly known as a health equity impact assessment (HEIA).

HEIAs distinguish themselves from HIAs by emphasizing the ways in which policies and programs disproportionately affect specific at-risk groups. Rather than simply acknowledging that certain populations are at higher risk of negative health outcomes due to inequities in education, economic opportunities, access to health care, and other social determinants of health, an ArchEPI HEIA would craft recommendations that attempt to lessen or remedy the social inequities alongside concerns about environmental exposure.[SR2.19]

For a more detailed explanation on how to integrate equity into a HIA, see Mahoney et al., *Equity-Focused Health Impact Assessment Framework*, 2004[27] (https://www.researchgate.net/publication/305018353_Equity-focused_health_impact_assessment_framework).

HIAs offer a useful framework for applying the larger scale data gathered in the first four steps of the Guyer framework (sections 2.2–2.5) to the unique assets and limitations of an individual project and site. In some cases, an HIA could also serve as the organizing framework for the entire ArchEPI assessment.

Appendix N provides technical guidance on how to develop and implement an HIA or HEIA as part of an ArchEPI project.

CORE COMPETENCY 2.22

Real Estate Development
Market Research Analysis

Facility Design, Construction, Operations
Programming and Analysis; Conceptualization

Sustainability
Integrative Services; Understanding Policy Landscape

Philanthropy
Planning

DEFINITION 2.4

Health Impact Assessment (HIA)
"[A]n analysis, evaluation, and assessment of the consequences and implications for public health of specific social or environmental interventions or processes. . . . A combination of procedures, methods, and tools by which a policy, program, or project may be judged as to its potential effects on the health of a population. Considered an opportunity to integrate health into all policies, HIA aims to influence the decision-making process, addressing all determinants of health, tackling inequities, and promoting participation and empowerment in health."

Porta, M., ed. *A Dictionary of Epidemiology*. Sixth Edition, IEA Oxford University Press; 2014.

CORE COMPETENCY 2.23

Epidemiology
Assessment and Analysis; Policy Development

STAKEHOLDER ROLES 2.18

Opportunity for local public health practitioners to perform this task, coach others, and/or provide quality control

---

STAKEHOLDER ROLES 2.19

Opportunity to center questions of equity and social justice in the project

2.6.a Core Competencies

Prioritizing and Recommending the Most Effective Policies and Strategies: Core Competencies

Field	Core Competencies
Epidemiology	• Assessment and analysis • Policy development
Real estate development	• Market research analysis
Facility design, construction, operations	• Programming and analysis • Conceptualization
Sustainability	• Integrative services
Philanthropy	• Planning

2.7. Step 6—Implementing and Evaluating Interventions

The final step in an ArchEPI assessment has two parts. First, the ArchEPI team should document which recommendations were implemented in the final design or facility operations policy. Second, the ArchEPI project budget should include funding to perform a post-occupancy evaluation (POE) of the effectiveness of the health interventions that were implemented.[SR2.20]

STAKEHOLDER ROLES 2.20

Opportunity for developers, local government, and community to publicly support ArchEPI recommendations

2.7.a. Making the Case for Implementing ArchEPI Recommendations

Given that the ultimate goal of an ArchEPI assessment is to implement its recommendations, it is fitting that we close this chapter by sharing a few tips on how to communicate the results effectively with stakeholders and decision-makers on the project team and in the community. The following list is adapted from the chapter on communications during a public health investigation in the US *CDC Field Epidemiology Manual*.[28]

CORE COMPETENCY 2.24

Epidemiology
Communication

Facility Design, Construction, Operations
Communication and Interaction

Sustainability
Communication and Corporate Social Responsibility

Philanthropy
Communication

2.7.a.i Frame the Project's Priority Health Concerns Appropriately[CC2.24]

ArchEPI communications (including the final report) should use language that emphasizes

- the environmental hazard that poses a high risk to climate, health, and equity,
- its relevance to the ultimate users of the site, and
- the proactive steps that can be taken through the design/policy development process to mitigate the risk.

Table 2.4 annotates communications recommendations from the *CDC Field Epidemiology Manual*[28] with an example from extreme heat, demonstrating how messaging that responds to different stakeholder groups' assessment of risk can motivate them to act in order to reduce that risk.

TABLE 2.4.

Factors Influencing Risk Perception, Annotated with Extreme Heat Examples

More Acceptable (i.e., Lower Priority) Risks	Extreme Heat Example	Less Acceptable (i.e., Higher Priority) Risks	Extreme Heat Example
Voluntary or involving choice	Stakeholders may believe that experiencing uncomfortably warm temperatures outside is a choice (and, therefore, *low priority*), because they expect buildings to separate them from the elements at all times (even during blackouts caused by extreme heat events).	Imposed on the affected population or not allowing choice	Stakeholders may perceive extreme heat as a *high-priority risk* if they are obliged to spend time outdoors during heat waves due to their occupation; their reliance on walking, cycling, or public transportation to move around; or their need to perform domestic activities like walking pets.
			Stakeholders who cannot afford to use air conditioning during extreme heat events because of high electricity costs may perceive extreme heat events as a *higher priority risk* than stakeholders who are not energy insecure.
Under a person's control	Stakeholders may perceive extreme heat as a *low-priority risk* if they believe that individuals can control their own exposure to warm temperatures by opening the window, lowering the thermostat, or driving where they need to go instead of walking.	Controlled by others	Stakeholders may perceive extreme heat as a *high-priority risk* if they feel pressure to work in uncomfortably warm workplaces where the employer controls the thermostat.
			Renters living in poorly maintained homes may also perceive extreme heat as a *high-priority risk* if they rely on owners and property managers to weatherize the building and provide air conditioning.
Associated with clear benefits to the stakeholder	Stakeholders may believe that the urban heat island (UHI) effect, which intensifies exposure to extreme heat events, is a *low-priority risk* if they benefit directly from the impervious surfaces that cause it, such as parking lots, roads, and freeways.	Associated with intangible or deferred benefits	Stakeholders may perceive the UHI effect as a *high-priority risk* if they view the benefits of roads and freeways as intangible in comparison with the immediate and tangible benefits that green spaces provide, such as lower air temperatures, reduced risk of flooding, cleaner air, opportunities for recreation, and improved mental health.
Naturally occurring	Stakeholders may be *less inclined to prioritize* design or operations strategies that mitigate the UHI and reduce the building's overall greenhouse gas emissions if they believe that climate change is a naturally occurring phenomenon.	Human made	Stakeholders may believe that *urgent action is needed* to reduce both the UHI and greenhouse gas emissions on-site if they believe that climate change is largely caused by society's reliance on fossil fuel combustion.
Generated by a trusted source	Stakeholders may perceive extreme heat as a *low-priority risk* if they rely on industry minimum standards that recommend maximizing impervious surfaces, for example, minimum parking requirements and dark colored composite roof standards.	Generated by an untrusted source	Stakeholders may perceive extreme heat as a *high-priority risk* if they are located in an environmental justice neighborhood where government, industry, or other landowners have increased impervious surface and reduced the tree canopy over time without community input.

(cont.)

TABLE 2.4. (cont.)

More Acceptable (i.e., Lower Priority) Risks	Extreme Heat Example	Less Acceptable (i.e., Higher Priority) Risks	Extreme Heat Example
Familiar	Stakeholders may perceive extreme heat as a *low-priority risk* if they are accustomed to experiencing multiple heat waves every summer.	New or exotic	Stakeholders may perceive extreme heat as an *urgent public health concern* if they experience a heat wave in a mild climate where, historically, extreme heat was an unusual phenomenon.
Affecting adults primarily	Stakeholders may perceive extreme heat as a *low-priority risk* if the information they receive about heat-related health risks primarily talks about occupational health, recreational exposure, and other exposures among able-bodied adults, because healthy adult bodies are better able to self-regulate their core temperature than the bodies of children and the elderly.	Affecting children primarily	Stakeholders working on projects serving children (such as schools) may be *highly motivated* to integrate strategies to reduce the UHI in the project design if they perceive children as a group who could be harmed by exposure to extreme heat, because children rely on their caregivers to keep them safe.

Source: Modified and reproduced with permission from the 2019 *CDC Field Epidemiology Manual*.[28]

STAKEHOLDER ROLES 2.21

Opportunity to work with developers, local government, and community groups to establish trust, credibility, and accountability with all key stakeholders

CORE COMPETENCY 2.25

Epidemiology
Community Dimension of Practice; Cultural Competency

Facility Design, Construction, Operations
Plan Implementation and Placemaking

Sustainability
Project Surroundings and Public Outreach

Philanthropy
Communication

2.7.a.ii Establish Trust and Credibility with Stakeholders

The ArchEPI approach to identifying site-specific environmental public health concerns and developing evidence-based design and operations recommendations for addressing them will be a new experience for many projects.[SR2.21] It is therefore essential that the ArchEPI team establish trust and credibility with all key stakeholders, so that ArchEPI recommendations are accepted and adopted to the greatest extent possible.[CC2.25]

Drawing again from the *CDC Field Epidemiology Manual*,[28] ArchEPI communications should use four attributes to build trust with the rest of the project team and with key stakeholders:

- empathy and caring
- honesty and openness
- dedication and commitment
- competence and expertise

Specifically, a communications strategy should follow the following steps:

1. *Start the message with an expression of empathy:* During an infectious disease outbreak, this step usually involves an acknowledgement that epidemics are frightening and unpredictable. However, empathy takes a slightly different tone within the context of an ArchEPI project. Rather than empathizing about the public health threat, it may be more effective to empathize with project team members who are feeling something that might be characterized as "new topic fatigue." Many built environment professionals feel that topics like green building and health and wellness are distractions from the core business of building and operating a real estate asset that meets both minimum building code requirements and the return-on-investment expectations of owners and their financial backers. Expressing empathy with the frustration that yet another topic has been added to the list of considerations ancillary to these two core project requirements can be a helpful way to open the door to a productive conversation with the team.

72 ARCHITECHTURAL EPIDEMIOLOGY

2. *Explain the public health threat:* This is the place to insert the public health message that was developed during the previous sub-section. It is important to avoid the use of jargon and use plain language to describe the public health threat to build rapport and credibility.

3. *Explain what is known and unknown:* It is vital that ArchEPI communications strike a balanced tone—not underselling or overselling information. It is true that many links between design or operations interventions and health outcomes have yet to be established. But the results of the project's literature review should provide sufficient evidence to show the current state of scientific understanding and which research questions are still pending.

4. *Explain the recommendations for design and/or operations interventions and why they have been selected by the ArchEPI team:* Simply stating what is known and unknown does not provide enough information to move forward with ArchEPI recommendations. People want to understand what the EPHIs means for them and how each priority environmental public health topic relates to recommended actions. This is the place for communicating the results of the HIA or HSA. It is important to use plain language and explain how each intervention is expected to contribute to protecting the health of building occupants and/or the surrounding community. Recommendations may be accompanied by suggestions for roles and responsibilities among the project team. Who will lead the design effort for converting a conventional roof into a combined vegetative and solar roof, for example? Who will research the design modifications required to connect a portion of the building air conditioning system to a solar-powered battery pack? Who will focus on improving building energy efficiency? Who will ensure that windows are operable and fitted with screens?

5. *Outline the ways in which the ArchEPI team is available to support the larger project team throughout the project delivery process:* Wrap up the communication by reiterating the urgency of the public health concerns that will be at least partially addressed if the project follows the ArchEPI assessment's recommendations. Explain how the EPHIs will be used to keep track of progress throughout the rest of the project. And walk through an ArchEPI timeline overlaid on the project schedule to explain how the ArchEPI team will support the team through project completion. See chapter 3 for additional details on this step.

2.7.a.iii Develop a Simple Phrase Summarizing the Main Outcomes from the ArchEPI Assessment

This suggestion is modified from the concept of a "Single Overriding Health Communication Objective," or "SOHCO (pronounced sock-O)," explained in the *CDC Field Epidemiology Manual*.[28] The idea is to boil down the complicated topics and relationships that are laid out in detail in the ArchEPI report into one or two sentences that explain in plain language

- the risk posed by the environmental hazards,
- their relevance to the ultimate users of the site, and
- the proactive steps that can be taken through the design/policy development process to mitigate risk of exposure and support quality of life.

Distilling this information into a soundbite length will help the project team talk about health in passing as it integrates ArchEPI concepts into each discipline working on the project team. If it is necessary to walk through the entire ArchEPI report every time the concept of health-promoting design recommendations is raised, the ArchEPI team will quickly find itself sidelined.

SOHCOs are designed to be repeated. The ideal SOHCO could be quickly refined to clarify its relevance to the landscape architect, adjusted again to address the HVAC system, and adapted further to support the larger design vision developed by the architect all in the same project team meeting.

2.7.b Documenting the Implementation of ArchEPI Recommendations and Evaluating Their Effectiveness

The most effective ArchEPI projects will front-load their work early in the project delivery process—during the visioning and schematic design phase. But the ArchEPI team should maintain a strategic presence throughout the design, documentation, and construction/implementation phase of the project to ensure that their recommendations have been integrated into the design or policy to the greatest extent possible.[CC2.26] For example, the ArchEPI team might join the larger project team meetings once a month or at major project phase milestones to report out on the extent to which their recommendations have been deployed. These reports also should identify specific aspects of the design or policy that could be modified to better integrate health recommendations into the core project. See chapter 3 for additional information about how to incorporate health metrics and the ArchEPI process in general into a typical design and construction project delivery process.

After the project is complete, a POE should be conducted to evaluate the effectiveness of the health promoting strategies that were incorporated into the design or policy.[CC2.27] This assessment could take place anytime from a few months after project completion to a year or more after occupancy. Depending on the public health issues studied, the ArchEPI team may need to take into account the latency periods or incubation periods of some health outcomes. And, ideally, the team would collect new data on several EPHIs to compare the baseline to the post-occupancy reality. If collecting pre- and post-health data is not realistic for the project (which is often the case), environmental exposure and environmental mediator indicators can be used as proxies. It can also be useful to collect qualitative data from building occupants to understand how they experience the building and whether they have noticed an improvement or deterioration in their health status. In many cases, collaborating with academic programs or scientific organizations can increase capacity for this step of the process without adding to the financial or time burden of the project. Similarly, design teams often conduct POEs to determine how occupants experience the design. Health questions could easily be added to these self-assessments as a part of the overall POE process.[SR2.22]

For more information about how to conduct a POE: The Center for the Built Environment at the University of California, Berkeley has developed an Occupant Indoor Environmental Quality Survey and Building Benchmarking Tool that could be tailored to topics covered by an ArchEPI assessment (https://cbe.berkeley.edu/research/occupant-survey-and-building-benchmarking/).

CORE COMPETENCY 2.26

Facility Design, Construction, Operations
Project Development and Documentation, Construction and Evaluation; Quality Control/Quality Assurance

Sustainability
Integrative Services

CORE COMPETENCY 2.27

Real Estate Development
Facilities Management; Property Management

Facility Design, Construction, Operations
Quality Control/Quality Assurance

STAKEHOLDER ROLES 2.22

Opportunity for the development team to demonstrate leadership in community benefit design

BOX 2.8.

Example—Comparison of Two Public Elementary Schools in Raleigh, North Carolina, USA

A study in Raleigh, North Carolina, USA, compared a public elementary school designed using a community-centric approach and co-located with a YMCA with a conventional elementary school in the same school district and designed by the same architecture firm a decade earlier.[29] A survey sent to teachers, administrators, and staff a year after the case school opened compared the experience in the two schools according to five themes drawn from the social determinants of health framework:[30] economic stability, education, health care, social and community context, neighborhood and built environment. Results from the 48 completed surveys (29 in the case school and 19 in the matched school) point to a positive association between a process that integrates school design and operations into the broader community on the one hand and improved self-reported scores of health and wellbeing on the other (table 2.5).

TABLE 2.5.
Results from Social Determinants of Health Post-Occupancy Survey of a Case Elementary School and a Matched Elementary School in the Wake County, North Carolina, USA, Public School System

	Case School	Matched School		Case School	Matched School
Education Access and Quality			**Physical and Mental Health**		
Diversity	74%	74%	Physical activity	74%	61%
Inclusion	74%	63%	Mental health	79%	50%
Sense of belonging	70%	42%	Social and emotional health	84%	56%
Social Connection and Community Engagement			**Economic Security (Upon Campus Re-entry after the COVID-19 Pandemic)**		
My school engages the community	62%	32%	General employee happiness	80%	42%
I feel connected to the community	62%	32%	Employee development	80%	71%
I believe the community feels connected to my school	62%	21%			

(cont.)

INTRODUCTION TO METRICS FOR BUILT ENVIRONMENT PROFESSIONALS **75**

TABLE 2.5. (*cont.*)

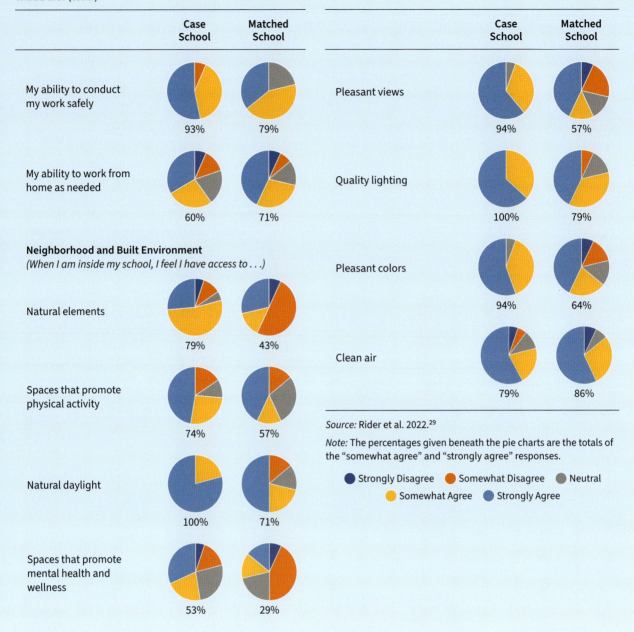

2.7.c Core Competencies
Implementing and Evaluating Interventions: Core Competencies

Field	Core Competencies
Epidemiology	• Communication • Community dimension of practice • Cultural competency
Real estate development	• Facilities management • Property management
Facility design, construction, operations	• Project development and documentation • Construction and evaluation • Quality control/quality assurance • Communication and Interaction • Plan implementation and placemaking
Sustainability	• Integrative services • Project surroundings and public outreach • Communications and corporate social responsibility
Philanthropy	• Communication

2.8 Conclusion

Prioritizing site-specific environmental public health concerns and deciding how the project team will measure progress in addressing them lies at the heart of the ArchEPI process. This chapter used the Guyer Problem-Solving Framework as a guide to implementing ArchEPI within the context of a building or facility operations project. Embedded within each of the six steps in the framework are technical skills and competencies that different members of the project team may possess and need to apply to move from one step to the next in the process.

However, before embarking on any of the analysis techniques above, the first order of business should be to consult available resources in case that work has already been performed by others.

The key to a successful ArchEPI project is the ability of the project team to balance rigor with speed. Rigor is needed to ensure that the project selects environmental public health concerns that are high priorities for the surrounding neighborhood and develops metrics that demonstrate how the project is contributing to achievement of those goals. Given the compressed schedule of most building projects, speed is necessary for the ArchEPI analysis to contribute to early conversations between the design team, owner, and community. The ultimate design (or operations protocol) following ArchEPI recommendations will leverage the environmental and population health attributes that are unique to the project location to create a positive ripple effect on the surrounding community.

Luckily, many projects will be able to use reports and data sets from public health, environmental justice, medical, climate change, air quality, and other sources rather than running new data-gathering activities themselves. Furthermore, the toolbox in this book was designed to reduce the burden of the ArchEPI process. Once the project team has settled on a short list of environmental public health topics to prioritize, they can apply the metrics and evidence-based design strategies in the toolbox directly to their projects instead of engaging in their own, project-specific analysis for every step in the process. One specific resource in the toolbox, table T.4, shares a crosswalk of evidence-based contributions that common green and healthy building strategies can make to climate change and community health goals.

Now that we have reviewed each step in the ArchEPI process, we turn our attention in chapter 3 to overlaying the ArchEPI method onto the project delivery process, so that critical information is delivered to the right audience at the right time.

DISCUSSION QUESTIONS

1. Explain the usefulness of correlation when causation is not known, particularly for questions about the relationship between changes to the built environment and health outcomes.
2. Identify three examples of EPHIs and three examples of related built environment interventions.
3. Explain what buffering is and give an example that explains how it might be useful for a building design or facility operations project.
4. What are the three parts of a SOHCO and why are they important to the ArchEPI Process?

Architectural Epidemiology Toolbox

Introduction

A successful application of architectural epidemiology involves two steps. The first step is to identify the site-specific environmental health priorities for a building project through data gathering, analysis, and community engagement as outlined in chapter 2. This toolbox is designed to support the second step: using evidence-based design and operations strategies to address the priority health concerns identified in step 1.

The toolbox is divided into two major health categories that are influenced by the built environment: community health conditions and climate change. Each section lays out the links between design/operations and health outcomes for five topics.

Community Health Conditions	Health Effects of Climate Change
• Cardiovascular disease	• Extreme heat
• Respiratory disease	• Flooding
• Obesity, diabetes, and hypertension	• Natural disasters / storms
• Cancer	• Air quality
• Mental health	• Vector-borne disease

An infographic summarizes each sub-section's health topic and shows how it affects the built environment, how design can help protect building occupants and neighbors from negative health outcomes associated with it, who is most vulnerable to experiencing negative health outcomes, and what are the highest priority health risks. Finally, a crosswalk table at the end of the toolbox (figure T.4) helps you easily identify the design and operations strategies that benefit more than one health topic.

After following this two-step approach, you will be well-positioned to prioritize design and operations strategies with the greatest potential to bring co-benefits and avoid co-harms to the surrounding neighborhood and community. Figure T.1 illustrates an example of how a project team can use the two parts of this book (chapter 2 and the toolbox) to develop a guiding vision (composed of co-impact pathways) that generates added value for multiple project objectives and stakeholder groups. Please read the referenced article to learn more about how to develop a co-benefit diagram for a specific project.

HEALTH EFFECTS OF COMMUNITY HEALTH CONDITIONS

KEY MESSAGES

1. Community health conditions are health conditions that are prevalent in many populations, leading to significant loss of productivity, financial instability, and premature death around the world—particularly among groups with physiological vulnerabilities and groups experiencing discrimination and marginalization.

2. The buildings and communities where people living with community health conditions spend their time influence disease distribution, progression, and treatment.

3. Health-promoting decisions made at each scale of development—community planning, real estate development, architectural and landscape design, interior design, and operations—can help advance local public health action plans targeting the highest priority diseases in their area.

4. A large body of scientific research and open data sets are now available. It is therefore increasingly feasible for individual project teams to identify which community health conditions are most relevant to the future occupants of a building and its surrounding neighborhood, as well has how those concerns dovetail with local, regional, and national health targets. Armed with that information, design teams can tailor health-promoting design strategies to support healthier outcomes for the diseases that are most relevant to the project site and the surrounding community.

Community health conditions are health conditions that are prevalent in many populations, leading to significant loss of productivity, financial instability, and premature death around the world—particularly among groups with physiological vulnerabilities and groups experiencing discrimination and marginalization. They are caused by a variety of infectious pathogens, non-communicable precursors, and strains on mental health.

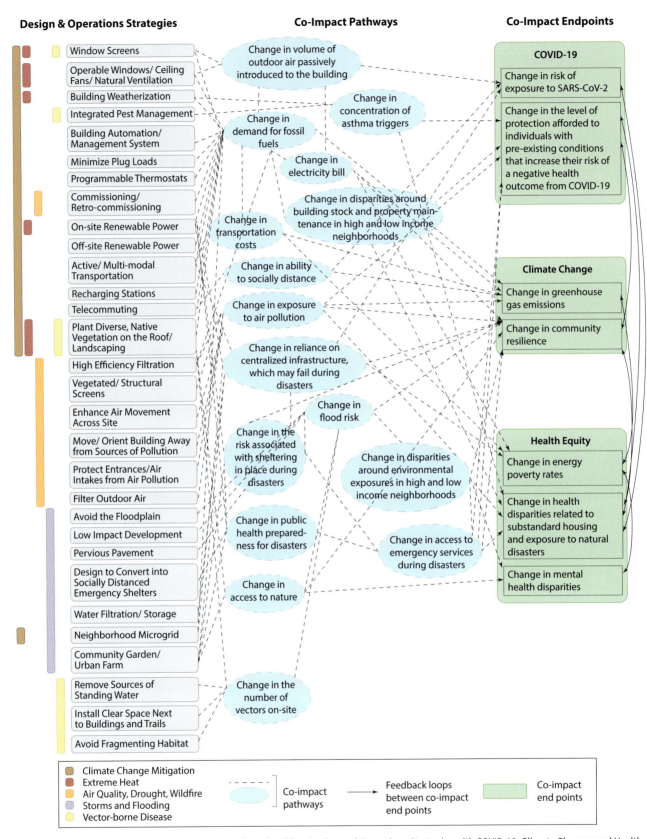

Figure T.1. Example of Co-Impact Pathways Linking Selected Building Design and Operations Strategies with COVID-19, Climate Change, and Health Equity Desired Outcomes

Note: The design strategies in the left-hand column are traced over to three desired project outcomes (i.e., reduce risk of COVID-19, climate change mitigation and adaptation, and promoting health equity) in the righthand column via co-impact pathways (organizing ideas that describe a set of design strategies all working towards a specific goal).

Source: Houghton 2021[1]

Infectious disease has played a prominent role in architecture and urbanism throughout the history of communal settlements. However, the incidence of both waterborne and airborne disease fell dramatically starting in the late 19th century. The sanitation movement dramatically reduced waterborne disease in high-income countries in the late 19th century through the 1920s. (See chapter 1 for more details and a summary of the intertwined history of architecture and epidemiology.) Starting in 1946, respiratory diseases like pneumonia, influenza, and tuberculosis began to fall down the list of the top 10 causes of death—replaced by chronic diseases like heart disease, stroke, and cancer.[2] The COVID-19 pandemic starting in 2020 reminded the global community that infectious disease is a perennial threat in every corner of the globe. As of December 2022, the World Health Organization (WHO) reported over 645 million confirmed cases and over 6.6 million deaths[3] (over 1 million of which occurred in the US[4]). Similarly, climate change related weather events (such as drought, flooding, and tropical cyclones) are a high-frequency reminder that waterborne diseases quickly spike after natural forces breach man-made water infrastructure.[5]

Chronic, or non-communicable, diseases are a pressing and intensifying public health crisis with strong links to the built environment. They account for close to 70% of deaths each year worldwide—more than all other causes combined.[6] And their impact on global health is projected to rise from 38 million deaths in 2012 to 52 million in 2030.[6] In the US, 1.6 million people died from the four most prevalent chronic diseases in 2017 (58% of all deaths).[7] The rising costs of chronic disease are so significant that the World Economic Forum has identified them as 1 of 13 global trends that could threaten social and economic stability if left unaddressed.[8] The WHO has identified chronic disease as a major barrier to poverty alleviation, because they reduce productivity and pose a disproportionate financial burden on families living in poverty—particularly in low- and middle-income countries.[6]

Approximately 40% of chronic disease deaths occur among people under the age of 70, and, therefore, might be prevented through proper medical care and behavior change.[6] In an effort to reduce chronic disease mortality among this population, the WHO launched "25 by 25" in 2012: an initiative with the goal of lowering the death rate from four high priority diseases among adults aged 30–70 years 25% by 2025.[9]

Chronic diseases are influenced by land use and building design. The WHO estimates that the burden of chronic disease attributable to environmental exposures increased from 17% in 2002 to 22% in 2012. Meanwhile, the burden of infectious, parasitic, neonatal, and nutritional diseases attributable to the environment fell from 31% in 2002 to 20% during the same period.[10]

The first four sections in the toolbox are devoted to these high priority diseases, which represent 82% (31.2 million) of deaths from chronic disease,[6] and can also be caused or exacerbated by communicable pathogens:

1. Cardiovascular disease
2. Respiratory disease
3. Diabetes, Hypertension, and Obesity
4. Cancer

The fifth section will address mental health challenges, which are often chronic conditions and can have a devastating effect on an individual's finances, social interactions, and physical health. In 2010, it was estimated that 700 million people suffered from mental disorders—40% of whom experienced major depression.[11] The WHO estimates that more than 21% of the total number of "years lived with a disability" (YLD) globally (26% in the US) are caused by mental illness.[12] Major depression falls within the top 10 causes of YLD for every country that has reported to the WHO.[13] Similar to chronic disease, mental illness is projected to rise in the future. For example, the prevalence of mental illness and substance use disorders in sub-Saharan Africa is projected to rise 130% between 2010 and 2050.[14] Depression is on track to displace ischemic heart disease as the leading cause of disease burden worldwide by 2030.[15]

While chronic disease and mental health challenges are often assumed to be concentrated in developed countries, the WHO estimates that low- and middle-income countries bear the burden of close to three quarters of total chronic disease deaths and over 80% of deaths under age 70.[6] Similarly, 80% of mental disorders occur in low- and middle-income countries.[16] Chronic diseases often cause disabilities, which reduce the number of years a person lives in good health (i.e., healthy life expectancy). For example, a study of 187 countries found that, while global healthy life expectancy increased by four years from 1990 to 2010, almost none of those gains were due to reductions in disabilities—particularly mental illness, musculoskeletal pain connected with obesity, and the side effects of diabetes (e.g., diabetic foot, neuropathy, retinopathy, amputation, and chronic kidney disease). Furthermore, the study found that, as overall life expectancy increased, the gap between life expectancy and healthy life expectancy also increased—mainly due to increased disability from chronic diseases. The comparison was particularly stark between high-income countries and low- to middle-income countries. For example, at age 50, men in Japan can look forward to another 25.6 years of healthy life on average, while men in Haiti have a 10.1-year healthy life expectancy at the same age.[17]

All of the conditions covered in the community health section of the toolbox are influenced by the design and operation of buildings, neighborhoods, and communities. Pearce et al. (2014)[18] refers to the built environment as a "cause of causes." In other words, design and operations influence the direct causes of chronic disease. One study estimates that environmental exposure accounts for more than 80% of deaths from chronic disease.[19] For example, poor diet and a sedentary lifestyle increase the risk of developing cardiovascular disease, respiratory disease, diabetes, hypertension, and obesity. The built environment behind that diet and lifestyle either creates conditions that promote healthier behaviors and reduce exposure to environmental hazards like air pollution and extreme heat, or it supports a physical context that increases the risk of building occupants' succumbing to chronic conditions. Table T.1 illustrates the difference between design choices related to diet and exercise at various geographic scales that contribute to either disease reduction or increased risk of chronic disease.

Each section in the toolbox will introduce a community health topic and its relevance both globally and in the US. It will then walk through the ways in which the natural, built, and social environments can influence the progression of the disease. Finally, it will present architectural and land use design strategies that have been shown in the scientific evidence to support efforts at reducing the burden of these diseases, particularly on vulnerable populations.

T.1 Toolbox—Community Health Conditions: Cardiovascular Disease

T.1.a Introduction

Cardiovascular and cerebrovascular diseases (which include heart disease and stroke) are the leading cause of death worldwide, resulting in 17.9 million deaths in 2016 (31% of global deaths), 75% of which occurred in low- and middle-income countries.[20] In the US, heart disease is the leading cause of death (23%; 647,457 deaths in 2017), with

TABLE T.1.

Examples of the Built Environment as a "Cause of Causes" of Cardiovascular Disease, Respiratory Disease, Diabetes, Hypertension, and Obesity

Cause of Causes: Design/Operations Strategies	Cause: Diet Protective	Cause: Diet Increase Risk	Cause: Exercise Protective	Cause: Exercise Increase Risk
Building	• One or more options to purchase fresh, healthy food • On-site farmer's market or agriculture	• No fresh, healthy food kiosks, restaurants in building	• Stairs • Fitness room, showers	• Elevator only option • Main entrance links building to garage/parking lot
Campus design/ operations	• Options to purchase fresh, healthy food in every building • On-site farmer's market or agriculture	• No fresh fruits and healthy meals available on campus	• Campus sidewalks/bike paths link to street • Walking trail	• No sidewalks or bike paths
Neighborhood design/ operations	• Three to five restaurants serving fresh, healthy food within 0.25 miles	• No restaurants serving fresh, healthy food within 0.25 miles	• Direct link from campus to neighborhood sidewalks, bike paths, transit network	• None or fragmented pedestrian, cycling, transit infrastructure
Community design/ operations	• One or more grocery stores within 1 mile	• No grocery stores within 1 mile	• Safe and comprehensive pedestrian, cycling, transit systems linking office campus to the rest of the community	• None or fragmented pedestrian, cycling, transit infrastructure

(Increasing Geographic Scale ↓)

Source: Adapted from Pearce et al. 2014.[18]

costs from medical care and lost productivity averaging $200 billion per year.[21] Strokes are the fifth leading cause of death (5.2%; 146,383 deaths in 2017), with costs averaging $34 billion per year.[21] The US Centers for Disease Control and Prevention estimate that one-third of cardiovascular and stroke deaths in the US (91,757 cardiovascular deaths per year; 16,973 stroke deaths per year) are preventable.[22]

T.1.b What Is Cardiovascular Disease?

Cardiovascular disease refers to damage to the heart and/or blood vessels. It includes mechanisms that narrow or block blood vessels and damage the heart muscle. If blood and oxygen flow is sufficiently slowed, it can lead to the death of tissue: a heart attack if it occurs to the heart muscle; a stroke if it occurs in the brain.[20]

Most forms of cardiovascular disease are caused by plaque build-up in the arteries, which can slowly block blood flow. Or, if the plaque ruptures, it can form a blood clot that restricts blood flow. A heart attack occurs when blood flow is restricted to the heart.[20] Almost 90% of strokes are caused by restricted blood flow to the brain.[21]

T.1.c What Are Its Symptoms?

Cardiovascular disease can cause a number of symptoms, depending on their severity (table T.2).

Heart attack symptoms include pain or discomfort in the chest, arms, left shoulder, elbows, jaw, or back; shortness of breath; nausea or vomiting; breaking into a sweat; and symptoms of faintness (e.g., feeling light-headed or dizzy and/or becoming pale). Symptoms of less acute heart disease include shortness of breath, fatigue, chest pain, and irregular heart beats. Chronic cardiovascular diseases are treated with a combination of medication and behavior modifications (e.g., no smoking, reduced alcohol consumption, healthy diet, exercise). More serious conditions may require surgery to open blockages in the arteries, repair heart tissue, or assist the heart in functioning properly.[20]

Symptoms of stroke include numbness on one side of the body, confusion or difficulty speaking or understanding speech, difficulty seeing or walking, loss of balance or coordination, severe headache without a known cause, and fainting or unconsciousness.[20] Similar to heart attacks, the initial course of treatment for strokes often involves a medication to dissolve the blood clot or blockage that caused the stroke. More intensive treatments include surgery to clear out the blockage and repair arteries and brain tissue. Stroke recovery often involves similar behavior modifications to heart disease, because the underlying risk factors are the same for both conditions.[23]

TABLE T.2.

Symptoms of Cardiovascular Disease and Stroke

Health Condition	Symptoms
Cardiovascular disease	• Chest pain • Faintness • Fatigue • Irregular heart beats • Nausea or vomiting • Pain or discomfort in the chest, arms, left shoulder, elbows, jaw, or back • Shortness of breath • Sweating
Stroke	• Confusion or difficulty speaking or understanding speech • Fainting or unconsciousness • Difficulty seeing or walking • Loss of balance or coordination • Numbness on one side of the body • Severe headache without a known cause

T.1.d Relationship with Climate Change

Climate change is increasing the risk of negative health outcomes from cardiovascular disease through increasingly frequent and intense heat waves; increased risk of disruption to medical care caused by severe storm events; and, deteriorating air quality—among other exposures that can exacerbate symptoms.[24]

T.1.d.i Heat

High temperatures can exacerbate chronic cardiovascular disease, leading to increased emergency department visits and increased mortality.[25(p46)] For example, a large-scale study in Europe found that daily cardiovascular mortality in five Mediterranean cities (Athens, Greece; Barcelona, Spain; Milan, Italy; Rome, Italy; and Valencia, Spain) increased 14.7%–34.7% among men 65 years and above and 38%–43.3% among women 65 years and above during heat waves from 1990–2002 and in 2004 compared with non-heat wave days.[26] Similarly, a study of 107 US cities from 1987–2000 estimated that cardiovascular mortality increased on average by 8.8% on heat wave days compared with non-heat wave days.[27]

T.1.d.ii Storms

Exposure to severe storms can place both physical and mental strain on people living with chronic cardiovascular

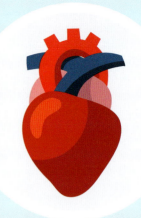

02 HOW DOES IT AFFECT THE BUILT ENVIRONMENT?

FOOD DESERTS
Neighborhoods without access to fresh, healthy food put residents at higher risk of cardiovascular disease.

SPRAWL, SINGLE USE DISTRICTS
This kind of environment increases traffic-related air pollution & reduces opportunities for physical activity.

UNSAFE BIKE/PED ENVIRONMENT
This kind of environment increases risk of cardiovascular disease by reducing opportunities for physical activity.

ON-SITE GROCERY/ FOOD PRODUCTION
Increases food security & access to fresh, healthy options.

COMPACT, MULTI-USE DEVELOPMENT NEAR TRANSIT & BIKE/PED INFRASTRUCTURE
Increases opportunities for physical activity.

NATIVE VEGETATION
Increases access to physical activity. Reduces urban heat island.

FILTRATION
Filters out pollutants from both outdoor & indoor sources.

LOW EMITTING MATERIALS
Reduces the concentration of pollutants generated indoors.

04 WHO IS MOST VULNERABLE...

ELDERLY
Body is less resilient & many elderly also have underlying health conditions.

HIGH CHOLESTEROL
Deposits in arteries can cause heart disease.

OBESITY, DIABETES, HYPERTENSION
Inflammation & damage to arteries can cause or exacerbate heart disease.

SMOKING
Increases plaque build up & thickens the blood.

MENTAL HEALTH
Can increase inflammation & lead to unhealthy behavior.

POVERTY
Increased risk of stress & reduced access to healthy food, opportunities for physical activity, medical care.

Toolbox Infographic T.1. Linkages among Cardiovascular Disease, the Built Environment Determinants of Health, Protective Design and Operations Strategies, the Groups Who Are at Highest Risk, and Related Negative Health Outcomes

01
CARDIOVASCULAR DISEASE

- Leading cause of death globally.
- Refers to damage to heart and/or blood vessels. Caused by reduced blood and oxygen flow.

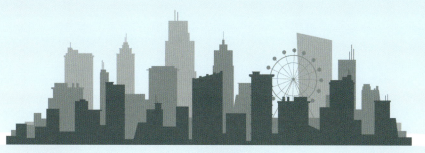

AIR POLLUTION
Exposure to both indoor & outdoor air pollution can damage the cardiovascular system through plaque formation & increasing risk of blood clots.

URBAN HEAT ISLAND
Exposure to high temperatures can exacerbate cardiovascular disease symptoms.

LACK OF RESILIENCE
Disruption to medical services & electrical equipment during power outages can trigger a life-threatening condition in cardiovascular patients.

03
HOW CAN DESIGN HELP?

WELL-MAINTAINED BUILDINGS
Reduces the risk of mold & other allergens; ensures filtration & emergency systems are working.

COOLING CENTER
Protects under-air conditioned residents.

ISLANDABLE SITES & MICROGRIDS
Design on-site energy, water, & food production to allow occupants to shelter in place when utilities are disrupted.

MINORITIES
Increased risk of stress & reduced access to healthy food, opportunities for physical activity, medical care.

DISABILITY & DEATH

DIABETES

HYPERTENSION

MENTAL HEALTH

... TO THE HEALTH RISKS? 05

Note: Many of the design and operations strategies in the infographic bring co-benefits to other topics in this toolbox as well. See figure T.4 for a crosswalk of all of the environmental health co-benefits.

disease. Disruption to medical services and electrical equipment due to flooding and power outages can transform a disease that is under control and minimally disruptive to daily life into a life-threatening condition.[28] The mental distress associated with dislocation and witnessing destruction and human suffering has also been found to exacerbate underlying cardiovascular conditions.[29] For example, New Orleans, Louisiana, USA, experienced a 10-fold increase in the number of cardiovascular deaths during Hurricane Katrina compared with an average week.[28] And, one hospital in New Orleans saw an increased rate of hospital admissions for heart attacks, particularly among late middle-aged men, up to three years after the event.[30]

T.1.d.iii Air Quality

Air quality can be compromised outdoors by mobile (i.e., traffic-related), stationary (i.e., industrial), or natural (i.e., wildfire) sources of airborne pollution. Indoors, it can be compromised by recirculating outdoor air, building materials that off-gas chemicals, and biological pathogens like mold. More detail is available in the air quality section of the toolbox. Both short-term and long-term exposure to air pollution can damage the cardiovascular system by initiating plaque formation and increasing the risk of blood clots.[31] Even short-term spikes in air pollution can increase the risk of heart attacks, strokes, and acute heart failure.[31] Exposure to traffic-related air pollution (TRAP; a combination of particulate matter, ground-level ozone (O_3), and gases like nitrogen and sulfur oxides) can harden artery walls.[31] A study of people >65 years in Denver, Colorado, USA—a city with relatively clean ambient air—found that an increase in ground-level O_3 was associated with heightened risk of cardiovascular hospitalization; sulfur dioxide was associated with increased length of hospitalization; and carbon monoxide (CO) was associated with risk of congestive heart failure.[32] A large-scale study of women in the US found that living less than 50 m (160 ft) from a major roadway increased their risk of sudden cardiac death by 38% compared with women living more than 500 m (1,600 ft) away.[33] Particulate matter is also a major cardiovascular health concern. The WHO estimates that 2.4 million deaths globally in 2016 were caused by exposure to fine particulate matter ($PM_{2.5}$) alone.[34] An increase of 10 μg/m³ in annual exposure to $PM_{2.5}$ has been found to increase cardiovascular mortality by 20% globally.[35] In the Netherlands, a large-scale study of over 30,000 Dutch residents found that long-term exposure to ultrafine particles (<0.1 μg) was associated with an 18% increased risk of cardiovascular disease.[36] And a 10 μg/m³ increase in annual exposure to nitrogen dioxide (NO_2) has been associated with a 13% increase in global cardiovascular mortality. Deaths from air pollution, like many environmental health conditions, are not distributed equally across the population. For both NO_2 and $PM_{2.5}$, mortality in Asia (58.8% increase from NO_2 exposure; 38% from $PM_{2.5}$ exposure) far outpaced mortality in North America (3% increase from NO_2 exposure; 4.7% from $PM_{2.5}$ exposure) and Europe (5.9% increase from NO_2 exposure; 18.8% from $PM_{2.5}$ exposure).[35]

T.1.e How Does the Built Environment Increase the Risk of Cardiovascular Disease?

Land use and building design decisions can increase the risk factors underlying cardiovascular disease in a number of ways. Car-centric planning configurations like urban sprawl can increase the risk of cardiovascular disease by making it difficult to have an active lifestyle. Walking, cycling, and using public transit can be dangerous in that kind of environment. The emphasis on single-use districts can lead to food deserts by concentrating all shopping in a few, centralized nodes that may be difficult to access by low-income residents or people living on the other side of town. Car-centric urban form also increases TRAP, which can damage the cardiovascular system. It also devotes large swaths of land to concrete and asphalt, which become urban heat islands. Exposure to high temperatures is a risk factor for people who are suffering from cardiovascular disease. Sprawling urban areas are often less resilient to extreme weather events because there may be only one or two evacuation routes out of a neighborhood or commercial district. Disruption to medical services and electrical equipment during power outages can lead to life-threatening crises for cardiovascular patients who depend on medical devices in their homes and places of work.

In terms of the indoor environment, poor indoor air quality can also exacerbate existing cardiovascular disease or trigger a health crisis in cardiovascular patients.

T.1.f How Can Design Help?

At the community planning scale, transitioning urban sprawl into a more dense, urban street fabric with accompanying sidewalks, protected bike lanes, and access to public transit can remove a significant barrier to physical activity. Interspersing dense, mixed-use nodes with parks and green space can further encourage active living and reduce exposure to extreme heat as a trigger for a cardiovascular episode.

Projects that include a community garden or urban farm, access to community-supported agriculture or a farmer's market, and retail selling fresh fruits and vegetables can all support healthy nutrition—the other primary pathway for promoting a heathy heart.

Reducing exposure to particulate matter and toxic chemicals in indoor air is another way to reduce the risk of exacerbating the symptoms of cardiovascular disease. Green building strategies like materials with low levels of volatile organic compounds (VOCs), enhanced filtration, integrated pest management, and green cleaning can all protect occupants from exposure to poor indoor air quality.

Projects located in regions where extreme heat events can lead to power disruptions may consider installing islandable renewable energy installations or microgrids with energy storage and designating a portion of the building as a cooling center, so that people with heart conditions have a place of respite away from the heat.

T.1.g Who Is Most Vulnerable?

Risk factors for cardiovascular disease stem from age (e.g., the elderly), disease precursors (e.g., blood cholesterol, obesity, diabetes, hypertension), behavioral factors (smoking), mental health conditions, and socioeconomic disparities (e.g., minorities, families living in poverty). It is a complex topic; when more than one risk factor is apparent, they can lead to a compounded result and markedly increase an individual's overall risk of disease or mortality.

T.1.g.i Elderly

Ageing is a significant risk factor for cardiovascular disease. For example, over half of the 41.7% global increase in deaths from ischemic heart disease from 1990–2013 is estimated to have been caused by population ageing, particularly in Asia.[37] As the body ages, it is less likely to resist stressors and rebound after cardiovascular events.[38] Older adults are more likely to suffer from multiple ailments such as hypertension, which are also risk factors for cardiovascular disease[39] and which are more likely to manifest as disabilities.[13] The majority of people diagnosed, hospitalized, and succumbing to cardiovascular disease are over 65 years of age. For example, 48% of adults in the US (121.5 million people) have at least one cardiovascular disease. That proportion rises to over 77% among people aged 60–79 years and 90% among people over 80 years. 64% of cardiovascular deaths in the US occur among people aged 75 and older.[40]

T.1.g.ii High Blood Cholesterol

According to the WHO, cholesterol is one of the top 10 leading risk factors for the global burden of disease.[41] It is a fatty, waxy substance that is produced by the body and used to build cell membranes and an array of molecules as diverse as Vitamin D, hormones like testosterone and estrogen, and fat-dissolving bile acids used to digest food. There are two types of cholesterol: low-density (LDL) and high-density (HDL). If too much LDL cholesterol circulates in the blood stream, it could be deposited on artery walls as plaque, constricting blood flow and thereby causing cardiovascular disease. Another type of cholesterol, HDL, helps to clean plaque off of artery walls, and is therefore beneficial in reducing the risk of cardiovascular disease.[42] Raised levels of cholesterol are estimated to cause 2.6 million deaths each year worldwide.[43] Europe and the Americas report the highest cholesterol levels—54% and 48%, respectively.[43]

T.1.g.iii Obesity, Overnutrition, and Sedentary Lifestyle

Obesity can increase the risk of cardiovascular disease in several ways. Obese individuals must increase their blood supply in order to circulate blood in fatty tissue. The result is a larger heart and increased strain on the heart as it pumps more blood to a larger volume of tissue. Fatty deposits around key organs like the heart can also reduce their ability to function normally, eventually leading to organ failure.[44] Obese individuals are also at higher risk of other risk factors for cardiovascular disease. For example, in the US, obese adults were more than 3 times as likely as normal weight adults to develop diabetes (18.5%, compared with 5.4%) and 50% more likely to develop hypertension (35.7%, compared with 19.8%).[45] Finally, obesity is a major cause of cardiovascular disease and mortality. A large-scale study in Norway found that the risk of cardiovascular mortality increased by 12% for each incremental increase in body mass index (BMI).[46] In the US, it has been associated with 112,159 excess cardiovascular deaths each year (13% of the total)[47] and a 64% increase in risk of stroke.[48] Globally, heart disease and stroke accounted for 76% of deaths caused by low levels of physical activity from 1990–2015. They also accounted for the majority of deaths caused by a poor diet.[41]

T.1.g.iv Diabetes

Diabetes refers to a chronic condition whereby the body either does not produce enough insulin or does not process it efficiently.[49] As a result, an excess of sugar circulates in the blood stream. Over time, the sugar can damage blood vessels and the nerves that control the heart and blood vessels, leading to cardiovascular disease. People with diabetes are more likely to develop heart disease younger than the population as a whole. They are also twice as likely to die from heart disease or stroke—which are the two leading causes of death among people diagnosed with diabetes.[50]

T.1.g.v Hypertension (High Blood Pressure)

Hypertension refers to blood pressure in the arteries exceeding 140/90 mmHg over a period of time.[51] One third of adults in the US have high blood pressure, but only half of them have it under control. Hypertension increases the risk of cardiovascular disease by hardening artery walls, which can decrease blood flow to the heart and/or brain. It can also burst or block arteries.[52] Hypertension alone is a more significant risk factor for cardiovascular death among women than all other risk factors combined and all but smoking for men.[21] In 2013, 27.7% of deaths from hypertension in the US listed cardiovascular disease as the underlying cause of death, and 9.2% listed stroke. This was a decrease from 34.2% (heart disease) and 14.9% (stroke) in 2000.[53] One study found that lowering blood pressure to normal levels could reduce the risk of cardiovascular-related death by as much as 30.4% among men and 38% among women.[54]

T.1.g.vi Smoking

Smoking increases the risk of cardiovascular disease in several ways. It can increase plaque build-up and decrease levels of "good" HDL cholesterol in the bloodstream. It also thickens the blood, making it easier to clot. And, finally, it can damage blood vessel linings, thicken blood vessels, and narrow their aperture.[55] Even low levels of exposure to tobacco smoke—including through secondhand smoke—can sharply increase the risk of cardiovascular disease.[56(pp356–59)] This is a particular concern for adult smokers (aged 40–50), because cardiovascular disease is the leading risk factor for smoking-related death among that age group.[56(p356)] Smoking also increases the risk of stroke by two to four times.[57]

T.1.g.vii Mental Health Conditions

Mental health conditions may increase the risk of cardiovascular disease both because they influence behavior (e.g., reducing adherence to healthy lifestyle choices like diet, exercise, and non-smoking) and because they have been associated with biological risk factors, such as inflammation, stress on the autonomic nervous system, and hardening of the arteries.[58] Depression has been identified as a risk factor for cardiovascular disease by the American Heart Association,[21] in part because it has been found to double the risk of recurrent cardiac events[59] and increase the risk of strokes by more than 30%.[60] This is a major public health concern, because one-fifth of cardiovascular patients in the US, Canada, and Europe report depressive symptoms—3 times higher than the general population[59]—and nearly one-third of stroke survivors are depressed.[61]

Anxiety can increase the risk of cardiovascular disease by 25% and increase the risk of cardiac death by 48%.[62] And chronic stress has been found to increase the risk of cardiovascular disease by 30%–50%.[63]

T.1.g.viii Minorities and Indigenous Populations

Minorities in the US face socioeconomic and geographic challenges that can make it difficult for them to follow heart healthy guidelines such as the "Life's Simple 7" goals developed by the American Heart Association. One study found that non-Whites were more likely than Whites to meet only two of the seven goals. These were non-smoking and normal cholesterol levels. On the other hand, non-Whites were more likely than Whites to be overweight or obese, less likely to exercise regularly, less likely to eat a heart healthy diet, more likely to be diagnosed with hypertension, and less likely to have normal blood glucose levels.[64] A study in China similarly found that a higher percentage of Hui and Mongolian minorities (23.1% and 21.1%, respectively) were more likely to demonstrate three or more risk factors for cardiovascular disease than the Han majority (16.6%).[65] In spite of disparities in risk factors among racial and ethnic groups in the US, deaths from cardiovascular disease are roughly the same percentage among Whites and African Americans (23.5% and 23.7%, respectively), with Hispanics experiencing a slightly lower percentage (20.3%). However, African Americans are at a higher risk of stroke onset and mortality than Whites in the US, with particularly large disparities at younger ages. For example, the rate of strokes among African American men aged 45–54 was 9.7 per 1,000 person-years from 1987–2001 compared with 2.4 among White men.[21] More than half of that excess stroke risk has been attributed to higher rates of high blood pressure among African Americans.[66] Indigenous communities also often have higher cardiovascular disease and mortality rates than the general population, because they do not receive the same level of public health and medical support as the general population. Furthermore, native populations that migrate throughout the year often live in remote areas and are more difficult to serve.[67] For example, the mortality rate from cardiovascular disease among Native Americans in the US remained more or less constant at 157 deaths per 100,000 while the overall mortality rate fell from 152 deaths per 100,000 in 1989 to 130.5 per 100,000 in 1998.[68] Similarly, ischemic heart disease is the leading cause of premature morality among Queensland Aboriginal and Torres Strait Islander populations in Australia—almost twice the number of years lost to the second leading cause, diabetes.[69]

T.1.g.ix Families Living in Poverty

Cardiovascular disease is a particular burden for families living in poverty, both in high-income countries like the US and in low- and middle-income countries. In the US, living in poverty has been associated with a number of risk factors for cardiovascular disease, including higher smoking rates (26.3% for adults living in poverty vs. 15.2% for adults living above the poverty line);[70] higher exposure to secondhand smoke (43.2% poverty vs. 21.2% higher income);[71] higher percentage that do not meet physical activity guidelines (58.2% poverty vs. 41.5% higher income);[21] almost twice the proportion of adults eating a poor diet (60.6% poverty vs. 35.7% higher income);[72] and, lower management of LDL cholesterol (21.9% poverty vs. 33.2% general population with high LDL levels).[73] People living in poverty in low- and middle-income countries are arguably even more burdened by cardiovascular disease, because it takes a heavy toll on working age people—slowing these countries' ability to develop and expand their economies. About 45% of cardiovascular deaths in low- and middle-income countries occur among people below the age of 70. And one study projects that the number of productive years lost among people aged 35 to 64 in Brazil, China, India, Russia, and South Africa from 2000 to 2030 will increase from 20.6 million to 33.7 million.[74]

T.2 Toolbox—Community Health Conditions: Respiratory Disease

T.2.a Introduction

Respiratory disease is a leading cause of disease, disability, and death worldwide, particularly in low- and middle-income countries. The COVID-19 global pandemic increased attention about both respiratory diseases and their relationship with indoor environments, because the SARS-CoV-2 virus—which causes COVID-19—primarily attacks the respiratory system. And, as an airborne virus, it is more likely to achieve high concentrations in poorly ventilated buildings. It is important to note, however, that SARS-CoV-2 can also harm the digestive system, the brain, the urogenital system, the central nervous system, and the circulatory system.[75] After its appearance in the US in early 2020, SARS-CoV-2 rapidly rose to become one of the top three causes of death, representing 12.2% of total deaths between March 2020 and October 2021—exceeded by only heart disease (20.1%) and cancer (17.5%). During pandemic surges in 2020, the seven-day running average of daily deaths from COVID-19 actually surpassed both heart disease and cancer. The scale of the pandemic remains hard to fathom. For example, 3,411 deaths were recorded in the US on December 9, 2020, representing more than two deaths per minute. And scientists estimate that the actual excess death rate may be up to 50% higher than the official accounts. Perhaps because of its scale, the pandemic also brought to light disparities in health outcomes that are tied to the way US society is organized. The elderly (particularly individuals over 85 years of age), people of color, and low-income individuals were at higher risk of severe disease and death than the general population—particularly in the early phase of the pandemic before a vaccine became available.[76–78]

An estimated six million people die of chronic obstructive pulmonary disease (COPD) or lower respiratory infections each year, more than any other condition except heart disease.[79] And COPD deaths are on the rise, increasing 11.6% from 1990 to 2015.[80] Lower respiratory infections are the leading cause of death among children under 5 years of age globally. They are responsible for 20% of deaths in that age category each year, equivalent to the death rate from premature birth and twice the death rate from diarrheal diseases and malaria.[81] Tuberculosis (TB) is the leading single cause of death from an infectious agent, resulting in more than 1.2 million deaths in 2018.[82] And, lung cancer is the leading cause of both new cancer diagnoses (2.09 million cases per year) and cancer deaths (1.76 million deaths per year) worldwide.[83]

Economic development is a major contributing factor to health outcomes from infectious respiratory diseases. For example, the death rate in 2017 among children under 5 years from acute respiratory infections in Africa was 11.5 per 1,000 live births, compared with 5.2 per 1,000 births in Southeast Asia, and 1.4 per 1,000 live births in the Americas.[81] Similarly, the 2018 death rate from TB among HIV-negative adults was twice as high in Africa (37 per 100,000 population) and Southeast Asia (32 per 100,000) than the global average (16 per 100,00).[81]

Acute lower respiratory infections lead to many millions of doctor visits and hospitalizations each year. It is estimated that up to 20% of the global population contract influenza each year. In Europe alone, 16.5 million cases of acute bronchitis are diagnosed each year. And, of the 3.4 million cases of pneumonia diagnosed each year in Europe, one million cases result in hospitalization.[84]

Chronic respiratory diseases are an ongoing health and economic burden for the people affected and their families. Asthma, the most prevalent, afflicts 358 million people worldwide,[80] many of whom are children.[85] It is estimated that over 174 million people have COPD.[80] And the prevalence of both diseases is on the rise. Prevalence of asthma increased by 12.6% from 1990–2015; and, prevalence of COPD increased by 44.2%.[80] In the US, close to 25 million people currently suffer from asthma,[86,87] and roughly the same number are estimated to suffer from COPD, although only 14.8 million have been officially diagnosed.[88]

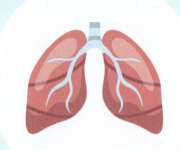

02 HOW DOES IT AFFECT THE BUILT ENVIRONMENT?

ALLERGY-TRIGGERING PLANTS
Plants producing allergenic pollen can trigger or exacerbate existing respiratory diseases like asthma and COPD.

URBAN HEAT ISLAND
Exposure to high temperatures can exacerbate respiratory disease symptoms.

ELECTRICAL GRID INSTABILITY
Power outages can be dangerous for patients requiring oxygen. In warm weather, they can allow for mold growth.

ENVIRONMENTAL TOBACCO SMOKE
Secondhand smoke can exacerbate existing conditions like asthma & increases risk of lung cancer.

NON ALLERGENIC LANDSCAPING
Plants that remove pollutants from the air but do not produce allergens.

ISLANDABLE SITES & MICROGRIDS
Design on-site energy, water, & food production to allow occupants to shelter in place when utilities are disrupted.

COMPACT, MULTI-USE DEVELOPMENT NEAR TRANSIT & BIKE/PED INFRASTRUCTURE
Reduce the need for car travel, a major cause of air pollution.

VEGETATIVE & STRUCTURAL BARRIERS TO EMISSION SOURCES
Reduce exposure to large & heavy air pollutants.

04 WHO IS MOST VULNERABLE...

CHILDREN
At higher risk for developmental & behavioral reasons.

ELDERLY
Body is less resilient & many elderly also have underlying health conditions.

CHRONIC DISEASE
Increased sensitivity to respiratory infections.

IMMUNO-COMPROMISED
Weak immune system reduces protection from exposure.

MENTAL HEALTH
Depression is common in COPD patients.

POVERTY
Increased risk of exposure & reduced access to medical care.

MINORITIES
Increased risk of exposure & reduced access to medical care.

Toolbox Infographic T.2. Linkages among Respiratory Disease, the Built Environment Determinants of Health, Protective Design and Operations Strategies, the Groups Who Are at Highest Risk, and Related Negative Health Outcomes

01
RESPIRATORY DISEASE

- Second leading cause of death globally & leading cause of death for children under 5.
- Refers to damage to the lungs, airways, or surrounding muscles.

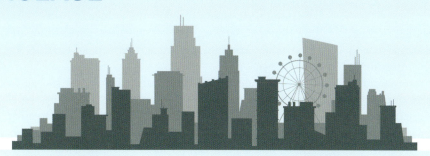

OUTDOOR AIR POLLUTION
Exposure to outdoor air pollution from traffic & point sources like industrial plants can stunt lung growth & damage airways, leading to COPD.

INDOOR AIR QUALITY
Emissions increase indoors when outdoor air is polluted. Paint, adhesives, sealants, interior finishes, & equipment can emit toxins. Exposure to radon and asbestos increases risk of cancer.

03
HOW CAN DESIGN HELP?

LOCATE ON SITE EMISSIONS (VEHICLES, SMOKING) AWAY FROM OPENINGS & AIR SUPPLY
Reduce the risk of pollutants entering the building.

INTEGRATED IAQ
Enhance ventilation & filtration to minimize outdoor air pollution & infectious disease. Install low VOC materials to minimize indoor emissions.

WELL-MAINTAINED BUILDINGS
Reduces the risk of mold, pests, high emitting cleaning products. Ensures filtration & emergency systems are working.

PRIMITIVE HOUSING
Indoor combustion increases risk of respiratory disease.

DISABILITY & DEATH

LUNG CANCER

HEART DISEASE

MENTAL HEALTH

... TO THE HEALTH RISKS? 05

Note: Many of the design and operations strategies in the infographic bring co-benefits to other topics in this toolbox as well. See figure T.4 for a crosswalk of all of the environmental health co-benefits.

Much of this suffering could be prevented by reducing exposure to air pollution and tobacco smoke and increasing access to proper medical care.[41,80] For example, the US Centers for Disease Control and Prevention (CDC) estimates that 40% of the 72,000 deaths from COPD each year could be prevented.[22]

T.2.b What Is Respiratory Disease?

Respiratory disease refers to damage to the lungs, airways, or muscles that pump air in and out of the lungs (such as the diaphragm).[89] Damage can be caused by infection or exposure to harmful chemicals (such as tobacco smoke, radon, asbestos, or indoor or outdoor air pollution).[89]

The five most common respiratory diseases and their associated symptoms are detailed below and summarized in table T.3.

COPD is a chronic, progressive disease of the air sacs in the lungs (e.g., alveoli) where oxygen is absorbed into, and carbon dioxide (CO_2) is exhausted from, the bloodstream. A person with COPD may experience damage to the walls between alveoli (a condition called emphysema) and/or irritation and inflammation to the lining of the alveoli, which results in the accumulation of thick mucus in the airways (a condition called chronic bronchitis). Mild COPD is treated in a similar manner as asthma—with a combination of lifestyle changes (such as not smoking) and inhaled medicines. More severe COPD may require oxygen therapy or surgery to remove portions of the lung that are so damaged that they reduce overall lung function.[90]

Asthma refers to a condition in which the airways into the lungs become inflamed and/or tighten, causing them to narrow and reduce the flow of oxygen. In many cases, inflammation is triggered as the body's immune system response to exposure to an airborne allergen, such as air pollution or pollen. While asthma is not usually curable, it can be treated with a combination of lifestyle changes (such as not smoking) and inhaled medicines that reduce inflammation and expand the airways to increase oxygen flow.[91,92]

Acute Lower Respiratory Infections refer to a suite of infectious diseases (both bacterial and viral) that impact the lung alveoli (such as pneumonia) and/or airways (such as bronchitis, influenza, and whooping cough).[84] Many of these conditions are transferred from one person to the next through contact with mucus that has been expelled from the patient through coughing or sneezing.[84] Pneumonia can be caused by bacteria, viruses, or fungi. The most common form of bacteria, *Streptococcus pneumoniae*, is present in most people's upper respiratory system, only causing an infection when the immune system is depressed.[93] Pneumonia causes the alveoli to become inflamed and fill up with fluid, which prevents them from absorbing oxygen.[94] Bronchitis causes the lung airways (e.g., bronchial tubes) to become inflamed, reducing airflow to the lungs and resulting in the production of excess mucus. It is usually caused by either an infection (usually viral) or by exposure to an irritant such as tobacco smoke, air pollution, or pollen.[95] Influenza (also known as the flu) is a highly infectious viral disease that affects both the respiratory system and other organs in the body.[96] Viral pneumonia is often caused by the influenza virus.[93] Viral respiratory infections are generally treated with fluids and rest, while bacterial infections may respond to antibiotic medicines.[94–96]

Tuberculosis (TB) is an infectious disease caused by the bacteria *Mycobacterium tuberculosis*. It usually settles first in the lungs, where it replicates and spreads to other organs, such as the lymph nodes, bones, kidneys, brain, spine, and skin. It can be spread from person to person through the air after an infected person coughs, sneezes, or talks. Normally, infection occurs after longtime exposure to the bacteria from a close family member, friend, or colleague. There are two types of TB. Latent TB refers to a person who has been infected with the TB bacteria but whose immune system is preventing the bacteria from replicating to the point of making the person sick. Active TB refers to patients who are experiencing symptoms and are contagious to others. It is estimated that one-quarter of the world's population (1.4 billion people) are infected, only 10 million of whom have been diagnosed with the active disease. People with latent TB may not develop active TB for years if their immune system remains in good condition. Most cases of active TB are treatable with medication. However, some strains are resistant to drug therapy, which can dramatically increase the difficulty of effectively treating the disease.[97]

Lung Cancer refers to cancers of the windpipe (e.g., trachea), airways (e.g., bronchial tubes), and/or air sacs (e.g., alveoli). It is caused by damage to cell DNA and mutations that cripple protective genes—both of which have been identified as outcomes of smoking tobacco.[92] Lung cancer is a deadly disease, resulting in the deaths of seven out of eight patients within five years of diagnosis. Up to 90% of cases are diagnosed too late to cure the disease. However, a combination of surgery, chemotherapy, and/or radiation are often used to slow the course of the disease and prolong life.[98]

T.2.c What Are the Symptoms?

COPD is notoriously underdiagnosed, in part because it can be asymptomatic.[90] One large-scale global study found major geographic disparities in diagnosis rates, ranging from 50% of COPD cases in Lexington, Kentucky, USA, going undiagnosed to over 98% of cases in Ile-Ife,

Nigeria.[99] As the disease progresses, common symptoms include an ongoing cough, a cough with a lot of mucus, shortness of breath (particularly during physical activity), wheezing, and tightness in the chest. More severe symptoms include swelling in the lower extremities, weight loss, reduced physical endurance, a rapid heart rate, and signs of low oxygen levels such as blue fingertips and deteriorated mental alertness.[90]

Asthma symptoms include intermittent "attacks" of wheezing, coughing, chest tightness, and shortness of breath. Asthma attacks can occur frequently or rarely, depending on the age of the patient, the types of triggers that set off an attack, and the severity of the disease.[91]

There are several types of acute lower respiratory infection with various symptoms:

- Symptoms associated with pneumonia include cough, fever, chills, and difficulty breathing.[94]
- Symptoms of bronchitis include coughing up mucus, a runny and stuffy nose a few days before the cough begins, fatigue, and wheezing.[100]
- Symptoms of influenza (e.g., flu) include high fever/chills; cough; sore throat; nasal congestion; fatigue; and, headache, muscle ache, and joint pain. Some cases of the flu, particularly among children, include nausea, vomiting, and/or diarrhea.[101]
- TB symptoms include cough, weight loss, fever/chills/night sweats, and symptoms related to the system function that has been attacked by the TB bacteria. For example, TB of the lungs is associated with coughing up blood or mucus.[97]
- Lung cancer symptoms include cough (including coughing up blood), shortness of breath, chest and/or bone pain, weight loss, and swelling in the extremities.[98]

T.2.d Relationship with Climate Change

Four climate-related natural disasters—extreme heat, flooding, storms, and poor air quality—can trigger or exacerbate chronic and infectious respiratory diseases.

T.2.d.i Heat

High temperatures can exacerbate chronic respiratory diseases, such as asthma and COPD, leading to increased emergency department visits and increased mortality during heat waves.[25(p46)] For example, the week of the 2003 European heat wave, respiratory deaths in Essen, Germany, increased 61% compared with average summer mortality. The week following the heat event, respiratory mortality increased to 77% above average.[102] Similarly, a study of 114 cities in the US found that hospital admissions

TABLE T.3.

Symptoms of Respiratory Disease

Respiratory Disease	Symptoms
Acute lower respiratory infection	• Chills • Coughing • Diarrhea • Fatigue • Fever • Headache • Mucus in the lungs • Muscle ache, joint pain • Nasal congestion • Nausea, vomiting • Shortness of breath • Sore throat • Wheezing
Asthma	• Coughing • Shortness of breath • Tightness in the chest • Wheezing
Chronic obstructive pulmonary disease	• Coughing • Low oxygen levels • Mucus in the lungs • Rapid heart rate • Reduced physical endurance • Shortness of breath • Swelling in the extremities • Tightness in the chest • Weight loss • Wheezing
Lung cancer	• Coughing • Muscle ache, joint pain • Shortness of breath • Swelling in the extremities • Tightness in the chest • Weight loss
Tuberculosis	• Chills • Coughing • Fever • Mucus in the lungs • Weight loss

for respiratory disease increased 4% among the elderly (65 years and above) during the 8 days following an extreme heat event.[103]

T.2.d.ii Flooding and Storms

People with chronic respiratory diseases or acute respiratory infections are vulnerable to both the direct and indirect impacts of flooding and storms. Respiratory patients with depressed immune systems are at higher risk of infection if they come in contact with floodwaters, which often contain a mixture of biologic pathogens and toxic chemicals.[104,105] If a flood disrupts power, it can exacerbate symptoms for patients on oxygen or ventilators.[104,106,107] Flooded roads can prevent patients from receiving routine medical treatment that is needed to keep their chronic conditions under control.[104,105,108,109] People who are rendered homeless by flooding or wind damage are at heightened risk of acute respiratory infections as a result of overcrowded living conditions, insufficient ventilation, and/or poor nutrition in emergency shelters.[110] For example, after Pakistan suffered heavy flooding in the summer of 2010, affecting more than 14 million people and causing over 1,400 deaths, the WHO reported more than 115,000 cases of respiratory tract infections—second only to skin infections (>143,000 cases).[111] This risk increased during the COVID-19 pandemic, particularly in 2020 before vaccines and therapeutics became widely available. For example, the daily new infectee rate in Croatia increased for about two weeks after a magnitude 5.3 earthquake displaced thousands of residents in Zagreb in spring 2020.[112] People with chronic respiratory diseases are also particularly sensitive to the aeroallergens that can accumulate in buildings within days of a flood if they are not promptly and thoroughly cleaned and dried.[113,114] For example, pediatric asthma symptoms spiked among victims of Hurricane Katrina (USA, 2005) both during the event—when 24% of evacuated children ran out of asthma medication or were concerned that they might run out—and 3 months afterwards—when 3% of children reported new asthma diagnoses and 40% of children self-reported that their asthma had worsened since the storm.[115]

T.2.d.iii Air Quality

Both outdoor and indoor air pollution can stunt lung growth in children and damage lung airways and alveoli, resulting in COPD. It can also trigger the onset or exacerbation of chronic respiratory diseases like asthma and COPD by triggering inflammation, restricted lung airways, and the production of excess mucus. It is also a major risk factor for lung cancer.[116] The most significant causes of outdoor air pollution are TRAP, point-source air pollution (such as pollution generated at industrial sites), and wildfires. Indoor air pollution is caused by recirculating pollutants that enter from the outdoors, chemicals off-gassed by building materials and furniture, and pollutants caused by poor maintenance, such as mold and mildew. More information is available in the air quality section of this toolbox. An increase of 10 µg/m³ in annual exposure to NO_2—a major traffic-related air pollutant—has been associated with a 2.4% increase in respiratory mortality worldwide; and, a similar increase in $PM_{2.5}$ has been associated with a 5% increase in respiratory mortality.[35] In Europe, it has been estimated that exposure to traffic-related particulate matter reduces life expectancy by 8.6 months.[117] And a global study estimated that exposure to traffic-related NO_2 resulted in four million new cases of pediatric asthma each year, accounting for 13% of new pediatric cases globally. The same study estimated 690 new cases each year in Lima, Peru; 650 new cases in Shanghai, China; and, 580 new cases in Bogota, Colombia; demonstrating the global reach of air pollution's health effects.[118]

T.2.e How Does the Built Environment Increase the Risk of Respiratory Disease?

The built environment can increase the risk of respiratory disease both directly and indirectly. Car-centric community planning can lead to increased exposure to traffic-related particulate air pollution, O_3, and allergy-triggering plants. Carbon dioxide emitted from tailpipes has been shown to increase the quantity of pollen produced by plants like ragweed. Neighborhoods downwind from industrial installations can also be exposed to harmful airborne toxins, which can cause or exacerbate a variety of health conditions including COPD, asthma, and lung cancer.

Inside the building, many finishing materials (e.g., paint, adhesives, sealants, composite wood, legacy materials containing asbestos) are manufactured using toxic chemicals that are emitted into the air over time. Indoor air can also be compromised if smoking is allowed inside or near entrances, if polluted outdoor air is introduced to the building, or if naturally occurring radon is allowed to accumulate inside the building rather than being vented to the outdoors.

When buildings fail to protect their occupants from climatic events (like extreme heat) or their effects (like power outages), they can increase the risk of injury and death among occupants with existing respiratory complaints.

T.2.f How Can Design Help?

Design solutions that promote respiratory health can be categorized into strategies that reduce or eliminate contaminants at their source and strategies that reduce occupant exposure. Community planning and zoning requirements that result in reduced car travel, lower emissions from industrial installations, and lower concentrations of allergenic pollen can benefit respiratory health at the community and regional scales. Master planners, landscape designers, and mechanical engineers can work together to locate on-site emission sources like delivery bays, carpool lines, and ambulance idling areas away from building openings and air supply vents. And the property can be protected (at least partially) from off-site emissions by constructing vegetative and structural barriers to emission sources like busy roads and industrial plants.

Inside the building, following green and healthy building protocols for ventilation, high-efficiency filtration, low-emitting building materials, integrated pest control, green cleaning, and building maintenance can dramatically reduce occupant exposure to respiratory irritants and infectious pathogens like SARS-CoV-2 or the influenza virus.

Finally, designs that enable ongoing operation of building utilities during power disruptions and after extreme weather events are particularly protective for occupants with chronic respiratory conditions.

T.2.g Who Is Most Vulnerable?

Vulnerability to respiratory disease may be associated with a person's physiology (e.g., developing organs for children; the ageing process for the elderly), pre-existing health conditions (e.g., chronic disease, mental health concerns, immunocompromised status), behavioral choices (e.g., smoking tobacco), socioeconomic determinants of health (e.g., marginalized communities, poverty, living in primitive housing), or a combination of factors.

T.2.g.i Children and the Elderly

Children and the elderly are particularly vulnerable to respiratory infections for both physiological and socioeconomic reasons. Children are vulnerable to long-term damage, because their respiratory system is still developing. They also have a 50% higher exposure rate, because they have a higher lung surface area per pound of body weight than adults.[119] They tend to spend more time outdoors and perform more rigorous activities on average than adults, which can increase their exposure to outdoor air pollution.[119] Exposure to tobacco smoke, indoor or outdoor air pollution, recurrent respiratory infections, and contracting a chronic disease like asthma can stunt lung growth, reducing lifelong lung function and accelerating lung deterioration later in life.[120,121] Children experiencing asthma and recurrent lower respiratory tract infections are also at a higher risk of developing COPD as adults.[92] This phenomenon is of particular concern, because acute lower respiratory infections account for almost half of pediatric doctor visits each year globally.[84] One study in the US found that 11% of asthmatic children in the study were diagnosed with COPD by age 26, far earlier than the typical diagnosis age of ≥40 years.[120] Health effects have even been found through exposure in the womb. For example, if pregnant people smoke tobacco or are exposed to poor outdoor air quality, their children are more likely to develop respiratory and cardiovascular diseases later in life.[121] Low birth weight is also a risk factor for developing asthma and COPD.[121]

Children in low- and middle-income countries are at particularly high risk of serious health consequences from respiratory diseases. For example, close to three-quarters of deaths among young children from the most common cause of acute respiratory infection in children (respiratory syncytial virus) occur in low- and middle-income countries.[122] Phase Three of the global childhood asthma study ISAAC found that children in North America had the highest rate of lifetime asthma (17.3%) compared with many low- and middle-income regions: for example, 10.8% in Africa, 7.4% in Eastern Mediterranean, and 5.6% in the Indian subcontinent. However, the percentage of new onset asthma cases with severe symptoms was higher in low- and middle-income regions (28.5% in Africa, 28.8% in Eastern Mediterranean, and 24.5% in the Indian subcontinent) compared with North America (19.5%).[123] Children in low- and middle-income countries are also more sensitive to poor air quality than children living in countries with a higher level of economic development.[92] Low-income women and children bear the highest health burden associated with exposure to poor indoor air quality caused by solid fuel combustion for cooking and heating.[124]

Similar to children, the elderly face both physiological and social risks associated with respiratory disease. On a physiological level, lung function in healthy adults generally plateaus around age 26 and begins to decline around age 50.[121] Most cases of COPD are diagnosed after age 40, which is when symptoms begin for many patients.[90] The chest wall becomes more rigid and less elastic through the aging process. The diaphragm and other respiratory muscles begin to lose strength. Lung airways become constricted.[125,126] And the lungs become more vulnerable to inflammation.[127] As a result, it becomes more difficult to clear fluids from the lungs—putting the elderly at higher risk of acute lower respiratory infections than younger adults.[128] They are also more likely to suffer from a depressed immune system and complications from other chronic diseases, which can exacerbate symptoms and reduce the effectiveness of medical treatment.[126,128] The elderly may also become socially isolated, which can lead to malnutrition (a risk factor for infectious disease) and delays in treatment.[92,128] Globally, over 90% of deaths from influenza each year occur among older age groups.[84] The elderly are also overly represented in the group of people who die from pneumonia each year.[94] For example, a major international study estimated that 6.8 million episodes of pneumonia among patients aged 65 years or older resulted in hospital stays in 2015, 1.1 million (13%) of whom died in hospital.[129] The average death rate from COVID-19 was 630 times higher for individuals 85 years and older compared with those 18–29 years of age in 2020.[77] The elderly are also more likely to be underdiagnosed and undertreated for acute asthma than younger adults.[125,126] A study in Brazil found that older adults who were diagnosed with asthma when they were children (12 years or younger) were more likely to be sensitive to environmental asthma triggers like dust mites than patients with later asthma onset (72% of patients diagnosed ≤12 years versus 38% of patients diagnosed ≥55 years).[130] Furthermore, a large-scale study in the US found that adults 55 years and older were more likely than younger adults to suffer from co-morbidities (particularly hypertension, diabetes, fluid and electrolyte disorders, and congestive heart failure), be hospitalized for acute asthma attacks, have longer hospital stays, receive higher hospital bills, and experience near-fatal asthma-related events. They were also five times more likely to die from the asthma event that resulted in their hospitalization.[131]

T.2.g.ii Chronic Disease and Pre-existing Mental Health Conditions

Chronic diseases increase the risk of respiratory disease, in part, because they complicate the effects of any illness. For example, individuals with poorly controlled diabetes are more susceptible to contracting active TB,[92] and chronic conditions like obesity and diabetes have been found to exacerbate the severity of respiratory diseases like asthma and pneumonia.[92] Because influenza affects many systems in the body, it is particularly dangerous for people with pre-existing chronic disease.[96] A study of elderly patients in the UK found that preexisting COPD quadrupled the risk of a patient with respiratory infection being admitted to hospital during winter months, while the presence of other chronic diseases (i.e., asthma, heart disease, diabetes, or cancer) tripled the risk. Patients with both COPD and another chronic condition were over six times more likely to be admitted to hospital with a respiratory infection than patients who were otherwise healthy.[132] Regarding mental health conditions, depression is common among patients diagnosed with COPD, possibly in part because inflammation plays a role in both diseases. For example, a study in Poland found a more than 20% increase in concentration of a protein associated with inflammation (IL-6) among patients diagnosed with COPD, depression, or both diseases compared with healthy adults.[133]

T.2.g.iii Immunocompromised Patients

Immunocompromised individuals are at higher risk of respiratory infections, because their bodies' defenses are weakened.[92] For example, pneumonia often occurs in people who are already suffering from a viral respiratory infection (such as influenza), are over age 65, or are recovering from surgery.[93] A more rare cause of pneumonia, from fungi, is often associated with people with compromised immune systems such as people with HIV/AIDS.[93] HIV also increases the risk of contracting pneumonia from *Streptococcus pneumoniae* by 20 times.[92] Globally, 8.6% of new cases and 17% of deaths from TB in 2018 affected people who had also been diagnosed with HIV.[82]

T.2.g.iv Smoking

Smoking is a common risk factor for all respiratory diseases.[90,91,94–98] Tobacco smoke destroys lung tissue, leading to emphysema. It also irritates lung airways, causing them to swell and produce excess mucus, which triggers chronic bronchitis.[92] Exposure to tobacco smoke can accelerate the decline in lung function among asthmatics.[92] It is responsible for more than 80% of lung cancer cases[98] and over one-fifth of all cancer deaths.[41] Up to three-quarters of patients with COPD are current or previous smokers.[90] And smoking can harm future generations. A grandmother who smokes increases the risk of asthma in both her own children and the children of her daughters, even if the daughters do not smoke.[134,135] Maternal and paternal smoking have both been associated with children developing COPD later in life.[121] The WHO estimates that over 7 million people die each year from smoking, 80% of whom live in low- and middle-income countries. An additional 1.2 million non-smokers die each year from exposure to secondhand smoke.[136] The all-cause death rate is three times higher among smokers than non-smokers, and their life expectancy is 10 years shorter.[137] However, a study in Japan estimated that exposure to secondhand tobacco smoke increased non-smokers' risk of lung cancer by 28%.[138]

T.2.g.v Minorities and Indigenous Communities

Disparities in exposure and access to medical care among minorities and Indigenous communities often place them at higher risk of respiratory disease and death than the majority population. In the US, African Americans have the highest rate of both diagnosis and death from tobacco-related cancers: 205.2 cases and 116.5 deaths per 100,000 from 2009–2013, compared with 193 cases and 99.7 deaths per 100,000 among Whites.[139] They are three times more likely than non-Hispanic Whites to have undiagnosed COPD.[140] And they are less likely than Whites to take protective measures such as receiving the flu vaccine each year.[141] African American children are more likely than White children to be hospitalized for respiratory infections—possibly because they are less likely to receive primary care services outside the hospital setting.[142] Indigenous populations in some parts of the world may be at higher risk of negative outcomes from respiratory disease due to a combination of socioeconomic, physiological, and cultural characteristics. For example, Indigenous populations in the remote areas of the Northern Territory in Australia have a higher prevalence of chronic respiratory disease and tuberculosis as well as lower lung cancer survival rates compared with the majority White population. Some population groups have also been found to be particularly sensitive to lung cancer. For example, Australian Indigenous populations are also more likely to contract an aggressive strain of lung cancer.[143] And people of Asian descent are more likely to contract lung cancer, even if they are non-smokers.[92]

T.2.g.vi Families Living in Poverty

People living in poverty are at higher risk of many respiratory diseases for environmental, socioeconomic, and behavioral reasons. They are more likely to be employed in occupations that expose them to airborne toxins. They are more likely to live in neighborhoods with high levels of air pollution. And they are more likely to be exposed to indoor air pollution in the home, particularly if they use solid fuels for cooking and heating. Tobacco use places a financial strain on low-income families by diverting income away from basic needs, such as rent and food.[136] People with lower socioeconomic status are also more likely to smoke tobacco (a risk factor for respiratory disease) and less likely to receive primary medical care (a protective behavior).[144] In the US, tobacco-related cancer and death rates increase as educational attainment and annual income decrease.[139] Chronic respiratory disease can also accelerate the cycle of poverty through direct medical costs and indirect costs such as lost productivity and school absenteeism.[145] For example, in the US, COPD was estimated to cost $32.1 billion in medical costs and $3.9 billion in absenteeism in 2010 alone.[145] Similarly, in the European Union, COPD was estimated to cost €23.7 billion in direct medical costs and €25.1 billion in lost productivity in 2011.[146] Meanwhile, asthma is estimated to cost $81 billion in lost productivity[147] and more than 10 million lost days of school each year in the US.[147] Finally, severe malnutrition in low- and middle-income countries has been associated with a fourfold increase in the risk of deaths among children under five years of age from acute lower respiratory infections.[148]

T.2.g.vii Primitive Housing

Roughly half of all households in the world and 90% of rural homes—representing 2.8 billion people, particularly in rural areas and in low- and middle-income countries—rely on fuels for heating and cooking that allow smoke to be present in living areas.[149] The health effects of exposure to indoor combustion products include heightened risk of COPD and lung cancer among adults, and pneumonia and asthma in children.[124] In 2012, the WHO estimated that 4.3 million people died prematurely as a result of exposure to solid fuels in the home.[149]

T.3 Toolbox—Community Health Conditions: Obesity, Diabetes, and Hypertension

T.3.a Introduction

While obesity, diabetes, and hypertension (i.e., high blood pressure) are three distinct conditions, they often appear together.[150] For example, over 40% of patients diagnosed with diabetes in the US are also obese.[151] And the risk of developing type 2 diabetes increases roughly 20% for every incremental increase in body mass index (BMI).[152] Obesity at the waistline has been associated with both type 2 diabetes and hypertension.[150] All three conditions are often associated with high-income countries because the Western diet and sedentary lifestyle are both contributing risk factors. However, the percentage of people reporting a sedentary lifestyle, high BMI, and/or high glucose levels (a sign of diabetes) have also risen in low- and middle-income countries where social and economic development have increased.[41]

The prevalence of obesity, diabetes, and hypertension is rising worldwide. The percentage of adults who are obese increased globally from 9% in 1980 to 12% in 2015. It doubled in 73 countries—particularly low- and middle-income countries in west Africa and southeast Asia.[153] Populations in the US followed a similar trend, albeit at a higher prevalence rate. The percentage of obese adults in the US almost doubled from 15% in 1976–1980[154] to 29% in 2015.[155]

The rate of diabetes prevalence increased almost 45% worldwide from 4,137.3 cases per 100,000 population in 1990 to 5,991 cases per 100,000 in 2013, surpassing ischemic heart disease (1,518.7 cases per 100,000 population), malaria (4,702.6 per 100,000 in 2013), and COPD (4,903.8 cases per 100,000 in 2013).[13] Low- and middle-income countries are experiencing the majority of rapid growth in diabetes prevalence, while growth has slowed or leveled off in high-income countries.[41] For example, roughly 650

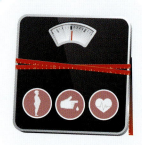

02 HOW DOES IT AFFECT THE BUILT ENVIRONMENT?

FOOD DESERTS
Neighborhoods without access to fresh, healthy food put residents at higher risk of obesity, diabetes, & hypertension.

SPRAWL, SINGLE USE DISTRICTS
This kind of environment increases traffic-related air pollution & reduces opportunities for physical activity.

UNSAFE BIKE/PED ENVIRONMENT
This kind of environment increases risk of obesity, diabetes, & hypertension by reducing opportunities for physical activity.

ON-SITE GROCERY/ FOOD PRODUCTION
Increases food security & access to fresh, healthy options.

COMPACT, MULTI-USE DEVELOPMENT NEAR TRANSIT & BIKE/PED INFRASTRUCTURE
Increases opportunities for physical activity.

NATIVE VEGETATION
Increases access to physical activity. Reduces urban heat island.

FILTRATION
Filters out pollutants from both outdoor & indoor sources.

LOW EMITTING MATERIALS
Reduces the concentration of pollutants generated indoors.

04 WHO IS MOST VULNERABLE…

CHILDREN
At higher risk for developmental & behavioral reasons.

ELDERLY
Body is less resilient & many elderly also have underlying health conditions.

SMOKING
Increases plaque build up & thickens the blood.

WESTERN LIFESTYLE
Can increase inflammation & lead to unhealthy behavior.

MENTAL HEALTH
Can increase inflammation & lead to unhealthy behavior.

POVERTY
Increased risk of stress & reduced access to healthy food, opportunities for physical activity, medical care.

Toolbox Infographic T.3. Linkages among Obesity, Diabetes, and Hypertension; the Built Environment Determinants of Health; Protective Design and Operations Strategies; the Groups Who Are at Highest Risk; and Related Negative Health Outcomes

01
OBESITY, DIABETES, HYPERTENSION

- Major risk factors for disability & premature death.
- Often develop in parallel, because they are all associated with the Western diet & sedentary lifestyle.

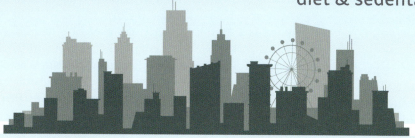

AIR POLLUTION
Exposure to air pollution can increase accumulation/transition of adipose tissue (obesity), increase insulin resistance (diabetes), & exacerbate inflammation (obesity, hypertension).

URBAN HEAT ISLAND
More sensitive to heat exposure & at greater risk of overheating.

LACK OF RESILIENCE
Disruption to medical services & increased stress during disasters increases risk of death (diabetes, hypertension.)

03
HOW CAN DESIGN HELP?

WELL-MAINTAINED BUILDINGS
Reduces the risk of mold & other allergens; ensures filtration & emergency systems are working.

COOLING CENTER
Protects under-air conditioned residents.

ISLANDABLE SITES & MICROGRIDS
Design on-site energy, water, & food production to allow occupants to shelter in place when utilities are disrupted.

MINORITIES
Increased risk of stress & reduced access to healthy food, opportunities for physical activity, medical care.

DISABILITY & DEATH

HEART DISEASE

RENAL DISEASE

MENTAL HEALTH

... TO THE HEALTH RISKS? 05

Note: Many of the design and operations strategies in the infographic bring co-benefits to other topics in this toolbox as well. See figure T.4 for a crosswalk of all of the environmental health co-benefits.

new cases of diabetes per 100,000 are diagnosed each year in the US. While this increases the total number of people living with diabetes each year, the rate of new cases has leveled off after falling from its height of 850 per 100,000 in 2007–2010.[156]

Finally, it is estimated that prevalence of hypertension among adults increased from 594 million in 1975 to 1.13 billion in 2015—two-thirds of whom live in low- and middle-income countries. Africa has the highest prevalence at 27% of adults. This is a major public health concern, because many people are unaware they suffer from hypertension until it causes a catastrophic health condition. According to the WHO, fewer than 20% of people suffering from hypertension have it under control.[157]

Both individually and as a cluster, these conditions are a major cause of disability and death worldwide. Individually, they represented three of the top five risk factors for disability in 2015.[41] And from 1990–2013, diabetes alone increased from the tenth to the seventh leading cause of years living in disability.[13]

Deaths from obesity, diabetes, and hypertension are on the rise. In 2015, 4.0 million deaths globally were attributed to high BMI, more than two-thirds of whom died from cardiovascular disease.[153] From 2005–2015, the percentage of global deaths from diabetes caused by high BMI increased 36% from 408,000 (12.3%) to 555,000 (14.0%).[41] And in 2016, almost 1.6 million people died of diabetes and roughly 900,000 died of hypertension worldwide, a significant increase from 944,000 and 619,000, respectively, in 2000.[158] While the Africa region experienced the highest number of deaths (1.6 million in 2016 and 944,000 in 2000), Southeast Asia and the eastern Mediterranean regions, both of whose death rates doubled during that period, experienced the fastest rate of increase.[158]

Finally, obesity, diabetes, and hypertension are also risk factors for cardiovascular disease.[22,159] A population scale study in the US found that controlling their diabetes could reduce the risk of cardiovascular mortality by 1.7% among men and 4.1% among women. Controlling hypertension could reduce cardiovascular mortality by 3.8% among men and 7.3% among women.[54] Furthermore, mortality risk increases substantially when a patient suffers from all three conditions.[150] A large-scale study in the US found that adults who were free from obesity, diabetes, and hypertension at 45 years of age lived 3, 6, and 10 (men) to 13 (women) years longer than their peers exhibiting 1, 2, or 3 of those risk factors, respectively.[160]

T.3.b What Are Obesity, Diabetes, and Hypertension?

T.3.b.i Obesity

Obesity refers to the accumulation of excessive body fat (also called adipose tissue), which can contribute to adverse health effects, including diabetes and hypertension.[161] The most common way to measure obesity, the body mass index (BMI), is calculated as the ratio of weight over height squared (kg/m^2). Normal weight is defined as a BMI of 18.5–24.9. Overweight is defined as a BMI of 25.0–29.9. And obesity is defined as a BMI of 30 or above.[161] The accumulation of adipose tissue is associated with higher levels of free fatty acids circulating in blood vessels, which can contribute to insulin resistance and, eventually, type 2 diabetes.[161] While lifestyle modifications (discussed more fully below) are the primary form of treatment for obesity, medications that reduce food cravings, and in severe cases, bariatric surgery to the digestive system may be recommended to make weight loss easier.[162] One large-scale study in Utah, USA, found that seven years after bariatric surgery, all-cause mortality among patients decreased by 40% compared to a control group, mortality from coronary artery disease decreased by 56%, mortality from diabetes decreased by 92%, and cancer-related mortality decreased by 60%.[163]

T.3.b.ii Diabetes

Diabetes is an umbrella term for diseases associated with difficulty regulating blood sugar (i.e., glucose) levels. Type 1 diabetes is primarily an inherited condition in which the body's pancreas does not produce a hormone (insulin) that is needed to break down sugar, so that it can be delivered to cells and converted to energy. Type 2 diabetes is a chronic disease in which the body stops using insulin efficiently and/or stops producing enough insulin to break down sugar and deliver it to cells. This section of the book focuses on type 2 diabetes, because the built environment can be designed to reduce the two primary modifiable risk factors associated with developing that form of the disease: obesity and physical inactivity.[49] Diabetes is diagnosed when glucose levels meet or exceed one of the following thresholds: 6.5% according to the A1C test, 126 mg/dL according to the fasting plasma glucose test, or 200 mg/dL according to the oral glucose tolerance test or the random plasma glucose test.[49]

T.3.b.iii Hypertension

Hypertension, also called high blood pressure, is a condition where blood flowing through the circulatory system places too much pressure on the walls of the body's blood vessels, which can harden the arteries and reduce the flow of blood and oxygen to the heart. It is diagnosed when blood pressure readings show ≥140 mmHg / ≥90 mmHg on two consecutive days. Obesity and diabetes are both risk factors for developing hypertension.[157]

Preventive and first-line treatment measures typically focus on the two modifiable risk factors that are common to all three conditions: increasing physical activity and improving the patient's diet.[150] For example, a population-scale study in suburban Beijing, China, found that adults who were physically active were 33% less likely to be overweight or obese, 13% less likely to have diabetes, and 8% less likely to have hypertension. And adults who ate a vegetarian diet were 21% less likely to be overweight or obese, 32% less likely to have diabetes, and 19% less likely to have hypertension.[164]

T.3.c What Are the Symptoms of Obesity, Diabetes, and Hypertension?

T.3.c.i Obesity

As total body tissue increases, the cardiovascular system must work harder to supply blood efficiently to all parts of the body, which can damage both the heart (leading to cardiovascular disease) and blood vessels (leading to hypertension).[161] The increased body mass in obese individuals can also create physical obstructions that make it more difficult to sleep, to breathe, to prevent acid reflux, and for major organ systems such as the kidneys to function properly. Adipose tissue can excrete substances that interfere with the normal functioning of the liver and the reproductive system. Finally, these excretions can establish a positive feedback loop with some types of cancer.[161]

T.3.c.ii Diabetes

The direct symptoms of type 2 diabetes include increased thirst and urination, increased hunger, fatigue, blurred vision, numbness or tingling in the feet or hands, sores that do not heal, and unexplained weight loss. The long-term health effects of elevated blood sugar levels can include damage to the cardiovascular system, nervous system, kidneys, gums and teeth, eyes, and feet.[49]

T.3.c.iii Hypertension

Many people suffering from hypertension have no symptoms until they experience a health crisis associated with the disease. Early symptoms include morning headaches, nosebleeds, irregular heart rhythms, changes to vision, and buzzing in the ears. More severe symptoms include fatigue, nausea, vomiting, confusion, anxiety, chest pain,

and muscle tremors.[157] Uncontrolled hypertension can cause severe damage to the cardiovascular system, leading to heart attack, heart failure, or stroke. It can also damage the renal system, leading to kidney failure.[157]

Table T.4 summarizes common symptoms associated with all three conditions: obesity, diabetes, and hypertension.

T.3.d Relationship with Climate Change

Individuals diagnosed with obesity, diabetes, and/or hypertension are more vulnerable to negative health outcomes after exposure to extreme heat events, poor air quality, floods, and severe storms.

TABLE T.4.

Symptoms of Obesity, Diabetes, and Hypertension

Health Condition	Symptoms
Obesity	• Damage to blood vessels • Damage to heart • Damage to kidneys • Damage to liver • Damage to reproductive system • Increased risk of cancer • Physical obstructions
Diabetes	• Damage to blood vessels • Damage to eyes, blurred vision • Damage to feet • Damage to gums and teeth • Damage to heart • Damage to kidneys • Damage to nervous system • Fatigue • Increased hunger, thirst, and urination • Numbness/tingling in hands and feet • Sores that do not heal • Unexplained weight loss
Hypertension	• Buzzing in the ears • Confusion, anxiety • Damage to eyes, blurred vision • Damage to heart • Damage to blood vessels • Damage to kidneys • Fatigue • Headaches • Irregular heart rhythms, chest pain • Muscle tremors • Nausea, vomiting • Nosebleeds

T.3.d.i Heat

Obese individuals are more sensitive than the general population to negative health outcomes after exposure to high temperatures.[165(p34)] Obesity is also a risk factor for other chronic conditions, such as cardiovascular disease and diabetes, that can be exacerbated by warm temperatures.[25(p46)] Diabetes, for example, reduces the body's ability to dissipate heat through dilating blood vessels in the skin and sweating. As a result, the body's core temperature may increase to unsafe levels, triggering a heat-related illness.[166] For example, a population-scale study in California, USA, from 1999–2009 found that hospital admissions for diabetes increased 6% when temperatures increased 10°F above average.[167] Another population-based study—in Brisbane, Australia—found that, from 2005–2013, hospital admissions for diabetes increased 6% and post-discharge deaths increased 68% during extreme heat events.[168] Finally, patients with hypertension are also at greater risk of overheating during heat waves; similar to diabetes, the damage to blood vessels that leads to hypertension can restrict blood flow to the skin, thereby slowing the body's efforts to lower its core temperature.[169]

T.3.d.ii Air Quality

A growing body of evidence has found that TRAP is associated with prevalence, exacerbation, and death rates from obesity and type 2 diabetes, in part, because it can influence the accumulation and transition of adipose tissue (leading to obesity) and increase insulin resistance—a risk factor for diabetes.[116] Populations in Europe and North America experience an 8%–10% increased risk of type 2 diabetes for every 10-μg/m³ increase in exposure to $PM_{2.5}$ or NO_2.[170] A large-scale study in Denmark found that adults living in the top quartile of exposure to NO_2 were more than twice as likely to die from diabetes than people living in the lowest quartile of exposure.[171] And, a study in Los Angeles, California, USA, found a 13.6% annual increase in BMI among children aged 5–11 years who lived within the top tenth percentile of TRAP exposure in comparison with children in the bottom tenth percentile.[172] Air pollution can also trigger or exacerbate inflammation, a risk factor for oxidative stress and hypertension.[116] A study of overweight and obese Latino children in Los Angeles, California, USA, found a correlation between higher exposure to $PM_{2.5}$ or NO_2 and two major contributing factors to the development of type 2 diabetes: insulin sensitivity and b-cell function.[173]

T.3.d.iii Flooding and Storms

Disruptions in medical care coupled with increased stress and anxiety during and after major storm events can exacerbate the symptoms of diabetes and hypertension and increase the risk of mortality.[29] For example, following Hurricane Katrina (2005), health and social service providers in Alabama and Mississippi, USA, found that patients with diabetes and hypertension struggled to keep their diseases under control in the absence of medications and appropriate nutritional options at shelters.[109] The health risks associated with major storms can continue on for months after the event. The risk of mortality from diabetes in Kauai, Hawaii, USA, was found to be 2.6 times higher than average during the 12 months following Hurricane Iniki (1992).[174]

T.3.e How Does the Built Environment Increase the Risk of Obesity, Diabetes, and Hypertension?

Car-centric community planning can increase the risk of obesity, diabetes, and hypertension by erecting barriers to active living and healthy eating. In particular, urban sprawl makes it difficult for people to safely walk, ride a bike, or use public transit to perform their daily activities. Land use patterns like sprawl also increase exposure to TRAP, which is a direct risk factor for all three conditions. The focus on expanding roadways to facilitate traffic flow can exacerbate the urban heat island effect by increasing the percentage of impervious surface. Sprawl is often characterized by single-use districts, which cluster household necessities like grocery stores in a handful of shopping centers, rather than distributing them throughout the community. That configuration can make it more difficult for low-income families to purchase fresh and healthy food, thereby increasing their risk of developing or experiencing triggering events for all three diseases.

Like other chronic diseases, people suffering from obesity, diabetes, and hypertension are at higher risk of negative health outcomes when they are exposed to extreme weather. So flood-prone infrastructure, fragile electricity grids, and other aspects of the built environment that could disrupt protective adaptations like air conditioning and electric-powered medical devices can lead to increased hospital admissions and death rates after exposure to heat events, floods, storms, and other disasters. Finally, the increase in mental stress associated with exposure to extreme weather—particularly if it leads to population displacement—is a risk factor for people diagnosed with diabetes or hypertension.

T.3.f How Can Design Help?

At the community design and master planning scale, land use zoning and transportation planning can reduce the risk of obesity, diabetes, and hypertension by enabling active modes of transportation and by promoting a variety of retail and commercial uses distributed throughout the community. The easier it is to access public transit, walking, and cycling routes, the more community members will use them. Similarly, if fresh and healthy food is available throughout the community at reasonable prices, community members are more likely to purchase them instead of processed foods with high fat, salt, and sugar content.

Building owners can promote a community's approach by filling in gaps in their neighborhood—for example, maximizing use of vegetation on the site level as well as the roof; providing bike racks and pedestrian amenities; and hosting a grocery store, community garden, or farmer's market on site. Buildings that include features such as indoor streets and monumental stairs, furniture encouraging movement (such as standing desks), and publicly available outdoor circulation routes can encourage physical activity for both building occupants and the surrounding community. Similarly, building design can support neighborhood and community efforts promoting resilience by hosting a cooling center and installing a microgrid or solar installation that can be islandable in the event of a power disruption. Finally, indoor air treatments like filtration and low emitting materials can protect occupants suffering from obesity, diabetes, or hypertension from exposure to indoor or outdoor air pollution.

T.3.g Who Is Most Vulnerable?

The risk factors for developing obesity, diabetes, and hypertension are complex and interrelated. Children and the elderly are vulnerable due to a combination of physiological and socioeconomic factors. The absence of physical exercise, a poor diet, and smoking are the three primary lifestyle factors contributing to the development of all three conditions. Pre-existing mental health conditions can create a positive feedback loop, particularly with obesity in children. Finally, societal disparities among minorities, Indigenous populations, and families living in poverty have also been found to contribute to an increased risk of developing these chronic diseases.

T.3.g.i Children

Childhood obesity is a growing trend worldwide, more than doubling from 2% in 1980 to 5% in 2015. And while prevalence rates in low- and low- to middle-income countries continue to hover around 2%, the trend lines in middle-, high- to middle-, and high-income countries show similarly marked increases over that period of time, with the highest prevalence of obesity in the highest income countries (~8% in 2015) and stepping down in concert with lower income brackets (~6.2% in high- to middle income countries; ~4.5% in middle income countries).[153]

A number of genetic, prenatal, and birth factors can increase the risk of an individual developing obesity during childhood, including parents with a high BMI, racial/ethnic heritage, maternal weight gain and/or diabetes while pregnant, smoking while pregnant, birth weight, formula feeding rather than breastfeeding, and Caesarian section delivery. Socioeconomic factors, such as parental education and income level, have also been found to be negative predictors of childhood obesity—obesity rates falling in families with higher educational attainment and/or higher income levels.[175]

Childhood obesity is influenced by the same two primary lifestyle factors as adults: poor diet and insufficient exercise. Children's diet is largely determined by adults—family caregivers in the home and school cafeteria options at school. If children live in a family or community that is food insecure, they may be more likely to be offered calorie-dense foods with little nutritional benefit rather than fresh, healthy options. Worldwide, children's increasingly sedentary lifestyle has been attributed to a combination of technology (i.e., television, computer games, smart phones, etc.), inadequate investment in physical education and sports programs at school, and reduced opportunities for active play at home—whether due to lack of access to outdoor space or a concern among caregivers regarding safety.[176]

While type 2 diabetes and hypertension are rare among children, obesity during childhood is a risk factor for developing both of these diseases as an adult.[176] For example, a study in the UK found that childhood obesity doubled the risk of cardiovascular death for participants later in life.[177] And, the rapidly increasing prevalence of childhood obesity has been associated with an increase in diagnosis of type 2 diabetes among adolescents.[176] For example, the proportion of diabetic children aged 0 to 19 years diagnosed with type 2 diabetes jumped from less than 5% in the 1980s to 30%–50% in some areas by the late 1990s.[178]

T.3.g.ii Elderly

As the body ages, it becomes both weaker and more brittle. When combined with chronic conditions, these changes can lead to or precipitate injury, disease, or death. The complex interactions among obesity, diabetes, and hypertension are exacerbated among the elderly, often affecting cardiovascular and kidney health in addition to the direct effects of these three chronic conditions.[179] In the case of hypertension, arteries and blood vessels become less flexible with age, which may reduce blood flow and increase blood pressure.[179] Roughly half of the increase in disability-adjusted life years caused by high blood pressure from 1990–2015, one-third of the increase in high fasting plasma glucose, and one-quarter of the increase in high BMI worldwide has been attributed to the global trend of an ageing population.[41] A study in India found that the prevalence of pre-hypertension and hypertension cases increased markedly with age, starting at around 20% among adults aged 25–34 and increasing to close to 100% diagnoses of either pre-hypertension or hypertension among adults aged 65 years or older. However, only one-third of all subjects in the study had their blood pressure under control.[180] Diabetes also increases the risk of mortality among the elderly. For example, a review of studies in Japan found that the absolute risk of death from cardiovascular disease among people in their 60s, 70s, and 80s was 4.2, 4.8, and 19.4 times higher, respectively, among diabetics than among non-diabetic participants.[181]

T.3.g.iii Sedentary Lifestyle and Poor Diet

Sedentary lifestyle and poor diet are the primary modifiable risk factors for obesity, diabetes, and hypertension. Using diabetes as an example, in 2015, 15% of global deaths attributed to a sedentary lifestyle were caused by diabetes. Diabetes also factored into deaths attributed to poor diets, including 8% of deaths associated with low consumption of whole grains; 7.5% associated with low consumption of nuts; and, 18.8% associated with high consumption of processed meats.[41] On the positive side, a study in Spain found that overweight or obese patients who lost 10% or more body weight during a 16-week intensive program to improve diet and increase physical exercise also experienced almost three times the improvement in blood pressure as patients who lost 5%–9.9% of their body weight during the program.[182]

Physical activity increases the amount of energy expended by the body, thereby reducing the risk of overnutrition—the precursor to increasing body mass.[183] For example, a study of overweight and obese young adults (aged 18–30 years) in Kansas, USA, found that exercising five days a week resulted in an average 5% weight loss over 10 months without any change in diet.[184] Physical activity can help regulate blood sugar levels and counteract two major side effects of diabetes—loss of muscular strength and joint stiffness.[185] For example, a study in Canada found that physical activity and musculoskeletal fitness were associated with 22% and 61% reduced odds of developing diabetes, respectively.[186] Physical activity has also been found to improve cardiovascular health, slowing the natural increase in blood pressure caused by ageing and preventing the development of hypertension.[159] For example, a large-scale study in the US found that, among healthy young adults aged 18–30 years, the least physically fit group was twice as likely to develop hypertension 15 years later than the most physically fit group.[187] And a study in peri-urban Uganda found that people engaged in sedentary work were 2.7 times as likely to have hypertension that people whose work required physical activity.[188]

T.3.g.iv Smoking

Smoking tobacco is a risk factor for developing childhood obesity, type 2 diabetes, and hypertension. Maternal smoking during pregnancy has been found to increase the risk of childhood obesity by over 50%.[189] Smoking also increases the concentration of blood sugar and disrupts the natural process of breaking down sugar within cells to create energy.[190] According to the US Surgeon General, smoking increases the risk of developing type 2 diabetes by 30%–40%.[191] And exposure to tobacco smoke is a major risk factor for hypertension. It has been found to disrupt normal cell functioning by increasing inflammation and damaging the heart and blood vessels, which can lead to hypertension.[192] Even after exposure to tobacco smoke ceases, blood pressure may remain high if the damage it caused to the blood vessels is permanent. Chemical interactions between smoking and anti-hypertension medications can also reduce the effectiveness of blood pressure treatment.[192,193]

T.3.g.v Mental Health Conditions

Mental health conditions can trigger positive feedback loops regarding obesity, diabetes, and hypertension. For example, children with attention-deficit hyperactivity disorder (ADHD) may become obese if their condition extends to their approach to food and eating.[194] For example, a population-level study in Germany found that overweight/obese children aged 11–17 years were twice as likely to receive an ADHD diagnosis than other children. Children with ADHD were twice as likely to be overweight or obese than their non-ADHD peers.[195] Similar results have linked a high BMI with internalizing disorders (such as depression, anxiety, and social isolation) and externalizing disorders (such as aggressiveness and rule-breaking) among children. On the one hand, there is a higher prevalence of these disorders among overweight and obese youth. And on the other hand, studies have found that the mental health disorder increases the odds of a child later becoming overweight or obese. For example, a study in the US found that normal-weight children aged 8–11 years who were treated for behavior problems were five times more likely than their peers to become overweight two years after the psychological diagnosis.[196] A similar feedback loop has been found between severe mental health conditions and diabetes. For example, patients suffering from schizophrenia have an almost 90% increased risk of developing type 2 diabetes than the general population;[197] and, a large-scale study of US military service members found that a diagnosis of posttraumatic stress disorder (PTSD) doubled the risk of developing type 2 diabetes three years later.[198] Finally, patients suffering from mental stress show a higher prevalence of hypertension than the general population. Likewise, patients who already suffer from hypertension respond to stressors with a higher spike in blood pressure.[199]

T.3.g.vi Minority and Indigenous Populations

Minority and Indigenous populations have been found to have higher rates of obesity, diabetes, and/or hypertension than the majority population in many countries due to a complex interplay of social and economic conditions that place them in harm's way. For example, in 2011 in the US, African American (38%), Hispanic (31%), Native American (39%), and Native Hawaiian and Pacific Islander (34%) adults were more likely than non-Hispanic White (27%) adults to report a BMI >30.[200] These disparities are likely a result of disparities in access to primary medical care, socioeconomic and lifestyle factors, and, in some cases, genetic factors. In the US, African Americans are also more likely than Whites to have high blood pressure. A population-scale study found that 71% of African Americans aged 45 years and above had hypertension, compared with 51% of Whites.[66] The study also found that while African Americans were more likely than Whites to be aware of and treat their hypertension, they were 33% less likely to have it under control.[66] Studies in Brazil have also found a higher rate of hypertension in people of African descent than among Whites.[199] Studies in the US indicate that minorities may face more barriers to leisure physical activity than Whites—placing them at a disadvantage in terms of modifying their behavior to reduce the risk of developing these three conditions. A review of studies in the US and Canada found that the major constraints preventing non-Whites from visiting parks and recreation areas on a regular basis are cost, transportation barriers, poor health, and lack of knowledge. The major barrier for Whites, on the other hand, was finding the time to go visit the park in question.[201]

In Australia, Queensland Aboriginal and Torres Strait Islanders are 4.7 times more likely to suffer from and 11.8 times more likely to die of diabetes than the non-Indigenous population. This extreme disparity in mortality rates has been attributed to a higher prevalence of diabetes and earlier disease onset (particularly for working age adults aged 35–64 years) among the Indigenous populations compared with non-Indigenous groups. Specifically, researchers attributed 67.8% of the burden of diabetes to high body mass among Indigenous populations and 31.8% to physical inactivity. High body mass was also the single most significant risk factor for the combined burden of disease among Queensland Aboriginal and Torres Strait Islanders. These results may be partially explained by lifestyle factors and/or reduced access to primary medical care associated with living in remote areas. The same study found that the risk of diabetes and cardiovascular disease (both of which are exacerbated by high BMI and low physical activity) increased twofold and 63%, respectively, among Indigenous groups who lived in remote areas compared with their peers living in major cities. Indigenous populations living in remote areas were also at higher risk of hypertension than their peers living in cities or their surroundings.[69]

T.3.g.viii Families Living in Poverty

People living in poverty are less likely to report regular physical activity—particularly leisure activities—for a variety of reasons. In the US, only 17% of adults in the highest income bracket report participating in no leisure-time physical activity, compared with 43% of adults in the lowest income bracket.[200] Low-income communities are less likely to have ready access to public amenities for recreation—such as parks—and are less likely to use them. They are also more likely to report that crime rates (real or perceived) prevent them from spending time outside in active pursuits. A review of studies in the US and Canada found that poverty was the single most significant barrier to visiting parks, with cost and distance from parks being the most significant reasons why low-income populations stay away—followed by fear, difficulties with transportation, not having a partner to participate in the visit, and poor health.[201] Several studies have also found a link between BMI and the perceived effect of physical activity among low-income workers. For example, a study of hotel room attendants in the US found that the participants who were educated about the health benefits of the physical activity they performed in the course of their work saw a reduction in body mass, blood pressure, body fat, waist-to-hip ratio, and body mass index over a four-week period compared with a control group, in spite of the fact that their physical activity and dietary habits remained constant.[202]

Restricted access to healthy food choices due to poverty is another risk factor for obesity, diabetes, and hypertension. A large-scale study in the US found that young adults (aged 24–32) who are food insecure were 67% more likely to have diabetes, 40% more likely to have hypertension, and 30% more likely to be overweight or obese.[203] International studies have similarly found that low- and middle-income countries are more likely to report high prevalence of both obesity and undernutrition, whereas high income populations are more strongly associated with obesity alone. This is because people living in poverty in low- and middle-income countries are both exposed to the risk factors for obesity common in high income countries (e.g., sedentary lifestyle, unhealthy diet) while also experiencing food insecurity.[204]

Finally, obesity, diabetes, and hypertension can help perpetrate the cycle of poverty by placing a significant financial burden on families who are already struggling to make ends meet. Taking obesity as an example, the total average annual health care expenditure in the US for managing the negative health effects of obesity is $1,360—higher than smoking ($1,046).[205]

T.4 Toolbox—Community Health Conditions: Cancer

T.4.a Introduction

Cancer is a major cause of death, disability, and economic hardship worldwide. It is the second leading cause of death globally. The WHO estimates that 9.6 million people died of cancer in 2018, roughly 70% of whom lived in low- and middle-income countries.[83] Roughly 20% of the world population and 30% of people living in industrialized countries are diagnosed with cancer during their lifetimes.[206] Lung cancer is the clear outlier—causing 4.5% of global deaths on its own.[10]

While many factors contribute to the onset and progression of different types of cancer—including genetics and behavioral factors—the WHO estimates that 36% of lung cancer deaths and 16% of other cancer deaths can be attributed to environmental factors globally.[10] That percentage rises to 46% in low- and middle-income countries.[207] And, the US Centers for Disease Control and Prevention estimate that one-fifth of cancer deaths in the US (84,443 per year) are preventable.[22]

T.4.b What Is Cancer?

Cancer refers to abnormal cell development that grows uncontrollably until it reaches beyond the limit of its originating tissue, sometimes circulating through the body and damaging multiple organ systems.[83] Most cancers are treated with surgery (to remove the cancerous growth), radiation treatment, and/or chemotherapy. However, unless the cancer is diagnosed early, it may not be possible to completely cure a patient. In those cases, treatment may be used to prolong life rather than rid the body of all cancer cells.[83]

There are many types of cancer. The following list and table T.5 review the most common cancers that are influenced by design and construction practices.

T.4.b.i Lung Cancer

Lung cancer is an umbrella term, referring to cancers of the windpipe (e.g., trachea), airways (e.g., bronchial tubes), and/or air sacs (e.g., alveoli). Cancer develops when DNA damage or mutations cripple protective genes that are active in the respiratory system.[92] A diagnosis of lung cancer often leads to poor outcomes. On average, 7 out of 8 patients die within five years of diagnosis, in part because up to 90% of cases are diagnosed too late to cure the disease. However, a combination of surgery, chemotherapy, and/or radiation are often used to slow its progression.[98] The WHO estimates that 17% of lung cancer cases are caused by exposure to household air pollution (particularly solid fuels); 14% from exposure to outdoor (i.e., ambient) air pollution; 7% from exposure to radon in the home; 7% from occupational exposure; and, 2% from exposure to secondhand smoke.[207]

T.4.b.ii Breast Cancer

Breast cancer refers to cancers originating in the breast tissue, usually in the lining of the milk ducts or within the milk glands.[208] It is the leading cause of both new cancer diagnoses (representing 25% of all cancers)[206(p363)] and cancer-related death among women, resulting in more than 625,000 deaths in 2018 (15% of all cancer-related deaths among women).[209] Women living in the highest income countries are twice as likely to receive a diagnosis of breast cancer than women living in low income countries, because more than 60% of disease risk factors are associated with behaviors more common in high income countries—such as physical inactivity, hormone replacement therapy, and alcohol consumption.[206(p362)] However, death rates are higher in low income countries, because the disease is often diagnosed at a later stage and treatment options are often less effective than in the highest income countries.[206(p363)] For example, almost 90% of women with breast cancer in the US survive at least five years after their initial diagnosis.[210]

T.4.b.iii Colorectal Cancer

Colorectal cancer refers to cancers of the colon and rectum, which make up the majority of the large intestine.[211] It is the third most common group of cancers among men and the second most common among women, representing roughly 10% of total cancer diagnoses worldwide[206(p393)] (8.3% in the US).[210] It is responsible for an estimated 700,000 deaths each year.[212] In the US 64.4% of people diagnosed with colorectal cancers are still alive five years after their initial diagnosis.[210] Colorectal cancer is more closely associated with high income countries and countries that are transitioning to higher levels of development where high levels of meat consumption and sedentary lifestyles are more common.[206(p393)]

T.4.b.iv Blood Cancer

Blood cancer is an umbrella term for cancers that develop in blood-forming tissue, such as the bone marrow. Common blood cancers include leukemia, lymphoma, and multiple myeloma.[213] Approximately 690,000 people died globally in 2018 from cancers of the blood.[209] A number of chemicals used in the occupational setting have been found to increase the risk of these cancers, including benzene; formaldehyde; pesticides and herbicides like diazinon, glyphosate (i.e., RoundUp), and malathion; solvents such as dichloromethane and trichloroethylene; chemicals used to manufacture rubber; and chemicals used in the petroleum refining process. Exposure to ionizing radiation is another risk factor for blood cancers.[207]

T.4.b.v Mouth and Throat Cancers

Mouth and throat cancers refer to cancerous growths in the lining of the mouth and throat.[214] They caused close to 360,000 deaths globally in 2018.[209] Asia bears a particularly heavy burden of mouth, nasopharynx, and hypopharynx cancers.[209] One-quarter of new diagnoses and one-third of deaths from mouth cancers occur in India. Other countries with higher than average incidence rates include Papua New Guinea, Bangladesh, Hungary, ad Sri Lanka.[206] While alcohol and smoking tobacco are the primary risk factors for this suite of cancers, construction workers may be at higher risk than the general population, because they may be exposed to diesel exhaust, isopropanol, polycyclic aromatic hydrocarbons, and/or sulfuric acid on the job site.[206]

T.4.c What Are the Symptoms?

T.4.c.i Lung Cancer

Symptoms include cough (including coughing up blood), shortness of breath, chest and/or bone pain, weight loss, and swelling in the extremities.[98]

T.4.c.ii Colorectal Cancer

The symptoms associated with colorectal cancers are generally related to the digestive system. For example, patients may experience diarrhea, constipation, or blood in their stools. They may also experience abdominal discomfort, such as bloating, feeling full, or cramps. And they may find that their appetite changes or that they lose weight without any known cause. They may also feel extremely tired.[215]

T.4.c.iii Breast Cancer

The symptoms of breast cancer include lumps in the breast or underarm; thickening, swelling, pain, or change in shape of the breast; pain, red or flaky skin, or discharge in the nipple area; and, dimpling or irritation of the skin on the breast.[216]

T.4.c.iv Blood Cancers

Symptoms of lymphoma include swollen lymph nodes, fever, night sweats, fatigue, weight loss, and pain if a cancerous growth presses against a nerve or gets in the way of normal bodily functions—such as chewing if the patient's cheek is swollen. Symptoms of leukemia include fever, fatigue, and easy bruising and bleeding. Symptoms of multiple myeloma include bone pain and easily broken bones.[215]

T.4.c.v Mouth and Throat Cancers

Symptoms of throat (pharynx) cancers include a chronic sore throat; a lump in the throat; ear pain or ringing in the ears; pain or difficulty swallowing; a change in the patient's voice; trouble breathing, speaking, or hearing; headaches; nosebleeds; unanticipated weight loss; and coughing up blood. Symptoms of lip and mouth cancers include persistent sores, white or red patches, bleeding, pain, numbness, and lumps or thickening of the lip or in the mouth. Additional symptoms include swelling of the jaw; difficulty chewing, swallowing, or moving the tongue or jaw; and a persistent feeling of pain or that something is stuck in the throat.[215]

T.4.c.vi Mental Health Concerns

Mental health concerns are a symptom that is common to most cancer diagnoses—in particular, depression and, to a lesser extent, anxiety. See the vulnerability section below for additional details about how mental health concerns manifest before, during, and after cancer treatment.

02 HOW DOES IT AFFECT THE BUILT ENVIRONMENT?

FOOD DESERTS
Difficulty accessing fresh, healthy food increases the risk of a number of cancers, including breast & colorectal.

SPRAWL, SINGLE USE DISTRICTS WITH UNSAFE BIKE/PED ENVIRONMENT
Increases traffic-related air pollution & reduces opportunities for physical activity, both of which are cancer risk factors.

OUTDOOR AIR POLLUTION
Exposure to diesel & industrial air pollution can increase the risk of cancer.

ENVIRONMENTAL TOBACCO SMOKE
Secondhand smoke increases the risk of lung cancer.

ON-SITE GROCERY/ FOOD PRODUCTION
Increases food security & access to fresh, healthy options.

COMPACT, MULTI-USE DEVELOPMENT NEAR TRANSIT & BIKE/PED INFRASTRUCTURE
Increases opportunities for physical activity.

VEGETATIVE & STRUCTURAL BARRIERS TO EMISSION SOURCES
Reduce exposure to large & heavy air pollutants.

LOCATE ON SITE EMISSIONS (VEHICLES, SMOKING) AWAY FROM OPENINGS & AIR SUPPLY
Reduce the risk of pollutants entering the building.

04 WHO IS MOST VULNERABLE...

CHILDREN
At higher risk for developmental & behavioral reasons.

ELDERLY
Body is less resilient & many elderly also have underlying health conditions.

SMOKING
10x–30x increased risk compared with non-smokers.

WESTERN LIFESTYLE
Can increase inflammation & lead to hormonal imbalance.

MENTAL HEALTH
Can increase risk of poor treatment outcomes. Cancer patients at higher risk of poor mental health.

POVERTY
Reduced access to medical care.

MINORITIES
Reduced access to medical care.

Toolbox Infographic T.4. Linkages among Cancer, the Built Environment Determinants of Health, Protective Design and Operations Strategies, the Groups Who Are at Highest Risk, and Related Negative Health Outcomes

01
CANCER

- 1 in 5 are diagnosed with cancer during their lifetime.
- 36% of lung cancer deaths & 16% of other cancer deaths can be attributed to environmental factors.

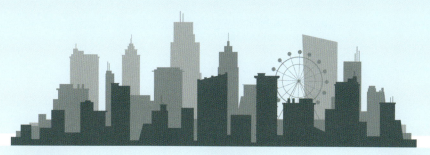

STANDING WATER - BREEDING SITES
Many cancer patients are immuno-compromised & therefore at higher risk of vector-borne disease.

INDOOR AIR QUALITY
Exposure to paint, adhesives, sealants, formaldehyde in composite wood, asbestos, and radon can increase the risk of cancer.

LACK OF RESILIENCE
Disruption to medical services & power outages during disasters increases risk of death among cancer patients.

03
HOW CAN DESIGN HELP?

INTEGRATED IAQ
Install low VOC materials, enhance ventilation & filtration to minimize indoor exposure to toxins.

WELL-MAINTAINED BUILDINGS
Reduces the risk of mold, pests, high emitting cleaning products. Ensures filtration & emergency systems are working.

ISLANDABLE SITES & MICROGRIDS
Design on-site energy, water, & food production to allow occupants to shelter in place when utilities are disrupted.

OCCUPATIONAL EXPOSURE
Risk of exposure during manufacturing, construction, demolition.

DISABILITY & DEATH

CHRONIC DISEASE

MENTAL HEALTH

... TO THE HEALTH RISKS? 05

Note: Many of the design and operations strategies in the infographic bring co-benefits to other topics in this toolbox as well. See figure T.4 for a crosswalk of all of the environmental health co-benefits.

TABLE T.5.

Symptoms of Common Cancers Associated with Environmental Determinants of Health

Cancer Type	Symptoms
Lung	• Chest, bone pain • Cough • Shortness of breath • Swelling in extremities • Weight loss
Colorectal	• Abdominal discomfort (e.g., bloating, feeling full, cramps) • Appetite loss, weight loss • Blood in stool • Constipation • Diarrhea
Breast	• Dimpling, irritation of breast skin • Lumps in breast, underarm • Pain, red or flaky skin, discharge in nipple area • Thickening, swelling, pain, change in shape of breast
Blood	• Bone pain, easily broken bones • Easy bruising, bleeding • Fatigue • Fever, night sweats • Pain around lymph nodes • Swollen lymph nodes • Weight Loss
Mouth and Throat	• Change in voice • Chronic sore throat, lump in the throat, pain or difficulty swallowing • Coughing up blood • Difficulty chewing, swallowing, or moving the tongue or jaw • Ear pain, ringing in ears • Headache • Nosebleed • Persistent sores, white or red patches, bleeding, pain, numbness, and lumps or thickening of the lip or in the mouth • Swelling of the jaw • Trouble breathing, speaking, or hearing • Weight Loss
All	• Mental health concerns (particularly depression and anxiety)

T.4.d Relationship with Climate Change

Cancer patients are particularly sensitive to the disruptions to medical care that can be caused by floods and severe storms. They are also often immunocompromised during and immediately following treatment, which can increase their vulnerability to disease when exposed to contaminated floodwaters or disease-carrying vectors. Finally, air pollution is a contributing factor to lung cancer among non-smokers, as well as a number of other less common cancers.

T.4.d.i Flooding and Storms

Patients undergoing cancer treatment are often immunocompromised. As a result, they are vulnerable to disease if they come in contact with contaminated floodwater or drinking water. Furthermore, disruptions to cancer care due to power outages, flooding inside the cancer center, or impassible roads can have dangerous consequences for patients undergoing active treatment.[104,105,115,217] For example, one-fifth of all oncology centers in Thailand (20 tertiary hospitals) were damaged after a major flood in 2011, disrupting cancer treatment for 40,000 patients.[218] A study of excess mortality during the two months following four hurricanes that hit Florida, USA, in 2004—Charley, Frances, Ivan, and Jeanne—attributed 19% of the increase to cancer-related deaths.[219]

T.4.d.ii Air Quality

Ambient air pollution is a well-established contributor to the development of lung cancer among non-smokers, as well as other chronic diseases,[220(p12)] even at concentrations lower than WHO guidelines.[221] There is also some evidence of a link between air pollution and bladder cancer, brain cancer, liver cancer, breast cancer, gastric cancer, and blood cancers.[222] According to the WHO, lung cancer accounts for 6% of global deaths caused by exposure to $PM_{2.5}$.[34] And a large-scale study in Japan found that lung cancer mortality in that country increased 24% with each 10 µg/m³ increase in ambient $PM_{2.5}$, 26% with each 10 ppb increase in sulfur dioxide, and 17% with each 10 ppb increase in NO_2 concentrations.[223]

T.4.d.iii Vector-Borne Disease

Immunocompromised cancer patients are more susceptible to developing a vector-borne disease or a secondary infection if they come in contact with a vector, because their body's defenses may not be able to effectively neutralize a pathogen once it is circulating in the body.[224] Immunocompromised patients who contract one of the four dengue serotypes are more likely to develop the more serious forms of the disease—dengue hemorrhagic fever or dengue shock syndrome—if they are re-infected with a second serotype. Cancer patients have also occasionally contracted dengue, Zika, and other vector-borne diseases through blood and organ transplants.[225]

T.4.e How Does the Built Environment Increase the Risk of Cancer?

The built environment can contribute to increased cancer risk either by increasing exposure to carcinogenic toxins or by decreasing access to behaviors that reduce the risk of developing cancer. Buildings expose their occupants to potentially harmful chemicals if they contain finish materials—such as paint and carpet—that emit volatile organic compounds (VOCs) or if smoking is allowed on the property. If the building is located downwind from a source of air pollution—such as an industrial plant or a freeway—occupants can be exposed both outside (directly) and inside the building (through outdoor air intakes). Land use decisions influence the amount of vehicular traffic (and the associated air pollution), where polluting installations are located, and whether or not building occupants will have an opportunity to engage in a physically active lifestyle with access to fresh and healthy food—two protective factors for many cancers.

Once an individual is diagnosed with cancer, his/her immune system may be compromised by the treatment regimen. Elements of the built environment that reduce its resilience to the effects of climate change can have devastating consequences if they increase cancer patient exposure to heat, flooding, or disease-carrying insects like mosquitoes. Furthermore, some cancer patients are dependent on electric medical devices, and extended power outages can increase their risk of hospital admission or death.

T.4.f How Can Design Help?

The two easiest ways for designers to reduce the risk of contributing to cancer prevalence in a community are (1) to ban smoking and vehicular idling on site, and (2) to specify building materials that do not contain or emit toxic chemicals. If a building is located in an area with poor outdoor air quality, efforts should be made to reduce pollution at the source by replacing generators and building equipment with combustion engines with electric models. Landowners can also work with the planning department to reduce traffic congestion in the neighborhood and encourage active and pollution-free modes of transportation. The project can also protect building occupants from exposure to outdoor air pollution by erecting vegetated and structural barriers between the pollution source and the building, moving outdoor air intakes away from pollution sources, installing high-efficiency filtration, and properly maintaining buildings. Sometimes the building itself can be used to separate outdoor activities from traffic-related air pollution on one side of the property. Building design can also promote behavior that reduces the risk of cancer—such as active living and healthy eating—by linking the property to larger community networks (e.g., transit lines, protected bike lanes, hike and bike trails) and by hosting a grocery store, community garden, and/or farmer's market on-site. Building projects can reduce the risk of poor outcomes among cancer patients during and after climate-related events by protecting them from power outages (by installing on-site renewable energy and water collection) and by properly maintaining the building to reduce the risk of exposure to mold, pests, and high-emitting cleaning products.

T.4.g Who Is Most Vulnerable?

Children and the elderly are vulnerable to developing cancer for physiological reasons. A number of behaviors also increase an individual's risk of developing cancer, such as smoking tobacco, as well as the two major contributors to obesity: overnutrition and a sedentary lifestyle. Mental health concerns have been found to increase the risk of developing some cancers. Poor mental health can also compromise treatment and the long-term physical health and quality of life of survivors. Finally, social and economic disparities place some groups at higher risk of cancer than the general population, including minority and Indigenous communities, poverty, and people who work in occupations that expose them to carcinogens.

T.4.g.i Children

Exposure to an environmental carcinogen during childhood can lead to a higher risk of developing cancer either during childhood or later in life, because the exposure occurs while the immune system and other organ systems are still developing.[226] Leukemia and other blood cancers are the most common childhood cancer in most parts of the world (representing 40%–60% of total cases); although children in sub-Saharan Africa are at a higher risk of developing non-Hodgkin lymphoma or Kaposi sarcoma.[206] Children living in low- and middle-income countries experience 82% of new cancer cases and 93% of cancer deaths globally. Furthermore, the mortality rate in African countries represents 60% of new cases, compared with 15% in the US—indicating an association between cancer rates and level of economic development.[206(p72)] Environmental exposures that have been associated with childhood leukemia include TRAP, pesticides, and low-frequency magnetic fields. For example, a population-based study in Denmark found that children who lived near high concentrations of traffic-related benzene pollution were 90% more likely to develop acute myeloid leukemia before age 15 than children who lived in areas exposed to lower than median levels of benzene pollution.[227] Children exposed to pesticides, insecticides, or herbicides in utero or in the home are up to two times as likely to develop leukemia as their peers.[228,229] While still inconclusive, there is mounting evidence that exposure to extremely low-frequency electromagnetic fields may double the risk of childhood leukemia for children living near high-voltage power lines.[229,230] Finally, children whose parents work with solvents or paint or smoke tobacco (before conception, mothers during pregnancy, or after birth) are at higher risk of a number of cancers, including childhood leukemia, hepatoblastoma, pancreatic cancer, and bladder cancer.[229]

T.4.g.ii Elderly

The risk of cancer increases with age, starting at 10 per 100,000 among children aged 0–14 years, rising to 150 per 100,000 among adults aged 40–44 years, and up to 500 per 100,000 by 60–64 years.[206] This increase may be partially explained by the natural ageing process. As the body ages, the rate of gene mutations that occur during the regular course of regenerating cells increases—increasing the risk of a mutation resulting in a cancerous cell. At the same time, the body's ability to repair mutated genes declines. Additionally, reduction in fertility changes the balance of hormones that are secreted, which has also been associated with an increased risk of tumor development.[231]

T.4.g.iii Obesity, Overnutrition, and Sedentary Lifestyle

Obesity, overnutrition, and sedentary lifestyle, coupled with smoking, may be the most important modifiable behaviors contributing to the development of cancer.[232] Overnutrition has been found to increase inflammation (an independent risk factor for some solid cancers[232]), suppress the immune system, increase circulating glucose and lipids (which can be used by cancer cells to speed their growth), and produce an hormonal imbalance that slows the body's natural process for destroying mutated cells.[232] Adipose tissue also produces and secretes some hormones, such as estrogen in obese postmenopausal women, which can increase the risk of developing breast cancer.[233] In addition to contributing to obesity, the Western diet (which is high in animal fat) and sedentary lifestyle have both been associated with accelerating the ageing process, an independent risk factor for cancer.[234] Taking colorectal cancer as an example, inflammatory secretions produced by fat deposits in obese individuals has been associated with increased risk of developing colon cancer.[235] The risk of developing colorectal cancer is estimated to increase 5% with every 5 kg/m^2 increase in body mass—particularly among overweight and obese individuals.[212] A large-scale study in the US found the risk of early onset colorectal cancer was almost double among women with a BMI ≥30 than among women in the normal range.[236] Furthermore, lack of physical activity—which is strongly influenced by land use design—has been estimated to contribute up to 20% of the burden of colorectal cancer worldwide.[212(p70)] And up to 30% of breast cancer cases have also been attributed to physical inactivity.[206(p367)]

T.4.g.iv Smoking

Smoking is the leading modifiable cause of lung cancer. The risk of developing lung cancer among smokers is 10–30 times the risk among never-smokers. In fact, the relationship is so strong that lung cancer rates rise and fall along similar trajectories as smoking rates—although lagging a few decades behind. While smoking has declined in high-income countries due to strong anti-smoking policies and social stigma, smoking remains strongly prevalent in many low- and middle-income countries. For example, lung cancer diagnoses and deaths have been declining in the US and the UK since the 1970s.[237] But diagnoses remain in the top 25 countries of the world at 35.1 per 100,000 in the US and 32.5 per 100,000 in the UK.[209] Worldwide, lung cancer deaths are expected to increase from 1.6 million in 2012 to 3 million in 2035, largely due to the continued popularity of smoking in low- and middle-income countries—particularly in Africa and the eastern Mediterranean region.[238]

T.4.g.v Mental Health Conditions

Mental health conditions have been found to contribute to the development of some types of cancer, the patient's prognosis, and his/her quality of life following a successful treatment. For example, a study in Australia found that patients suffering from depression, neuroses, or alcohol and drug disorders were 20% more likely to be diagnosed with cancer. Once diagnosed, men suffering from mental illness were found to have a 50% increased risk of mortality, and women experienced a 30% increased risk of mortality. These disparities may be associated with evidence that patients with mental illness receive later stage diagnoses, are less likely to receive surgery or radiotherapy, often do not receive adequate medical care upon discharge from the hospital, and may be less likely to adhere to guidance on how to continue treatment at home.[239] For example, patients suffering from depression are three times less likely to comply with their medical regimens.[240] These results are troubling, because many cancer patients develop depression while undergoing treatment. A large-scale study in Germany found that 24% of cancer patients experienced depression—five times the rate of the general population.[241] Cancer survivors are also almost twice as likely as adults without cancer to report poor mental health after treatment ends, particularly during the first 1–3 years of recovery.[242] Fear of recurrence and a sense of abandonment as medical care and social support wane after the completion of a treatment regimen have been found to contribute to post-treatment mental distress.[243] This is particularly true among cancer patients who are younger, less well educated, lower income, without immediate family, or suffering from non-cancer-related chronic disease.[242-244] In fact, patients with both cancer and other chronic diseases are six times as likely to claim a psychological disability.[242] Finally, some evidence points to a disparity between urban and rural areas. A large-scale study in the US found that cancer survivors living in rural areas were 23% more likely than survivors living in urban areas to report mental distress. Rural cancer survivors were also 15% more likely to suffer from two or more non-cancer medical conditions, 66% more likely to be unemployed because of their poor health status, almost twice as likely not to have health insurance, and 64% more likely to live below the federal poverty line—all of which are factors that can contribute to mental distress.[245]

T.4.g.vi Minorities and Indigenous Communities

In many countries, minorities and Indigenous communities are at higher risk of negative outcomes from cancer, because they receive lower levels of medical care due to socioeconomic barriers and/or because their communities are located in remote areas far from medical hubs.[246] In the US, for example, even though cancer survival rates increase among African Americans as their socioeconomic status increases, the gap in African American versus non-Hispanic White mortality rates also increases as socioeconomic status rises.[246] Indigenous populations in Australia, on average, receive later cancer diagnoses and have lower survival rates than the White population. These numbers may reflect the Indigenous population's lower average socioeconomic status and the higher proportion of Indigenous communities located in remote areas compared with the majority White population.[247] For some cancers, such as lung cancer, it may also reflect a genetic factor that makes some individuals more susceptible to aggressive strains of the disease.[143] Similarly, Chinese immigrants to Singapore, Malaysia, the US, Israel, Sweden, and the UK have demonstrated higher rates of nasopharyngeal cancer than the majority populations in those countries.[248] And, in the US, a disproportionate number of cases of liver cancer occur among people of Asian, Pacific Islander, and Hispanic backgrounds.[246]

T.4.g.vii Families Living in Poverty

Cancer care is notoriously expensive. It is therefore more difficult for patients living in poverty to access cancer treatment or long-term care after the cancer has been controlled or eliminated.[242] Low-income patients are also less likely to have ready access to primary medical care. And they are therefore more likely to be diagnosed when the disease has already progressed beyond the point of effective treatment.[242] A population-level study in the US found a 31% increased risk of mortality among all cancer patients and a 40% increase among women living in high-poverty neighborhoods.[249] The financial effects of cancer treatment are particularly burdensome for working age adults. A study of breast cancer survivors in the US found that cancer patients' average annual wages fell $3,500 during the first five years following diagnosis, while a comparison group of women without breast cancer experienced an average annual increase of $1,800.[250] Furthermore, a population-level study in western Washington State, USA, found that cancer patients were 2.65 times more likely than the general population to file for personal bankruptcy, and bankruptcy rates among working age cancer patients were two to five times higher than rates for patients over age 65.[251] A follow up study found an almost 80% increased risk of mortality among cancer patients who filed for bankruptcy compared with cancer patients who did not.[252] And a study in Switzerland found that families who had taken care of child cancer patients had lower household incomes and a 10% increased risk of poverty than families without childhood cancer survivors.[253] The financial burden of treating cancer can have long-term physical and mental health consequences. A population-level study in the US found that 28.7% of cancer survivors reported a financial burden associated with paying for their medical care. Compared with survivors who did not report a financial burden, this group reported lower physical and mental health status, were almost two times as likely to suffer from depression and were 3.5 times as likely to worry about cancer recurrence.[254] The financial burden of cancer is even more pronounced in low- and middle-income countries, where cancer diagnosis of one family member can perpetuate the cycle of poverty for the entire family. For example, a large-scale study among impoverished families in rural Heilongjiang Province, China, found that 86% of cancer patients living below the poverty line reported that their cancer diagnosis was the primary cause of their economic hardship, compared with 56% of the total population living in poverty. Given the extremely high cancer prevalence rate among people living in poverty in Heilongjiang Province—1,233.1 per 100,000 in men and 1,479.1 per 100,000 in women, compared with 666 per 100,000 among urban populations in China and 440 per 100,000 among rural populations—cancer clearly plays a role in slowing economic development in the region.[255]

T.4.g.viii Occupational Exposure

More than 20 chemicals commonly used in occupational settings have been designated as carcinogens, such as exhaust from diesel-powered motors, hexavalent chromium, silica dust, coke or aluminum production, and paint.[207] Occupational exposure to toxic chemicals is estimated to cause between 2% and 8% of all cases of cancer, worldwide.[256] In addition to the more common cancers listed in the section above, occupational exposure in construction-related industries to toxic chemicals has been found to increase the risk of a long list of other cancers, depending on the chemical or substance involved, for example melanoma (43% increased risk of diagnosis among outdoor workers[257]), bladder cancer (21% increased mortality risk among painters[258(p391)]), and liver cancer (35% increased mortality risk from exposure to vinyl chloride[259]). According to a population-scale study in the UK, 5.3% of cancer deaths in 2012 were caused by occupational exposure. Primary exposures included asbestos (lung cancer, mesothelioma), shift work (breast cancer), mineral oils (lung cancer, bladder cancer), silica (lung cancer), diesel engine exhaust (lung cancer, bladder cancer), painting (lung cancer, bladder cancer), environmental tobacco smoke among non-smokers (lung cancer), and welding (lung cancer).[260] Cumulative exposure to benzene at work has been found to increase the risk of leukemia by 64% for low levels of exposure (<40 ppm-years), 90% for medium levels of exposure (40–99.9 ppm-years), and 262% for high levels of exposure (>100 ppm-years).[261] Occupational exposure to high concentrations of formaldehyde (i.e., ≥4 ppm) has been associated with a 35%–78% increase in risk of leukemia.[262] Occupational exposure to wood dust has been found to increase the risk of nasopharyngeal cancer by 50%.[263] A number of occupations associated with the building industry have also been associated with an increased risk of larynx cancer, including painters (40% increased risk) and bricklayers and carpenters (30% increased risk).[264] There is also some evidence to support increased risk of breast cancer after exposure to polychlorinated biphenyls (a chemical that is used in electrical equipment and hydraulic systems and can persist in the environment for decades after its release)[265] or ethylene oxide (a sterilizer used in healthcare settings).[266] Finally, disruptions to the body's natural sleep cycle (or circadian rhythm) has been associated with increased risk of breast cancer. Circadian disruptions caused by night-time shift work have been associated with up to a 48% increase in risk of breast cancer.[267]

T.5 Toolbox—Community Health Conditions: Mental Health

T.5.a Introduction

Mental health is a large and complex topic covering many types of illness—some mild and some severe. More than 10% of the world population (792 million people) is estimated to live with one or more mental health condition. The two most common conditions are anxiety (3.8% of the population; 284 million people) and depression (3.4% of the population; 264 million people).[268] According to the 2016 Global Burden of Disease study, mental and substance use disorders are the leading cause of YLD worldwide, accounting for 150,476,000 YLDs in 2016—almost one-fifth of the total from all causes and a 13% increase since 2006. In comparison, all infectious diseases combined accounted for only 12.5% of the total (101,472,000 YLDs).[269] In spite of their heavy burden on human health and society, mental health conditions are woefully undertreated, even in high-income countries. For example, a global study found that only 14% of patients in lower- to middle-income countries, 22% in upper-to middle-income countries, and 37% in high-income countries received treatment for their condition.[270]

Many factors contribute to the development or exacerbation of a mental health condition, including genetics, experiences during childhood, participation in social networks, and physical health status. However, the WHO estimates that 20% of the disability-adjusted life years attributed to anxiety disorders, 12% attributed to depressive disorders, 12% attributed to childhood behavioral disorders, and 6% attributed to dementia (including Alzheimer's) were caused by modifiable environmental risks.[10]

T.5.b What Is Mental Health?

This section of the toolbox will focus on three common groups of mental health conditions that can be influenced by changes in the design and operations of the built environment.

T.5.b.i Cognitive Ability

Cognitive ability is generally studied as the rate of cognitive development during childhood and the rate of cognitive decline in old age.[271] Diagnosis in children often relies on a development scale to determine whether or not a child is lagging behind other children in their age group.[272] The most common cognitive diagnoses among the elderly are dementia and Alzheimer's.[273] Dementia refers to a state in which so many neurons have stopped connecting to other parts of the brain that an individual finds it difficult to perform daily life and activities on his/her own.[273] Alzheimer's disease is a form of dementia that is characterized by neurons losing the ability to connect with each other in the brain, abnormal clumps of neurons, and tangled bundles of neurological fibers. It is the most common form of dementia among the elderly, ranking among the top five causes of death in that age group in the US.[274]

T.5.b.ii Mood Disorders

Mood disorders such as stress, PTSD, anxiety, and depression refer to mental health conditions that are excessive and ongoing versions of emotional responses that everyone experiences at some point in their lives, such as the anxiety that motivates a student to study for a test or the sadness that follows the death of a loved one. The body is designed to experience these sensations periodically.[275] In fact, over 70% of adults worldwide report having experienced at least one traumatic event in their lives.[276] It is when an individual is not able to rebound after a negative stimulus and instead experiences acute stress, anxiety, or depression on a daily basis that the response shifts into the realm of a mental health disorder.[275]

Mood disorders affect the size, hormonal activity, and connectivity between neurons in the amygdala, hippocampus, and thalamus—portions of the central brain that control mood and process memories.[275] Studies have found that patients diagnosed with mood disorders have a smaller hippocampus and suppressed neuron activity in that region of the brain.[277-279] Antidepressants, on the other hand, have been found to increase the rate of neuron growth and connections there.[275]

Mood disorders are common mental health conditions among adolescents and adults. Over 30% of adolescents (aged 13–18) and 19% of adults in the US have experienced an anxiety disorder at some point in their lives. In 2017, 13% of adolescents (aged 12–17) and 7% of adults in the US reported experiencing a major depressive episode during the previous year. Mood disorders often occur in concert with each other and with chronic physical health conditions. Taking PTSD as an example, 3.6% of adults in the US have experienced PTSD at some point during their lives.[280] Over 50% of PTSD cases occur alongside mood, anxiety, or substance-abuse disorders.[281] And, a population-scale study in Canada found that PTSD diagnosis increased the odds of depression 10-fold, panic attacks more than 5-fold, asthma 2-fold, hypertension 1.5-fold, heart disease 1.7-fold, stroke 2-fold, and diabetes 1.6-fold, among many other mental and physical health conditions.[282]

T.5.b.iii Behavioral Disorders

Behavior disorders refer to a suite of conditions that are more common among children than adults and often occur together, including ADHD, oppositional defiant disorder (ODD), and conduct disorder. In each case, the individual with the condition acts in a way that disrupts social, learning, and/or work settings.[283] A child who experiences multiple behavioral disorders is at increased risk of future antisocial behavior, substance abuse, and diagnosis of bipolar disorder.[284] In the US, 4.6% of children aged 4–17 have been diagnosed with either ODD or conduct disorder. The prevalence of ADHD is the most commonly diagnosed condition of the three, increasing 42% from 7.8% in 2003 to 11.0% in 2011.[280]

T.5.c What Are the Symptoms?

T.5.c.i Cognitive Ability

Children are routinely tested at the pediatrician's office and at school for developmental delay and related mental health conditions, such as autism spectrum disorders. Symptoms may include delays in the development of gross and fine motor skills, as well as speech delays.[283] Symptoms of dementia and Alzheimer's include depression, apathy, agitation, argumentativeness or aggression, delusions, hallucinations, executive dysfunction, repetitive vocalization, shadowing and wandering, and resistance to care.[285]

T.5.c.ii Mood Disorders

Generalized anxiety disorder is diagnosed as a condition that has lasted at least six months where the patient experiences excessive and difficult to control anxiety and worry on most days about many events or activities. The patient also presents with at least three of the following symptoms: restlessness or feeling on edge, easily fatigued, difficulty concentrating, irritability, muscle tension, or difficulty sleeping.[286]

To be diagnosed with depression, a patient must report either a depressed mood or a loss of interest or pleasure in daily activities during the previous two weeks and at least three of the following: unexplained weight loss, weight gain, or marked change in appetite; slower thought processes and slower physical movements; fatigue; feelings of worthlessness or guilt; reduced ability to concentrate or make decisions; or death or suicide ideation. Both conditions cause significant distress or disrupt the patient's

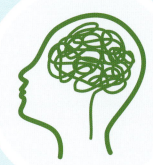

02 HOW DOES IT AFFECT THE BUILT ENVIRONMENT?

OUTDOOR AIR POLLUTION
Exposure to outdoor air pollution can damage the central nervous system & cause inflammation & oxidative stress in the brain, risk factors for poor mental health.

SPRAWL, UNSAFE BIKE/PED ENVIRONMENT
Reduced access to green space & opportunities for physical activity & social connection. Increased exposure to traffic related air pollution & noise pollution. All are mental health risk factors.

ACCESS TO OUTDOOR ACTIVITIES
Areas without access to outdoor activities can increase the risk of social isolation, depression, anxiety, & behavioral disorders.

PLACE BARRIERS & LOCATE EMISSIONS SOURCES AWAY FROM OPENINGS/AIR SUPPLY
Reduce the risk of pollutants entering the building.

COMPACT, MULTI-USE DEVELOPMENT NEAR TRANSIT & BIKE/PED INFRASTRUCTURE
Physical activity & social interaction can benefit mental health.

ON-SITE GROCERY/ FOOD PRODUCTION
Increases food security & access to fresh, healthy options. Can foster a sense of community.

NATIVE VEGETATION/ OUTDOOR ROOMS
Can bolster mental health by increasing access to nature & physical activity.

04 WHO IS MOST VULNERABLE...

CHILDREN
At higher risk for developmental & behavioral reasons.

ELDERLY
Body is less resilient & many elderly also have underlying health conditions.

CHRONIC DISEASE
Symptoms & treatments increase risk of poor mental health.

POVERTY
Financial pressures can increase the risk of anxiety, depression, & substance abuse.

MINORITIES
Social exclusion & marginalization increase the risk of poor mental health.

RURAL POPULATIONS
Reduced access to care, cost barriers, social stigma.

Toolbox Infographic T.5. Linkages among Mental Health, the Built Environment Determinants of Health, Protective Design and Operations Strategies, the Groups Who Are at Highest Risk, and Related Negative Health Outcomes

01 MENTAL HEALTH

- 10% of the world population live with 1+ mental health condition.
- 1 in 5 anxiety disorders & 1 in 10 depressive disorders are attributable to environmental conditions.

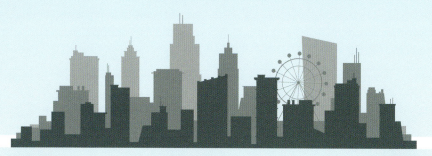

URBAN HEAT ISLAND
Absence of vegetation & exposure to high temperatures can exacerbate symptoms of mental illness.

LACK OF RESILIENCE
Disruption to medical services, displacement, & increased stress during disasters increases risk of mental health concerns.

INDOOR ENVIRONMENT
Dark, enclosed spaces without access to daylight, views, ventilation, & low emitting finishes & cleaning products can trigger or exacerbate mental health conditions.

03 HOW CAN DESIGN HELP?

ISLANDABLE SITES & MICROGRIDS
Can reduce mental stress of disasters by ensuring continuity of essential energy, water, & food until utilities are restored.

DAYLIGHT & VIEWS OF NATURE
Can contribute to sense of wellbeing, ability to focus, & productivity.

INTEGRATED IAQ
Enhanced ventilation & filtration minimizes outdoor air pollution & infectious disease. Low VOC materials minimize indoor emissions.

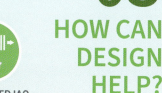

DISABILITY & DEATH   **CHRONIC DISEASE**   **CANCER**

... TO THE HEALTH RISKS? 05

Note: Many of the design and operations strategies in the infographic bring co-benefits to other topics in this toolbox as well. See figure T.4 for a crosswalk of all of the environmental health co-benefits.

ability to function in social, occupational, or other areas of daily life. And neither anxiety nor depression can be attributed to substance abuse or physical health conditions, such as hyperthyroidism.[286]

PTSD is a condition that is triggered by exposure to a traumatic event(s) that the patient re-experiences through vivid, intrusive memories that trigger strong emotions. The patient perceives themselves to be under heightened threat and avoids thoughts, situations, and activities that might trigger recurring memories. Similar to other mood disorders, the symptoms persist for several weeks and disrupt the patient's ability to participate in daily activities and social interactions.[287]

T.5.c.iii Behavioral Disorders

ADHD is characterized by developmentally inappropriate levels of inattention, hyperactivity, impulsivity, or a combination.[286] ODD is characterized by a child frequently losing his/her temper, defying adults, refusing to comply with rules, acting in a negative and aggressive manner, consciously annoying others, and blaming his/her behavior on others.[286] Conduct disorder is characterized by children consistently violating social norms and rules, ignoring the rights of others, destroying property, acting aggressively towards other people or animals, and acting deceitfully.[286]

Table T.6 summarizes common symptoms associated with impaired cognitive ability, mood disorders, and behavioral disorders.

TABLE T.6.
Symptoms of Mental Health Conditions

Mental Disorder	Symptoms
Impaired Cognitive Ability	
Developmental delays in children	• Delays in gross, fine motor skills • Speech delays
Dementia	• Apathy • Agitation • Argumentativeness • Aggression • Delusions • Depression • Executive dysfunction • Hallucinations • Repetitive vocalization • Resistance to care • Shadowing and wandering

TABLE T.6. (cont.)

Mental Disorder	Symptoms
Mood Disorders	
Anxiety	• Difficulty concentrating • Difficulty sleeping • Easily fatigued • Excessive and difficult to control anxiety and worry • Irritability • Muscle tension • Restlessness or feeling on edge
Depression	• Death or suicide ideation • Depressed mood or a loss of interest or pleasure in daily activities • Fatigue • Feelings of worthlessness or guilt • Reduced ability to concentrate or make decisions • Slower thought processes and slower physical movements • Unexplained weight loss, weight gain, or marked change in appetite
Post-traumatic stress disorder	• Avoid triggering situations • Perception of heightened threat • Triggered by exposure to a traumatic event(s) that the patient re-experiences through vivid, intrusive memories that trigger strong emotions
Behavioral Disorders	
Attention deficit hyperactivity disorder	• Hyperactivity • Impulsivity • Inattention
Oppositional defiant disorder	• Acting in a negative and aggressive manner • Blaming his/her behavior on others • Consciously annoying others • Defying adults • Losing temper • Refusing to comply with rules
Conduct disorder	• Acting deceitfully • Acting aggressively towards other people or animals • Consistently violating social norms and rules • Destroying property • Ignoring the rights of others

T.5.d Relationship with Climate Change

Climatic events—particularly heat waves, air pollution, and flooding and storms—can both trigger new mental health conditions and exacerbate pre-existing mental health conditions.

T.5.d.i Heat

Heat exposure can impair the central nervous system, reducing cognitive functions such as attention, memory, and processing information.[288] It can also exacerbate the symptoms of mental illness, thereby increasing the risk of injury or death.[289] In fact, mental illness is the most significant pre-existing health condition increasing the risk of mortality during an extreme heat event—raising an individual's risk by a factor of 3.6 compared with the population as a whole.[290] A retrospective study of the New York State psychiatric hospital found that the risk of mortality during heat waves for inpatients was twice the rate among the general population.[291] And a review of deaths during the 2003 heat wave in Paris found that elderly inhabitants with a pre-existing mental illness were almost 6 times as likely to die during the event than their peers.[292] The increased vulnerability among some mental health patients—such as people with Alzheimer's disease, dementia, psychosis, schizophrenia, or developmental disabilities—may be partially explained by their reduced capacity to protect themselves by adapting to the changing environment (e.g., increasing water intake, wearing appropriate clothing, or changing their daily routine to stay out of the heat).[290,293] Anti-depressant and anti-psychotic medicines can also increase the body's vulnerability to heat stress by interfering with the primary mechanisms used by the brain to regulate body temperature.[289] People experiencing homelessness (PEH) are particularly at risk of death or injury during heat waves, because of a combination of higher rates of mental illness and living conditions that are exposed to the elements. Studies in high-income countries have found substantially higher rates of alcohol and drug dependence, personality disorder, post-traumatic stress disorder, traumatic brain injury, depression, and psychosis among PEH populations compared with the general population.[294] While less information is available from low- and middle-income countries, it appears that severe mental illness is also a significant concern among PEH in those regions of the world.[295] Finally, increases in ambient temperature have been found to increase the risk of subjective measures of mental health. For example, a population-scale study in China found that each 1 °C increase over the daily average temperature was associated with a 15% decline in self-reported mental health status—particularly related to feeling nervous, upset, hopeless, or meaningless.[296]

T.5.d.ii Air Pollution

Air pollution is a mix of airborne particles, gases, and metals that are generally emitted outdoors by motor vehicles, industrial installations, or wildfires and indoors by building materials and biological pathogens like mold. Some airborne pollutants have been found to damage the central nervous system through direct damage to neurons or the blood–brain barrier or by disrupting hormone regulation and/or gene expression (particularly for "clock" genes, which control the body's circadian rhythm).[297] Exposure to particulate matter can cause inflammation and oxidative stress in the brain,[298] which has been found to contribute to the deterioration of nerve cells and the olfactory, respiratory, and blood–brain barriers.[299] Ground-level O_3 can damage neurons, interfere with hormonal regulation, cause motor and memory deficits, and (among children born to mothers who were exposed to O_3 while pregnant) interfere with brain development.[299] Sulfur oxides have been found to suppress brain activity, particularly related to spatial learning and memory.[300] NO_2 and VOCs like polycyclic aromatic hydrocarbons (components of tailpipe exhaust) have been found to damage neurons.[301,302]

If damage to the central nervous system is severe enough, it can lead to reductions in both self-reported and clinical measures of mental health and wellbeing. For example, a population-based study in China found that the increase in air pollution from 2007–2014 accounted for 22.5% of the decline in self-reported happiness over that same period. The same study found that depressive symptoms increased 33.6% as air quality deteriorated from Category 3 ("unhealthy for sensitive groups") to Category 4 ("unhealthy") on the US Environmental Protection Agency's (EPA's) air quality index scale.[303] Similarly, a population-scale study in the US found the number of self-reported "poor mental health days" among adults increased alongside increases in the concentration of air pollution, particularly at low altitudes.[304]

Studies measuring the effect of poor air quality on general psychological distress and depression have found similar results. For example, a population-scale study in the Netherlands found that people living in areas with high concentrations of $PM_{2.5}$ were 8% more likely to be diagnosed with psychological distress than the population as a whole.[305] A similar study in the US found that each 5 unit increase in $PM_{2.5}$ exposure was associated with a 0.46 point increase in the K6 test for psychological distress (based on a 20-point scale, where higher scores indicate higher levels of psychological distress).[306] A study of six cities in Canada found that daily emergency department visits for depression increased 15.5% under 0.8 ppm CO conditions and 20% under 20.1 ppb NO_2 conditions during warm weather and 7.2% under 19.4 µg/m³ PM₁₀ (coarse particulate matter) conditions during cold weather.[307]

Finally, exposure to air pollution has been associated with several severe mental illnesses. The chronic inflammation and oxidative stress caused by prolonged exposure to particulate matter has been associated with accelerating both cognitive decline in general and the onset of Alzheimer's and Parkinson's disease in particular.[298] A large-scale study in Denmark found that the risk of developing schizophrenia increased more than 3-fold among children who were exposed to high levels of ambient benzene or CO at birth. Risk was 5.5 times higher among children whose birth homes were located in highly trafficked areas and were therefore exposed to high concentrations of particulate matter, NO₂, and other traffic-related air pollutants.[308]

T.5.d.iii Flooding and Storms

Flooding and storms can exacerbate mental health conditions in two major ways. First, similar to other chronic diseases, mental health patients may experience a disruption in medications and medical care after a major storm or flooding event. Second, the stress and trauma associated with surviving the event may exacerbate symptoms among existing mental health patients, particularly related to PTSD.[104] The psychological toll is only heightened if a storm victim is displaced from home and/or experiences disruptions to work or school. Taking Hurricane Katrina (2005) as an example, residents of New Orleans, Louisiana, USA, who suffered from depression before the hurricane were 19 times more likely than the general population to report poor mental health one year after the event.[309] Mental health patients continued to face a critical shortage of qualified providers a year after the event in spite of the fact that cases of stress, depression, and PTSD had skyrocketed.[310] And residents who self-identified as minorities and low income reported severe mental health outcomes, particularly if they experienced a high number of stressors during the hurricane (e.g., no food or water, physical danger, disruption of medicine or medical care, separation from children or family members who might be in danger). A study of low-income African American women found that the percentage of participants with serious mental health concerns doubled from 7% pre-Katrina to 14% post-Katrina, perceived stress increased 50% from 20% to 30%, and perceived poor health status increased 50% from 13% to 19%. High levels of hurricane-related loss, stressors, and property damage were also associated with poor mental health outcomes—particularly PTSD.[311]

T.5.e How Does the Built Environment Increase the Risk of Mental Health Conditions?

Land use policies that lead to sprawl expose community members to both toxins and behavioral challenges that can increase the risk of poor mental health. Outdoor air pollution caused by TRAP and industrial pollution can damage the central nervous system and cause inflammation and oxidative stress in the brain, both of which are physiological risk factors for poor mental health. Car-centric areas reduce community access to green space and opportunities for physical activity and social connection that could counteract risks to mental health. Car-centric land use policies also result in increased impervious surface, which contributes to the urban heat island effect. Exposure to extreme heat has been found to exacerbate symptoms of mental illness and can have a harmful effect on people taking psychotropic medications. Infrastructure that is not resilient to climate-related extreme weather events unnecessarily increases the risk of poor mental health among victims of displacement and disruption to medical services. Finally, indoor environments that do not provide access to daylight, views of nature, enhanced ventilation, and low-emitting building materials and cleaning products can trigger or exacerbate mental health conditions.

T.5.f How Can Design Help?

At the master-planning and community-planning scales, design can reduce exposure to mental health triggers like air pollution and fragile infrastructure. Building-scale interventions include promoting community scale efforts, as well as erecting vegetative and structural barriers to protect occupants from sources of air pollution, flood risk, etc. Developing a comprehensive plan to protect occupants and the surrounding neighborhood in the event of a natural disaster can support mental health by reducing anxiety around a future disaster. Increasing access to nature and local food production can both enhance positive mental health and foster a sense of community. Finally, providing an indoor environment that both does not trigger negative mental health conditions through poor ventilation and high-emitting materials and further promotes a sense of wellbeing, focus, and productivity through ample access to daylight and views of nature can have a profoundly positive effect on all building occupants.

T.5.g Who Is Most Vulnerable?

Mental health conditions can arise at any time of life, although they often manifest during adolescence and in old age. People with pre-existing mental or physical health conditions are particularly vulnerable to developing some mental illnesses, such as mood disorders. Socioeconomic and demographic factors, such as living in poverty or identifying with a minority group, have been found to increase the risk of some mental health conditions. Finally, location has been identified as a risk factor for some mental health conditions—particularly absence of green space and challenges unique to rural areas such as reduced access to care.

T.5.g.i Children

Environmental exposures during pregnancy and in early life can permanently impair a child's cognitive development, leading to lifelong consequences. Children are particularly vulnerable to exposure to toxins, because their brains are still developing and the barriers in their lungs that will protect them as adults from absorbing particles into the bloodstream are also under development. Children are exposed to a higher concentration of airborne toxins, because their ratio of breathing to body mass is higher than adults. They are also often physically located closer to the source of toxins: the floor and outside.[312] Using air pollution as an example, a series of studies of children in New York City whose mothers were exposed to high concentrations (>2.26 μg/m³) of polycyclic aromatic hydrocarbons (a component of tailpipe exhaust) while pregnant found that exposure was associated with damage to DNA and impaired fetal growth before birth; slower cognitive and motor skills development at ages 1, 2, and 3; lower IQ scores at age 5; and higher rates of anxiety, depression, and attention deficit disorder at age 6–7.[301] A study in Spain found that increases in air pollution were associated with lower levels of cognitive development during the first two years of life.[313] A study in London, UK, found that exposure to high levels of TRAP at age 12 increased the odds of developing major depressive disorder at age 18 by 20%.[312] And a growing body of research has begun to establish a link between exposure to particulate matter and NO_2 either during pregnancy or early in life and an increased risk of diagnosis along the autism spectrum.[297] Furthermore, a large study of children in South Korea found that a 1 μg/m³ increase in exposure to PM_{10} and NO_2 corresponded to an 18% and 3% (respectively) increased risk of diagnosis for ADHD. Finally, children living in the highest tertile of exposure were at two to three times higher risk of developing ADHD than children living in the lowest tertile.[314]

T.5.g.ii Elderly

Part of the ageing process includes the slow reduction in functioning nerve cells (or neurons) in the brain. It is therefore not surprising that the rate of dementia is higher among the elderly than among younger, healthy adults. In fact, a study of individuals aged 90 years and above found that the rate of dementia diagnosis doubled every five years starting at age 90—exceeding 40% by age 100.[315] The risk of dementia increases in elderly patients if they also suffer from other mental health conditions. For example, one study found that among individuals over 90 years of age the risk of dementia increased 5-fold if they were diagnosed with another mental health condition, 8.4-fold if they were diagnosed with two additional mental health conditions, and 60-fold if they were diagnosed with three or more mental health conditions.[316] Feelings of loneliness and depression are also common among the elderly and have been found to increase with age, due in part to increasing social isolation[317]—which can be ameliorated or exacerbated by land use and building design decisions. Finally, exposure to air pollution may accelerate cognitive decline among the elderly. For example, a study in Chicago, Illinois, USA, of adults aged 57–85 years found that an increase in exposure to $PM_{2.5}$ and NO_2 were associated with cognitive decline equivalent to aging 1.6 years and 1.9 years, respectively.[318]

T.5.g.iii Chronic Disease

The relationship between chronic disease and mental health is so intertwined that it can be difficult to determine for any given individual whether developing a chronic disease increased the risk of poor mental health or whether it was the other way around. Regardless, it is clear that mental health conditions disproportionately affect patients with all types of non-communicable diseases. In some instances, there may be a physiological reason. For example, inflammation plays a role in the progression of both chronic diseases like cardiovascular disease, hypertension, and COPD, as well as depression.[58,133] A population-based study in Baltimore, Maryland, USA, found that participants with pre-existing depression experienced three times the risk of hypertension as non-depressive participants.[319]

In other cases, social stigma may play a role.[194] For example, a large-scale study of kindergarteners in the US found that girls who were overweight were 1.8 times more likely than their healthy weight peers to be identified by teachers as having behavior problems and 1.5 times more likely to be identified by teachers or parents as exhibiting symptoms of anxiety or depression.[320] A large-scale, school-based study in China found that boys who perceived themselves to be overweight or obese—irrespective of their measured BMI—were 1.6 times and girls were almost 2 times more likely to be diagnosed with a mental health condition than children who perceived themselves to be a normal weight.[321]

The persistence of chronic diseases and the intensity of their treatment regimens can also take a toll on mental health. For example, cancer patients experience depression at four to five times the rate of the general population during treatment[241,322] Cancer survivors are also twice as likely as non-cancer patients to report poor mental health status within two years after treatment ends.[242] The rate of depression among cardiovascular patients is three times higher than the general population.[59] And a study in the UK found that individuals with diabetes were 1.7 times as likely to suffer from anxiety and depression than the general population.[323] Furthermore, the combination of cancer and one or more pre-existing chronic disease increases the odds of a cancer patient claiming psychological disability by a factor of six.[242]

T.5.g.iv Minorities and Indigenous Populations

Minorities and Indigenous populations often experience higher rates of mental illness than the majority population, as a result of social exclusion and marginalization. For example, a population-scale study in the US found that non-Hispanic African American adolescents with depression were three times more likely to be obese than their peers.[324] Indigenous and immigrant groups are particularly at risk in societies that expect cultural assimilation from all members of society.[271] A study of Queensland Aboriginal and Torres Strait Islanders in Australia found a 50% higher rate of mental disorders among Indigenous versus non-Indigenous populations. Mental health conditions represented almost 30% of the total non-fatal burden of disease among Indigenous groups, representing almost half of the non-fatal burden of disease among young people, aged 15–30 years.[69]

T.5.g.v Families Living in Poverty

Living in poverty increases the risk of anxiety, depression, and substance abuse—particularly among the unemployed. Financial pressures can be mentally and emotionally taxing, because they exacerbate poverty by limiting access to opportunities and by making it more difficult to rebound after being confronted with difficult situations—such as a natural disaster or a life-threatening illness.[271] The cumulative economic burden of mental health conditions is daunting. The World Economic Forum (WEF) estimates that mental health conditions will lead to $16 trillion in lost economic output from 2011 to 2030, equivalent to one-quarter of the global gross domestic product in 2010.[325] Families living in poverty and populations in low- and middle-income countries experience the heaviest burden, because treatment may be inaccessible due to institutional or financial constraints. According to the WHO, the median number of mental health workers and mental health beds per 100,000 population is < 1 and 7, respectively, in low- and middle-income countries, compared with 72 and 50 in high-income countries. Low- and middle-income countries also allocate less than 2% of their medical care budget to treating mental health conditions.[326] Populations with access to mental health services often face prohibitively expensive medical bills. The WEF estimates that the combined direct and indirect cost of caring for mental health conditions worldwide will increase from $2.5 trillion to $6.0 trillion from 2010 to 2030.[325] Among the elderly, who are often living on fixed incomes, financial strain may further increase their already heightened risk of some mental illnesses. For example, a study in Slovakia and the Netherlands found that people aged 65 and older with low or medium levels of income were 1.75 times more likely to report poor mental health than their wealthier peers. The risk increased to 2.26 times their peers if they were experiencing financial strain.[327]

T.5.g.vi Absence of Green Space

People who live and work in areas with little or no green space have been found to be more susceptible to a number of mental health conditions. For example, a population-scale study in China found that each 0.05 point decrease in the Normalized Difference Vegetation Index surrounding a participant's home increased his/her risk of deteriorated mental health status by 19%—particularly in relation to depression and nervousness.[296] A population-scale study in the UK found that increasing levels of vegetation around a participant's residence reduced his/her risk of developing major depressive disorder.[328] Access to green space is also associated with improved mental health among children. For example, a study of 7- to 10-year-old children in Barcelona, Spain, found that an incremental increase in green space play time was associated with a 4.8% reduction in all behavior mental health problems, including a 2.7% reduction in hyperactivity and inattention, an 8.2% reduction in emotional difficulties, and a 15.4% reduction in peer relationship problems. Access to the beach (i.e., "blue space") was also protective, reducing the risk of total behavior problems by 3.9%. And proximity to green space both at home and at school were associated with a 4.5% reduction in total behavior problems and a 7.7% reduction in diagnosed ADHD.[329]

Many times, the absence of green space is accompanied by additional mental health stressors, such as traffic-related noise and air pollution. A population-based study in the Netherlands found that exposure to all three stressors—absence of green space, traffic noise, and air pollution—increased the risk of psychological distress by 18%, whereas no association was found between increased psychological distress and reduction in green space alone.[305] And a follow up to the Barcelona study of schoolchildren found that up to 60% of the cognitive benefits of green space in its analysis may be attributable to the role vegetation plays in reducing exposure to TRAP.[330]

T.5.g.vii Rural Areas

Rural areas, particularly in high-income countries like the US, have a higher percentage of residents who are older, less affluent, and suffering from one or more chronic disease[331-333]—all of which are risk factors for mental health conditions. A study in the US of rural African Americans (a group who is at high risk due to both location and demographics) found that participants who reported poor physical health and material hardship were 13% and 10% (respectively) more likely to experience depressive symptoms and 23% and 20% more likely to experience psychological distress than their healthier peers.[334] Individuals who live in rural areas may be at higher risk of untreated mental health conditions due to a combination of reduced access to mental health care, cost barriers (because many mental health services and medications are not covered by health insurance), disappointment with the level of service, and social stigma.[335,336] For example, one study found that rural mental health patients in the US visit their providers less often than their urban counterparts, even if they are actively using medication to control their condition.[337]

HEALTH EFFECTS OF CLIMATE CHANGE

KEY MESSAGES

1. Climate change has been identified by leaders in environmental science, public health, and real estate as one of society's most pressing challenges.

2. In each of these industries, climate change amplifies existing vulnerabilities by increasing the intensity and/or frequency of exposure to environmental challenges that have historically impacted a given area. It also creates new vulnerabilities by introducing environmental hazards that lie outside of local experience.

3. The built environment is uniquely positioned to safeguard community health from environmental stressors, as experienced historically. However, in order to safeguard health in changing climatic circumstances, real estate development and design practices will need to shift from basing decisions on historical records of temperature, humidity, precipitation, extreme weather, and environmental pests to projections of future conditions.

4. A growing body of research is refining our understanding of which green building strategies are most protective of human health under different environmental conditions. By proactively implementing the strategies that are most responsive to the combined environmental and community health needs of a project site, developers, designers, and facility managers can enhance health and wellness on-site and in the surrounding community while simultaneously protecting a valuable real estate asset from climate-related damage.

Climate change is caused by the build-up of CO_2 and other heat-trapping greenhouse gases (GHGs) in the Earth's atmosphere. The GHG effect has resulted in warming temperatures,[338(pp74–75)] which have thrown the Earth's entire climate system off balance. Climate change has been called a "wicked problem," because its impacts on the natural and built environment, economy, human health, and society are complex and interdependent.[339] Its effects are felt most at the local level,[340] but global cooperation will be necessary to halt its progression.[341(pp71–73)]

Climate change is experienced not only through warmer summers in regions with historically mild weather patterns. There is strong historical evidence that climate change is both amplifying existing extreme weather hazards (such as heat waves, cold snaps, flooding, wildfires, and drought) and introducing new hazards in many parts of the globe.[342]

The health effects of climate change are wide ranging, encompassing both direct and indirect health outcomes.

Rising temperatures are causing more frequent and intense heat waves, which can lead directly to heat-related illness and death and indirectly to a temporary spike in all-cause mortality.[343(pp720–21)] For example, 70,000 excess deaths have been attributed to the extreme heat wave in Europe in 2003, particularly among the elderly (75 years and older).[344]

Warmer air can hold larger quantities of water, which can intensify precipitation events. This means that, when it rains, more precipitation falls over a shorter period of time, leading to intensified flooding events.[345] The direct health effects of flooding include flooding-related injuries and drownings. Indirect health effects include the mental health consequences when houses are flooded out and communities disperse.[343(pp721–22)] For example, in 2017, Hurricane Harvey severely damaged the homes of 20% of residents in 24 counties along the Texas Gulf Coast, USA (with a total population of more than 7 million people)—mostly due to flooding. About 30% of residents who had experienced severe damage to their home and 34% who had not returned home almost a year after the event reported a decline in their mental health post-Harvey.[346]

Warming temperatures are often correlated with deteriorating air quality, particularly in terms of increasing the production of ground-level O_3.[343(pp727-29)] Emerging research shows a compounding effect of heat and O_3 exposure on overall mortality rates, as well as emergency department visits for cardiovascular and respiratory disease.[347] Increases in CO_2 emissions from cars has also been linked with increased production of asthma-triggering pollen counts.[348,349]

Climate change has been increasingly linked with the intensification of extreme weather events in the US[350] and around the world.[342(pp208-22)] More than 61 million people globally were affected by natural disasters in 2018, most notably the 23 million people affected by flooding in Kerala, India, which reported a death toll of 504.[351] In the US, the average number of natural disasters exceeding $1 billion (so-called "billion-dollar storms") has been increasing since 1980. The average of number of billion-dollar storms for the period 2016–2018 was more than double the long-term average.[352]

Vector-borne disease is perhaps the clearest example of climate change as a wicked problem playing out at the local level. Disease-carrying insects, rodents, and other animals (i.e., vectors) are shifting their habitat in response to the complex interplay of changing temperatures, changing precipitation patterns, and changing habitats caused by both natural and human factors. In some cases, these changes have led to increasing exposure to a human population that had previously thought of a disease, such as Lyme disease, as an endemic but low-level threat. In other cases, vectors are exposing new populations to the diseases they carry.[343(pp722-25)] Climate-fueled changes in weather patterns have also increased the risk of exposure to some diseases, such as Zika, by increasing the number of opportunities for disease transmission each year. In the case of Zika, the longer summer and increased number of heavy precipitation events caused by climate change in the southern US and Caribbean has increased the number of breeding cycles the main carrier mosquito, *Aedes aegypti*, can fit into a breeding season. The warmer weather has also shortened Zika's gestation period inside the mosquito. So, it is able to transmit the disease several days earlier than previously.[353,354]

This portion of the toolbox will address the health effects of exposure to all five of these climate change-related environmental challenges in detail:

1. Heat
2. Flooding
3. Air quality
4. Disasters
5. Vector-borne disease

Each section will lay out the science linking the environmental challenge with climate change. It will identify the groups who are most vulnerable to experiencing negative health outcomes after exposure. And it will review the state of the scientific literature linking the built environment with negative and positive health outcomes within the context of the environmental challenge.

T.6 Toolbox—Health Effects of Climate Change: Extreme Heat

T.6.a Introduction

Heat-related deaths have long outstripped deaths from other extreme weather events in the US[355] and are second to the death toll from earthquakes on a global level.[351] From 2006–2010, roughly 670 deaths per year in the US were directly attributed to heat exposure, more than the 662 total deaths attributable to exposure to floods, storms, or lighting combined.[356] Worldwide, an annual average of 10,414 deaths were attributable to extreme temperatures from 2000–2017—compared with 46,173 from earthquakes, 12,722 from storm events, and 5,424 from flooding events.[351]

The most generic definition of a heat wave, developed by the World Meteorological Society, defines it as a period of unusually hot weather during warm seasons of the year and lasting at least three consecutive days.[357] However, it is not possible to set a single definition for all regions, because health outcomes will vary depending on population demographics, whether or not the population is acclimatized to warm temperatures, humidity levels, and environmental factors such as access to air conditioning and the extent of vegetation and tree canopy.[358-360]

T.6.b Health Effects of Extreme Heat

When the human body is exposed to extreme heat, its ability to regulate its internal temperature is reduced, leading to conditions such as heat cramps, heat exhaustion, heat stroke, and hyperthermia.[25(p46)] This is particularly true if nighttime temperatures remain warm, because the body does not have a chance to recover from daytime exposure.[25(p46)] The point at which this breakdown occurs depends on an individual's age, socioeconomic status, the predominant weather in his/her region, and, of course, characteristics of the built environment.[25(p46)] Exposure to heat can exacerbate chronic conditions, such as heart disease, respiratory diseases like asthma, and complications related to diabetes. Individuals suffering from mental disorders are also at heightened risk of hospitalization and/or suicide.[293,361-365]

Temperatures even slightly exceeding the optimal range have been associated with increased heat-related illness and death rates if the combination of factors is right.[366-368] Time of year is also important. Heat waves occurring earlier in the summer[369] before the population has acclimated to the change have resulted in more hospital visits and deaths than heat waves later in the season.[370]

T.6.c Relationship with Climate Change

As GHGs have accumulated in the Earth's atmosphere, more heat has been prevented from dissipating into outer space, leading to warmer ambient temperatures across the globe.[338(pp74-75)] Average global maximum and minimum temperatures have both increased by more than 0.18°F (0.1°C) per decade since 1950.[342(p188)] By 2100, global annual average temperatures are projected to increase by 1.6°F–9.72°F (0.9°C–5.4°C) relative to the period 1850–1900.[371(p1056)] In the US, average annual temperatures have increased by 1.2°F–1.8°F (0.7°C–1.0°C) since 1895,[372(p186)] with climate models predicting an increase of 2.8°F–11.9°F (1.6°C–6.6°C) relative to 1976–2005 by 2100.[372(p195)] Furthermore, the number of warm temperature extremes is on the rise, while the number of cold temperature extremes is declining, both in the US,[372(pp189-92)] and globally.[342(p209)] It is important to note that not all regions are warming at the same rate. Temperatures in the Arctic, for example, are projected to rise more than two times faster than the global average.[371(p1055)] The annual average temperature in Alaska is projected to increase 12°F (6.7°C) by 2100.[372(p195)]

Both the Intergovernmental Panel on Climate Change (IPCC)[371(p1066)] and the US National Climate Assessment[372(p197)] predict that the frequency and duration of heat waves will continue to increase throughout the US and across the globe as annual average temperatures continue to rise. Furthermore, even in regions with moderate annual average warming trends, temperature extremes are projected to increase substantially due to the increasing variability in seasonal temperatures.[371(p1066)] By 2050, the average temperatures of both extreme heat events and extreme cold events in the US are projected to increase at least 11°F (6.1°C).[372(p197)] By 2100, under a low-emission scenario, 48% of the world population is projected to be exposed to potentially deadly levels of combined heat and humidity at least 20 days per year, up from 30% today.[373]

Annual heat-related deaths are expected to rise in the US to the thousands or tens of thousands by 2100[374-381] as a result of climate change. Exposure to the mix of ambient air temperature and humidity that has led to increased mortality in the past is projected to rise by 48%–74% by 2100 worldwide.[373] And climate projections estimate increasing numbers of vulnerable populations exposed to extreme heat if global annual average temperatures rise even to the 2°C (3.6°F) threshold set by the Paris Agreement:[382] 410 million to 2.4 billion if temperatures rise by 1.5°C (2.7°F) over pre-industrial levels and 506 million to 3.2 billion if temperatures rise to 2.0°C (3.6°F) over pre-industrial levels.[383(p246)]

T.6.d How Does Extreme Heat Affect the Built Environment?

Compromised infrastructure is often extreme heat's most visible (and, therefore, most reported) effect on the built environment. It is often possible to feel the difference in temperature between urban heat islands (areas of town with a lot of concrete/asphalt and little vegetation) and neighborhoods where parks and trees are abundant. As temperatures rise, electrical lines sag and sometimes spark, which can touch off wildfires. Roads and airport tarmacs buckle and become unusable. And the public's increased use of air conditioning can lead to brownouts and blackouts, which can leave vulnerable groups at risk of exposure to dangerous temperatures.

High temperatures also combine with outdoor air pollution to increase the risk of asthma attacks among people with chronic respiratory disease. Indoors, emissions increase from paint, carpet, composite wood, and other finish materials containing VOCs when temperatures rise. People often stay indoors during heat events even when the power goes out. So, they are more likely to be exposed to high concentrations of aerosolized chemicals that can harm a range of organs, including the heart, the lungs, and the endocrine system.

If extreme heat is treated culturally as an unmanageable fact of life, then it can lead to an assumption among community planners, real estate developers, and architects that community members prefer to spend time indoors. That assumption can become a self-fulfilling prophecy—leading to a reduction in investments in programmed outdoor spaces like sidewalks, parks, and hike and bike trails. Even in communities that attempt to mitigate the urban heat island effect and encourage outdoor activity, the warming climate has been found to place stress on native plant and animal life in many regions of the world. Invasive species and vector-carrying animals like mosquitoes and ticks are expanding their habitat into stressed ecosystems that previously were too cold for them to thrive. Aquatic plants and animals are often particularly hard hit in a warming ecosystem, because waterways warm and experience more concentrated pollution as they evaporate in the heat (which is often accompanied by another effect of climate change—drought).

Finally, extreme heat compromises the food system at many scales. The warming climate has been shown to

02 HOW DOES IT AFFECT THE BUILT ENVIRONMENT?

URBAN HEAT ISLAND
Exacerbates thermal gain and re-radiation by dark & impervious surfaces.

ACCESS TO OUTDOOR ACTIVITIES
It can be dangerous to spend time outdoors during heat waves.

STRESS ON PLANT & ANIMAL LIFE
It can slow plant and animal growth & increase the risk of disease.

FOOD INSECURITY
Food spoils more quickly and plants have lower yields in extreme heat.

WATER QUANTITY & QUALITY
Evaporation can compromise drinking and recreational water.

LIGHT COLORED ROOFS & PAVEMENT
Reflects solar radiation instead of absorbing and re-radiating it.

COMPACT, MULTI-USE DEVELOPMENT NEAR TRANSIT & BIKE/PED INFRASTRUCTURE
Reduces the need to increase impervious surface streets.

NATIVE VEGETATION
Evapotranspiration cools the air, reducing the effects of the heat event.

BUILDING INSULATION
Protects occupants from solar heat gain passing through walls.

04 WHO IS MOST VULNERABLE...

CHILDREN + ELDERLY
Difficulty with thermoregulation. Dependent on others for safety.

PREGNANT WOMEN
Thermoregulation. Premature birth.

CHRONIC DISEASE
Increased sensitivity to heat.

POVERTY + MINORITIES
Risk of exposure in poorly maintained buildings & reduced access to medical care.

UNSHELTERED
Higher risk of exposure to the elements.

OUTDOOR WORKERS
Higher risk of exposure during the heat of the day.

Toolbox Infographic T.6. Linkages among Extreme Heat, the Built Environment Determinants of Health, Protective Design and Operations Strategies, the Groups Who Are at Highest Risk, and Related Negative Health Outcomes

01 EXTREME HEAT

- Increase in average annual temperature.
- Increase in number, frequency, duration, and severity of heat waves.

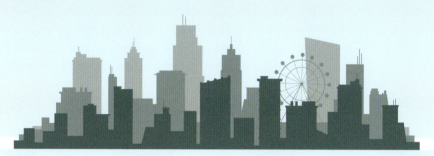

DISEASE-CARRYING VECTORS
Insect life cycle speeds up in heat, increasing risk of disease transmission.

AIR POLLUTION
Heat + air pollution increases the risk of asthma attacks in vulnerable groups.

INDOOR AIR QUALITY
Emissions increase when temperatures rise; and more time indoors increases exposure.

ELECTRICAL GRID INSTABILITY
Excess A/C use during heat events can lead to brown- & blackouts.

03 HOW CAN DESIGN HELP?

ENERGY EFFICIENCY MEASURES
Assists A/C by reducing heat waste inside buildings.

ON-SITE RENEWABLE ENERGY
If connected to A/C, can protect occupants when power goes out.

WELL-MAINTAINED BUILDINGS
Protects occupants from solar heat gain passing through walls.

COOLING CENTER
Protects under-air conditioned residents.

HEAT-RELATED INJURY & DEATH

HEART DISEASE

RESPIRATORY DISEASE

OBESITY/ DIABETES

MENTAL HEALTH

INFECTIOUS DISEASE

... TO THE HEALTH RISKS? 05

Note: Many of the design and operations strategies in the infographic bring co-benefits to other topics in this toolbox as well. See figure T.4 for a crosswalk of all of the environmental health co-benefits.

reduce agricultural yields for many products. It also requires more irrigation, which increases the stress placed on surface water sources. As temperatures rise, more foods must be refrigerated, which increases production expenses and increases the risk of spoilage before products reach the retail market. Extended periods of extreme heat also increase food insecurity among low-income households, because food spoils more quickly in warm weather.

T.6.e How Can Design Help?

Building and land use design can help protect people from the negative health effects of climate change in two ways. First, mitigation efforts reduce exposure to extreme heat by counteracting the urban heat island effect. At a community-planning scale, this approach translates into districts with compact, multi-use development interspersed with parks and green space and connected with public transit and active transportation infrastructure like sidewalks and protected bike lanes. At the building scale, designs that maximize use of vegetation, shading, and either light colored or vegetated roofs can help lower temperatures on and around the property.

The second opportunity to protect building occupants from extreme heat events is to reduce their exposure inside the building. Designs that maximize insulation, exterior shading, and energy efficiency measures will keep the building cooler for longer even if the heat wave triggers a utility blackout. Well-maintained buildings are another essential component of this strategy, because they help keep the cool air inside rather than leaking out through cracks in the envelope or forcing the mechanical system to work overtime because filters are clogged or ductwork is dirty. For net-zero buildings (i.e., buildings that generate as much power as they use) and projects located in regions with a fragile power grid, additional measures that will help future proof the building and increase the safety of occupants include installing islandable renewable power generation on-site and designating an area of the building as a cooling center for people who do not have air conditioning. The cooling center is also an opportunity for the building owner to demonstrate a commitment to social equity by opening the facility up for public use during heat events.

T.6.f Who Is Most Vulnerable?

The groups who are most likely to experience health setbacks during extreme heat events are the young,[369,384] the elderly,[369,384] pregnant people,[385–387] people suffering from chronic disease,[384] obese individuals,[165(p34),384] people living in poverty,[384] minorities, and people exposed to unsafe environmental conditions (such as people experiencing homelessness[384] and people living without access to air conditioning[27,356,385,388–390]).

T.6.f.i Children and the Elderly

The closer an individual is to the age extremes (whether young or old), the less their body is able to control its internal temperature and acclimatize to changing weather patterns.[369] It is therefore easier for these groups to suffer both hyper- and hypo-thermia. Both groups also often depend on caregivers to provide mobility and keep them out of harm's way.[27,356,385,391–393]

T.6.f.ii Pregnant People

Pregnant people are more sensitive to the physiological effects of extreme heat than the general population. Exposure to heat waves while pregnant has been associated with a heightened risk of preterm births, low birth weight, and infant mortality.[385–387]

T.6.f.iii Pre-existing Mental and Physical Health Conditions

Exposure to extreme heat, particularly over time, can also exacerbate underlying health conditions, such as heart disease, respiratory diseases (like asthma), and complications related to diabetes.[25(p46)] Furthermore, obesity (defined as individuals with a body mass index of 30 or above) is both a condition that can lead to all three of these chronic diseases and a risk factor in itself for increasing an individual's sensitivity to exposure to warm temperatures.[165(p34)] Finally, suffering from a mental illness could increase the risk of death during heat waves by up to a factor of 3.6.[290] This vulnerability may be partially explained by the fact that a disproportionate number of people experiencing homelessness suffer from mental illness.[394] Furthermore, some medications treating mental health concerns can interfere with the body's ability to regulate its temperature, increasing the risk of heat-related illness during extreme heat events.[395] For example, over half of the heat-related deaths associated with a heat wave in Wisconsin in 2012 were among people who were taking medication to treat mental illness.[396]

T.6.f.iv Minorities

While no race or ethnicity has been found to be physiologically more sensitive to the health effects of heat exposure, minorities in the US, particularly non-Hispanic African Americans, are at a higher risk of injury or death during and after heat waves due to the complex relationship between chronic disease, socioeconomic status, and the legacy of environmental injustices in many majority-minority neighborhoods.[27,356,385,389,397] Studies in Australia[397] and the UK[398] have treated minorities with linguistic and cultural differences from the majority populations as sensitive populations; however, additional research is needed to understand the similarities and differences between minority status in the US and in other parts of the world.[399]

T.6.f.v Poverty and Exposure to Unsafe Environmental Conditions

Living in poverty can expose individuals and families to heat-related risk factors if they do not have affordable access to environmental adaptations such as weatherized buildings and air conditioning.[27,356,385,388–390] Outdoor workers, such as construction and landscape workers, whose job involves significant physical exertion have been found to be at higher risk of heat-related illness and death during heat events[392,400,401] unless accommodations are made at the work site to allow for cooling down during breaks.[293] Finally, people experiencing homelessness are possibly the least protected group, particularly given the fact that many combine their exposure to the elements with other health risk factors such as psychiatric illness, chronic disease, and/or social isolation.[394]

T.7 Toolbox—Health Effects of Climate Change: Flooding

T.7.a Introduction

Flooding affects more people each year than any other natural disaster. Almost half of the deaths and one-third of economic losses attributed to natural disasters over the past few decades globally were caused by flooding.[402] In the US, flooding is both frequent and costly. 4,824 flooding events were recorded in 2018 in all but four US states (Hawaii, New Mexico, North Dakota, and Utah), resulting in 84 deaths, over $500 million in property damage, and over $400 million in damage to crops.[403]

T.7.b Definition

Flood forecasting models set warning thresholds based on a combination of hydrological, meteorological, topographic, structural, and social elements.[402] Given the complexity of predicting flooding vulnerability, the definition of an extreme precipitation event is tied to local precipitation data, such as a set threshold (i.e., 12 inches/30.5 cm over a 24 hour period) or a percentage increase (usually 90th, 95th, or 99th percentile) over average precipitation rates recorded at the local weather station.[357] This section of the toolbox addresses extreme weather events that include heavy rainfall but not wind. It will make passing references to the effects of hurricanes/tropical cyclones. For a more in-depth discussion of extreme weather events that combine precipitation with strong winds, please turn to section T.9 ("Disasters").

T.7.c Health Effects of Flooding

Flooding can lead to both direct and indirect health effects (table T.7). Direct exposure to flooding—often caused by traveling through or near floodwaters—can lead to injuries from floodwater debris, animal bites, electrocution, hypothermia, motor vehicle accidents on slippery roads, or drowning in extreme cases.[104,404–408] From 1986–2015, an average of 81 people died annually in the US as a direct result of flooding, making it the second leading cause of death from weather events after extreme heat.[409] Globally, an average of 5,424 people die and millions are affected each year as a direct result of flooding disasters.[351] The WHO estimates that climate change will exacerbate a rapid rise in deaths from coastal flooding over the coming decades in many regions of the world, particularly in North America and Asia.[410]

The aftermath of flooding is often characterized by polluted water and flooded buildings—leading to indirect health effects.

Stormwater runoff may be contaminated with fertilizers, herbicides, fungicides, and insecticides from agricultural lands; heavy metals, persistent bioaccumulative toxins, and other pollutants from mining and industrial facilities. Stormwater turbidity can strain municipal water treatment facilities or even temporarily put them out of commission.[411(p113)] Exposure to water that has been contaminated with sewage (i.e., combined-sewer overflows), chemicals from flooded agricultural or industrial sites, roadway runoff, and other pollutants can cause eye, ear, nose, throat, skin, and/or gastrointestinal infections.[104,408,412,413(p160)] Combined sewer overflows or direct contact with raw sewage are a particular concern in both developing and industrialized countries. The US EPA estimates that at least 23,000–75,000 sanitary sewer overflows occur each year in the US.[414] In 2014 alone, 1,482 combined sanitary and storm sewer overflows in the Great Lakes region resulted in an estimated 22 billion gallons of untreated sewage contaminating the Great Lakes Basin in the northern US and southern Canada.[415] In 2018, 79 out of 189 countries reported the percentage of domestic wastewater in their countries that was safely treated that year (Sustainable Development Indicator 6.3.1). Some of the highest reporting countries included Singapore at 100%, South Korea at 98.5%, the US at 89.9%, France at

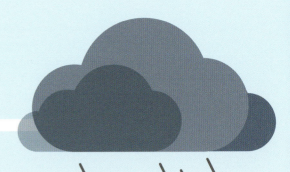

02 HOW DOES IT AFFECT THE BUILT ENVIRONMENT?

 ACCESS TO OUTDOOR ACTIVITIES
It can be dangerous to spend time outdoors during flooding events.

 STRESS ON PLANT & ANIMAL LIFE
It can slow plant and animal growth & increase the risk of disease.

 FOOD INSECURITY
Food supply can be disrupted after flooding events. Risk of spoilage.

 WATER QUANTITY & QUALITY
Flooding can increase nonpoint source pollution in waterways.

 PROVIDE MULTIMODAL EVACUATION ROUTES
Reduces the risk of getting trapped during evacuation if cars are not the only option.

 ON-SITE FOOD PRODUCTION
Increases food security for residents sheltering in place during an event or if supply is disrupted to grocery stores.

 NATIVE VEGETATION
Reduces the risk of flooding by absorbing & slowing stormwater flow across site.

 AVOID FLOOD-PRONE LOCATIONS
Avoid flood risk by locating the building outside of floodplains.

04 WHO IS MOST VULNERABLE...

 CHILDREN
Dependent on others for safety.

 ELDERLY
Frail with underlying medical conditions. Dependent on others for safety.

 PREGNANT WOMEN
Stress of displacement can increase the risk of premature birth.

 CHRONIC DISEASE
Home medical equipment may rely on electricity.

 POVERTY
Risk of exposure in poorly maintained buildings & reduced access to medical care.

 MINORITIES
Risk of exposure in poorly maintained buildings & reduced access to medical care.

 FLOODPLAINS
Risk of exposure to floodwater; getting trapped or drowning during evacuation.

Toolbox Infographic T.7. Linkages among Flooding, the Built Environment Determinants of Health, Protective Design and Operations Strategies, the Groups Who Are at Highest Risk, and Related Negative Health Outcomes

01 FLOODING

- Increase in rainfall intensity.
- Change in seasonal patterns of rainfall.

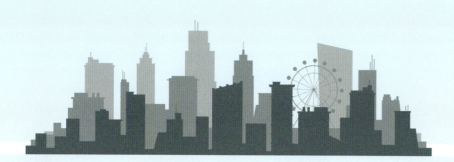

DISEASE-CARRYING VECTORS
It can trigger mosquito eggs to hatch & bring humans in contact with animals.

INFRASTRUCTURE DAMAGE
It can temporarily overwhelm & permanently damage infrastructure.

STRUCTURAL & MOISTURE DAMAGE
It can cause structural damage and mold growth in buildings.

EXPOSURE TO FLOODWATERS
They are often contaminated with chemical pollutants & waterborne pathogens.

03 HOW CAN DESIGN HELP?

CAPTURE, TREAT, REUSE WATER
Reduces the risk of waterborne disease during boil water notice.

ON-SITE RENEWABLE ENERGY
If connected to A/C, can protect occupants when power goes out.

PROTECT ENTRIES & SYSTEMS FROM WATER INTRUSION
Protects building from chronic flooding.

... TO THE HEALTH RISKS? 05

DISPLACED
High risk of negative mental & economic health.

RECOVERY WORKERS
Risk of exposure to floodwaters & flood debris.

RESPIRATORY DISEASE
FLOOD-RELATED INJURY AND DEATH

INFECTIOUS DISEASE
TOXIC CHEMICAL EXPOSURE
MENTAL HEALTH

UNDER- & MALNUTRITION

Note: Many of the design and operations strategies in the infographic bring co-benefits to other topics in this toolbox as well. See figure T.4 for a crosswalk of all of the environmental health co-benefits.

85.5%, and Australia at 73.4%. Some of the lowest reporting countries included Somalia at 0.7%, Lebanon at 13.4%, Argentina at 22.5%, and Turkey at 35%.[416]

As annual air temperatures have increased, temperate regions like the US Midwest have begun to see warmer water temperatures in rivers and lakes—accompanied by an increase in waterborne pathogens (which proliferate in warm water) and harmful algal blooms (HABs) which are caused by a combination of warmer water and fertilizer runoff from lawns and agricultural operations.[411(p113)] From 2007–2011, 458 human cases and 175 animal deaths were reported in the US from freshwater HAB-associated illnesses.[417] However, the real number of cases was likely higher given the fact that the US EPA estimates 30 to 48 million people in the US are currently at risk of exposure to HABs via their source of drinking water.[418] The risk to human health is even greater in regions that lack a water quality monitoring system. A case study of Ukerewe Island, Tanzania, which does not have a HAB monitoring program in spite of high nutrient loads in Lake Victoria, found that the rate of gastrointestinal illness among people who drink untreated lake and river water was 8.4 times higher than among groups who drink well water and 45.2 times higher than among people who drank treated municipal water.[419] As the climate and nutrient concentrations change, it is estimated that the length of an average HAB occurrence in the contiguous US will increase from seven days per year today to 16–23 days in 2050.[420]

Exposure to contaminated floodwaters is a serious health risk around the world but particularly in low- and middle-income countries. Flooding can overwhelm and contaminate the potable water and sanitary sewer systems, in addition to the stormwater system.[421(pp161–63)] Disrupted potable water supplies can lead to dehydration (particularly if the flooding occurs during warm months) and unsanitary conditions (which increases the risk of infectious disease).[422] In the US, 12–19 million cases of waterborne gastrointestinal disease are reported each year,[423–425] 97% of which can be traced to eight pathogens[426] that are benefiting from the trend of warming water in lakes and rivers[421(p160)] in temperate regions: norovirus, rotavirus, adenovirus, *Campylobacter jejuni*, *Escherichia coli* O157:H7, *Salmonella enterica*, *Cryptosporidium*, and *Giardia*.[426] While the numbers from the US are worrying, they pale in comparison with low- and middle-income countries, where unsafe water is the third highest risk factor for early death and disability.[41] In fact, access to treated potable water is such a fundamental public health concern worldwide that United Nations Sustainable Development Goal 6.1 seeks to increase the percent of the global population using safely managed drinking water services from 70.6% in 2017 to 100% in 2030.[427]

Moisture intrusion can foster mold growth in homes and workplaces within 48 hours of the flooding event,[428,429] potentially triggering or exacerbating chronic respiratory diseases.[113,114,429–435] If the flood causes a power outage or disables a building's heating, ventilation, and air conditioning system, the build-up of humidity and moisture can quickly lead to deteriorated indoor air quality.[436(p81)] Particularly during warm months (such as hurricane season), a flood immediately followed by a power outage can provide ideal conditions indoors for the proliferation of a mix of airborne contaminants, ranging from mold to dust mites to building materials' off-gassing VOCs like formaldehyde.[429–435] Loss of power is also associated with an increase in hospital visits due to CO poisoning, which can occur if backup generators or other combustion appliances are used indoors.[437,438]

It is estimated that 8%–20% of respiratory infections (such as acute bronchitis) and 4.6 million cases of asthma in the US are caused or exacerbated by the presence of dampness or mold in the home.[113,114] If moisture intrusion is not addressed quickly, a single flooding event can severely and permanently compromise indoor air quality even in buildings that previously had enjoyed low levels of airborne contaminants. For example, a case study in Khabarovsk in eastern Russia found a jump in asthma hospital visits among children and teenagers in the months following catastrophic river flooding in late summer 2013.[439] Two retrospective studies in New Jersey, USA, following Hurricanes Irene (2011) and Sandy (2012) found a marked increase in sensitivity to mold allergens after the hurricanes—increasing from 65% of patients before the hurricanes to 95% afterwards—and a statistically significant increase in sensitivity to both dust and dander (from 66.3% to 77.3%) and pollen (50.9% to 59.9%). Allergy patients were also younger and more likely to suffer from chronic lower respiratory diseases like asthma and chronic rhinitis after exposure to the hurricane.[440,441] A study in Bangkok, Thailand, also found changes in allergic sensitivities after a major flood in 2011. In that case, children's sensitivities to American cockroach, Bermuda grass, Johnson grass, and *Cladosporium* spp. declined after the flood, but their sensitivities to dog and *Alterneria* allergens increased over the same period.[442]

If standing water remains after a flooding event—particularly following a dry spell—it can support larval development and increase risk of mosquito-borne diseases several weeks later.[443–446] For example, an outbreak of dengue in Cairns, Australia, in late 2008 – early 2009 has been attributed to a combination of unseasonably heavy rainfall 1.5 months before the outbreak (potentially triggering eggs to hatch), unseasonably warm weather during the period when the first wave of larvae were maturing into adult mosquitoes (enhancing transmission of the disease to humans), and continued wet weather throughout the epidemic (providing sufficient moisture to support ongoing cycles of mosquito reproduction). In the end, 931 people were confirmed as infected with dengue and one person died of the disease.[447]

Malnutrition can be an indirect health effect of flooding if floodwaters disrupt food transportation routes, contaminate local food supplies, and/or destroy local crops. Disruptions in transportation routes tend to impact urban areas by creating food shortages or causing increased pricing. Communities along the Gulf Coast of the US experienced a scarcity of grain in the aftermath of Hurricane Katrina, because the storm surge temporarily incapacitated the barge transportation network.[448] In rural areas, the impact of a destroyed crop can lead to economic hardship, food insecurity for the farmer and his/her family, and mental distress.[448,449] A study of rural villages in the Jagatsinghpur district of India found that children who had been exposed to recurrent flooding were more likely to be underweight or malnourished than their peers in villages that had not been flooded.[450]

Finally, devastating floods can strain mental health if individuals lose loved ones, property, employment, and/or social networks.[104,404,408] In fact, a case study in Lewes, southern England, found that psychological distress was the most statistically significant health outcome among adults following a catastrophic flood in 2000—possibly even inflating some flood victims' perceptions of physical ailments, such as earache and gastroenteritis.[451]

T.7.e Relationship with Climate Change

Flooding is associated with a number of climatic events. Perhaps the most dramatic example is flooding in conjunction with hurricanes. In 2019, the IPCC expressed high confidence that human-caused climate change is associated with the increasing intensity of hurricanes that have been experienced over the past 30 years.[452] Three hurricanes that hit the Caribbean and the US in 2017 (Harvey, Irma, and Maria) cost the region $245.4 billion, more than $100 billion more than the global annual average cost of natural disasters.[453] Disparities between high-income and low-income countries were on particular display that year, where Cyclone Ockhi resulted in a much lower economic burden in India and Sri Lanka (estimated US$920 million[454]) but the second highest number of deaths by event (911 deaths).[453] The third highest death count that year (834 deaths) was attributed to a flood in India, Nepal, and Bangladesh that was not connected to an organized cyclone but still affected almost 27 million people in those countries.[453]

The IPCC reports that the global mean sea level rise accelerated over the decade from 2006–2015 due to a combination of historic ice loss from the Greenland and Antarctic ice sheets, loss of glacier mass, and the expansion of oceans as their temperatures warm.[452] Coastal cities along the East Coast of the US from Maine to Florida have begun to experience regular flooding during high tide due to rising sea levels caused by climate change.[455,456] Additionally, sea level rise has been attributed to a 33% increase in flooding after rain events in Miami, Florida, USA, from 2003 to 2013.[457]

River flooding is also a growing concern. Studies of regions as different as the US Midwest[458] and the African Sahel[459] have attributed increased flood risk near rivers to climate change and land use decisions that, together, increase streamflow. Finally, catastrophic flooding is often the unfortunate circumstance ending the severe droughts that have been exacerbated by global warming—adding another layer of suffering on top of the challenges caused by months or years of inadequate rainfall. For example, both drought and flooding are projected to increase by 50% in California by 2100.[460] Climate models predict that, by 2050, global river flooding will increase substantially in frequency, the number of people impacted, the quantity of crops destroyed, and overall flooding risk.[461]

Climate records for many regions in the world show a less dramatic change in total annual precipitation caused by climate change over the past 50 years than changes in annual average temperature.[342] However, seasonal trends tell a different story, because rainfall is not distributed equally across the year. As temperatures rise, the warmer air absorbs larger quantities of moisture, resulting in heavier rainfall especially in late winter and early spring. The redistribution of rain events can lead to flooding in the spring—disrupting planting season—and drought in the summer and fall, disrupting harvest.[462] The historical climate trends recorded by the Kentucky Climate

TABLE T.7.

Direct and Indirect Health Effects of Exposure to Floodwaters

Exposure	Health Effects
Direct	- Drowning[218,411,459,460] - Electrocution[104] - Hypothermia[218,411] - Injuries from a motor vehicle accident[218,460,461] - Injuries from debris, animal bites[104,411]
Indirect	- Deteriorated mental health[104,411,415] - Eye, ear, nose, throat, skin, and/or gastrointestinal infection[104,415] - Respiratory disease[113,114,436–442] - Under- and mal-nutrition[455–457] - Vector-borne disease[450–453]

Center show an appreciable increase in the 30-year average annual air temperature in western Kentucky since the 1970s compared with relatively stable total inches of rainfall. However, average precipitation during spring months follows the upward trend of average air temperature more closely (figure T.2). Similarly, 81% of weather stations in northeastern Europe show that spring flooding has shifted earlier—up to a week or more—over the past 50 years due to earlier spring snowmelt, whereas the Mediterranean coasts in Spain and France have shifted towards later flooding, due to the timing of strong precipitation and saturated soils.[463]

While climate models are not as accurate at estimating future changes in annual precipitation as changes in temperature, they predict more intense rain events with a high level of certainty.[464] Furthermore, 300–400 million people living in coastal flood zones around the world are projected to be exposed to a high risk of flooding due to sea level rise by 2060.[465] Coastal cities in Asia are particularly at risk. In 2000, over 70% of global populations living in 100-year low-elevation coastal floodplains were located in Asia, many in urban areas experiencing rapid population growth. By 2060, this population is projected to double in size.[465]

Modifying the built environment to absorb more rainfall on-site in areas experiencing heavier and heavier rainfall events and protecting coastal areas against sea level rise will be essential to protecting these areas from chronic flooding and associated risks to human health and the economy.

T.7.f How Does Flooding Affect the Built Environment?

Roughly 10% of the world population currently lives in low-lying coastal zones. It is estimated that by 2050 more than 800 million people in 570 coastal cities around the world will be at risk of constant flooding due to sea level rise.[466] Many communities in the interior—away from the coast—are also located next to rivers or lakes and are thereby at risk of periodic flooding. For example, roughly 25% of the population in Hungary live in floodplains surrounding the Danube river and its major tributaries.[467] In both cases, impervious areas introduced by development in the form of roads, buildings, and parking can disrupt the pathway that rain would normally follow after contact with the ground—either being absorbed or moving downhill to a river or other body of water.

Land use and building design decisions can reduce (or mitigate) these conditions—thereby minimizing the severity of flooding when it occurs—by returning the land to as close an approximation as possible of pre-development perviousness and by slowing the movement of stormwater, so that it has the opportunity to be absorbed into the ground rather than rushing into water bodies, which may already be at capacity.

Many countries have developed infrastructure and public safety protocols to reduce the risks of flooding to human health and the local economy following the United Nations Sendai Framework for Disaster Risk Reduction (https://www.unisdr.org/we/coordinate/sendai-framework).

T.7.f.i Exposure to Floodwaters

According to one estimate, floodplains occupy more than 13 million square kilometers (5 million square miles) of land area globally, representing between 6% (North America) and 13% (Africa) of a continent's total land mass.[468] The US Federal Emergency Management Agency (FEMA) estimated that over 17,800,000 people lived within a FEMA designated flood hazard area in 2011.[469] People living, working, and visiting these locations are at enhanced risk of exposure to flooding due to climate change.[105,368,470] The US National Climate Assessment identifies heavy precipitation and flooding as a major hazard for roads and bridges, often making them impassable for days or weeks at a time.[471] One study estimates that the annual damage from flooding in the US will double if global temperatures warm by 3°C (5.4°F).[472] Another study estimates that the number of hours of travel delay on flooded roadways caused by high tides along the East Coast of the US will increase from 100 million hours annually today to 1.2 billion hours in 2060.[473]

The two major pathways to flooding exposure are (1) being trapped inside of a structure and (2) traveling on or near flooded roadways. In the US, the majority of deaths from flash flooding take place in a vehicle (60%) or when someone is swept up by the floodwaters (20.5%). Only 8.4% of fatalities take place inside a permanent building or mobile home.[474] However, building condition continues to be a major risk factor associated with flooding, particularly in low- and middle-income countries. A case study of the 2012 flood in Lokoja, Nigeria, reported similar findings to US statistics in that most of the deaths occurred outside the home when residents (mostly children) were caught unawares at the beginning of the flood. However, there were two major differences from the experience in the US, both of which stem from the relative poverty of Lokoja residents. Most deaths occurred outside of a vehicle. And many of the buildings that were destroyed were poorly constructed and (in some cases) occupied before they were completely constructed.[475]

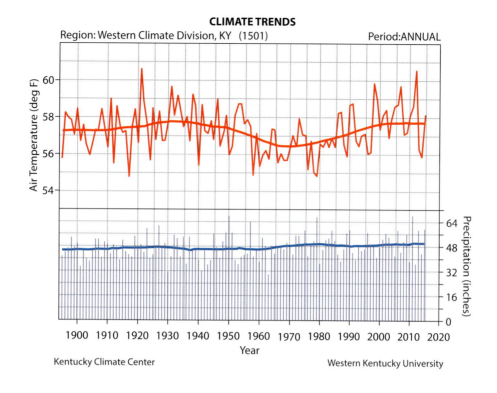

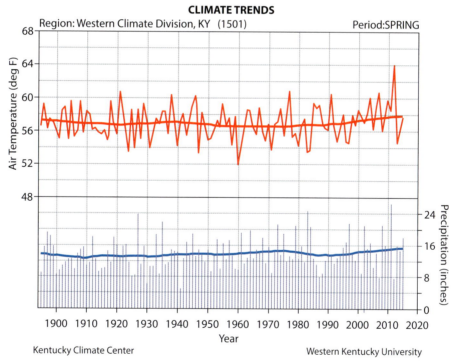

Figure T.2. Historical Climate Trends for Precipitation and Air Temperature in Western Kentucky, USA: Annual and Spring Months

Note: Heavy line displays 30-year moving average

Source: Climate and Health Addendum to 2015 Green River Community Health Assessment. 2016. Green River District Health Department, Owensboro, Kentucky, https://healthdepartment.org/wp-content/uploads/2016/06/GRDHD-2016-CHA-Addendum-Climate-Risks-and-Associated-Negative-Health-Effects-9-2016-CHA-Addendum-2016-1.pdf. *Data Source:* Kentucky Climate Center, Department of Geography and Geology, Western Kentucky University. Accessed May 3, 2016.

T.7.f.ii Flood-Related Structural and Moisture Damage

Flooding can cause structural damage and/or moisture intrusion, both of which can have short- and long-term effects. Heavy rainfall can damage a building's roof and/or facade, leading to moisture intrusion that can create conditions for mold growth, attract pests, and rot structural elements like wood beams.[476] Damage to building foundations and walls can be caused by floodwaters that are deep and/or moving at a high velocity (particularly if they are carrying heavy debris).[477,478] A study looking at the most important mechanisms for structural failure from flooding in the Netherlands found that, while the depth and velocity of floodwaters closest to the source of the flooding (a levee breach, in this case) put structures in that area most at risk of wall failure, the real risk of damage was contingent on the kinds of floating debris swept up in the floodwaters.[479]

While structural damage is arguably the most immediate threat to safety, moisture damage can lead to long-term health consequences if it is not addressed within a few days after the flood—particularly in warm weather. If building finishes and contents are not dried out within 72 hours of the storm, the moisture damage caused by flooding can cause so much damage to absorptive materials like drywall, carpets, curtains, and furniture that owners may be forced to remove and replace all building finishes and contents.[476,480,481] A case study measuring levels of mold and endotoxins before, during, and after the drywall and furnishings were removed and replaced in three houses in New Orleans, Louisiana, USA, flooded by Hurricane Katrina found unhealthy concentrations at baseline that matched or exceeded levels found in some industrial and agricultural environments. The level of endotoxins remained high in one of the houses even after the intervention, demonstrating the difficulty of eliminating this problem once it begins—although the investigators suspected that their post-intervention reading had detected dead bacteria in the household dust.[482]

T.7.f.iii Resilience of Utilities and Infrastructure to Flooding

When flooding disrupts transportation networks and key public services—such as electricity, telephone, internet, and water—a flooding event that might have been mildly disruptive to daily routines quickly transforms into a major catastrophe. This is particularly true in industrialized countries, where modern buildings, for the most part, are not designed to function "off the grid."[483] For example, after two days of heavy precipitation in May 2010 caused a 1,000-year flood in Nashville, Tennessee, USA—resulting in 31 deaths and $1.5 billion of property damage—50 roads were closed, one of two water treatment plants went offline, and 36,000 Nashville Electric Service customers lost power including the entire central business district.[484(p36)]

If evacuation is anticipated to occur on foot, pedestrian evacuation routes should be designed to minimize risk of exposure to floodwaters. A case study analysis in Japan found repeated examples of pedestrians being swept away by floodwaters while walking to designated shelters. The same study found that a number of designated shelters in the Edogawa Ward in Tokyo—70% of which is below sea level—would be inaccessible during a flooding event, because the surrounding roads are prone to flooding.[485]

T.7.f.iv Water Quantity and Quality

The damage to human health and property caused by a flooding event is largely determined by the extent to which water is not absorbed into the ground or channeled away from human settlements. If that excess water is contaminated, it poses an even greater danger to people and property. Because, as discussed above, floodwaters can contain anything from eroded soil to animals, debris, chemicals, human waste, biological pathogens, or a mix of all of the above. For example, in a case study of Mexico City, residents in lower income neighborhoods reported an ongoing need to clean out their homes and streets after flooding events, because floodwaters combining stormwater with raw garbage washed down from neighborhoods at higher elevations.[486] Suburban sprawl can also exacerbate flooding events and compromise water quality in wealthy regions such as the Washington, DC, USA, metro area. Researchers have identified the 60% increase in urban sprawl surrounding nearby Chesapeake Bay from 1990 to 2000 as a probable cause of the increasing levels of nitrogen contaminating the bay that were observed starting in the early 2000s.[487]

T.7.f.v Disease-Carrying Vectors

Floods can lead to three waves of surges in disease-carrying animal populations (known as "vectors" in public health parlance). During the flood itself, rodents, cockroaches, and other vectors may enter buildings or encounter evacuees passing through floodwaters as they attempt to escape drowning. The second wave occurs a few weeks after the flood. During warm months of the year, and particularly if the flood ends a dry spell, the rain event could trigger dormant mosquito eggs to gestate, leading to a bloom of mosquitoes two to three weeks after the event. The third phase is longer term. If moisture intrusion is not addressed quickly and thoroughly in flooded buildings, the ongoing moist environment can attract pests to buildings that previously had been pest-free.[444,445] Increased exposure to disease-carrying vectors is a growing concern in many regions around the world, as the climate continues to shift towards more frequent droughts followed by flooding events. The confluence of climate change, demographic shifts, rapid urbanization, and cyclic weather patterns like El Niño have led to increased exposure in the Americas to the mosquito that is the main transmitter of serious diseases like dengue, Zika, chikungunya, and yellow fever—*Aedes aegypti*.[488(p545)]

T.7.f.vi Access to Outdoor Activities

The extent to which community inhabitants have access to an interconnected network of parks and green spaces can impact both their exposure to floodwaters and their level of awareness regarding alternative evacuation routes. Interconnected vegetated spaces can act as a secondary stormwater distribution system, moving stormwater away from areas with the most intense rainfall or choke points (like rivers and streams), so that the region as a whole experiences less extreme flooding. Many times, these networks are also programmed for outdoor activities, such as walking, cycling, or sports. Combining flood control with increased access to nature is particularly important in low-income neighborhoods in the developing world. The World Bank estimates that the size of urban slums around the world will double by 2030 (increasing from 1 billion currently to 2 billion inhabitants) and that most of that growth will occur in floodplains and low-lying coastal areas that are vulnerable to flooding.[489]

T.7.f.vii Stress on Plant and Animal Life

The relative health of vegetated areas in and around cities and towns is a major factor in how successfully these areas absorb stormwaters—thereby protecting buildings and grey infrastructure. For example, a study of five cities on three continents (Bogotá, Colombia; London, UK; Chennai, India; Guayaquil, Ecuador; and, Jakarta, Indonesia) found that all of them depend on upstream water storage in peri-urban and rural areas to reduce urban flooding risk. Repeated and increasingly severe flooding, along with the other impacts of climate change, is reducing the ability of these upstream natural areas to continue to buffer the effects of heavy precipitation on the urban areas downstream. The study also found that only a small percentage of the upstream storage capacity was protected, ranging from 0% upstream of Chennai to 33% upstream of London.[490]

The natural ecosystem also suffers when exposed to contaminated floodwater. Much of the turbidity in floodwater—particularly in rural areas—is combination of topsoil and synthetic fertilizers.[491(p237)] For example, it is estimated that 75% of the turbidity in water bodies in England and Wales is caused by erosion of farmland.[492] When agricultural land loses topsoil, farmers are forced to use more chemicals—fertilizer, pesticides, herbicides, etc.—to make up for lost productivity. These chemicals then wash away in future floods, increasing the chemical burden placed on land downstream.[493(p92)] The Upstream Thinking (http://www.upstreamthinking.org) program run by the South West Water utility in the UK offers one systems-level solution to this problem. The utility provides technical expertise and grants to 750 farms and 1,300 hectares of moorland in southwest England that are upstream from water catchment areas to help farmers reduce the release of sedimentation, fertilizers, pesticides, and other pollutants into the region's potable water supply.

T.7.f.viii Food Insecurity

Severe flooding can temporarily disrupt customer access to grocery stores and store access to their supply chains.[448(p191)] A study of the 2011 flooding in Bangkok, Thailand, which left some neighborhoods underwater for up to 2 months, found that, while critical infrastructure—such as the power grid, water treatment plants, and hospitals—experienced relatively little flooding, supermarkets and grocery stores in some neighborhoods remained closed for the entire duration of the flood.[494] Residents living in "food deserts" (defined by the US Departments of Agriculture, Treasury, and Health and Human Services as locations with a poverty rate of 20% or more where at least one-third of residents live more than one mile from a supermarket or large grocery store) run a particularly high risk of exhausting their food supplies before access is restored. In 2006, 13.5 million people in the US lived in a food desert, mostly in urban areas.[495] More than 9% of households worldwide—684 million adults—are food insecure, according to the United Nations Sustainable Development Goals (Indicator 2.1.2, 2015–2017 three-year average).[427]

T.7.g How Can Design Help?

T.7.g.i Avoid Developing in Flood-Prone Locations

Locating new developments outside of the floodplain is the first step in protecting future occupants from the negative health consequences associated with flooding. Some jurisdictions have begun to restrict the use of private land in areas that are at high risk of flooding. For example, in response to major spring floods in 2017 and 2019, the Canadian province of Quebec instituted a policy prohibiting construction in areas that were flooded in 2017 and 2019 and/or located in the 0- to 20-year floodplain. The policy also restricts construction in the 20- to 100-year floodplain.

In regions with strong legal protections for private landowners, buyout programs often accompany stricter legislation regarding land use in flood zones. For example, after experiencing three 500-year floods in three years, more than $110 million has been set aside in the Houston, Texas, USA, metropolitan area to fund a voluntary buyout program to remove homes that have repeatedly flooded.[496] These lands will be used to increase stormwater capacity in the metropolitan area. And in many cases, they will be converted to dual use as parks and recreational areas,[497] which will benefit a city that, according to The Trust for Public Land, has only 2.5 parks per 10,000 residents (compared with 8.7 in Atlanta, Georgia).[498]

In some port cities, like Kolkata, India; Dhaka, Bangladesh; Shanghai, China; and, Miami, Florida, USA. the combination of sea level rise, subsidence, rapid population growth, and increased impervious surface may make it difficult to identify locations that are NOT flood prone by mid-century.[499] In those regions especially, it may be necessary to elevate buildings high enough off the ground to protect inhabitants and property during flooding events. Some of these cities are looking to the history of the 1900 hurricane that leveled Galveston, Texas, USA, and killed more than 6,000 people. After that event, the city took the extraordinary step of raising 2,000 buildings and the sewer, water, and gas mains from 8 to 16.5 feet in elevation in an effort to protect residents from damage in future storm surge events. A 3-mile long, 17-foot tall concrete seawall was also constructed on the side of the island facing the Gulf of Mexico.[500]

T.7.g.ii Increase Vegetation and Reduce Impervious Surfaces

This strategy dovetails with the previous strategy, because avoiding development in floodplains implies retaining vegetation in those areas. In general, converting impervious surfaces—such as roadways, surface parking lots, and sprawling buildings—into "green" (i.e., vegetated) infrastructure and pervious pavement (i.e., pavement that allows water to percolate through it rather than simply flow over it) can mitigate flooding by slowing down the speed at which stormwater moves off-site.[501] For this reason, cities as diverse as Chicago, Illinois, USA;[502] Colombo, Sri Lanka;[501] Singapore;[501] and, Rio de Janeiro, Brazil[503] have embraced the concept of combining traditional "grey" (i.e., concrete and steel) stormwater infrastructure networks with a complementary network of vegetation on or next to roads, parking lots, and building roofs. Even the US Federal Highway Administration has begun to address the impact of impervious roadways on flood risk by incentivizing the use of permeable pavement on secondary roadways in its sustainable best practices toolkit, INVEST (criteria PD-24 Permeable Pavement).[504]

If properties are connected to a network of linear parks and hike and bike trails, community members gain access to an alternative transportation network that could be useful for evacuation purposes during a flooding event. The educational signage and park education programs in these green infrastructure networks can be used educate the community about the dangers of flooding and how to protect themselves and their family—including options for evacuation routes.[505] For example, the Kobe City Master Plan (Japan), which lays out an interconnected network of "green spaces" and "green axes," was explicitly designed to increase both flood control and the number of evacuation routes and safe zones available to city residents in the event of a natural disaster.[506]

T.7.g.iii Provide Multimodal Evacuation Routes

Reports of New Orleans, Louisiana, USA, residents blockaded in the city after Hurricane Katrina[507] are a stark reminder that the way streets, bridges, and other infrastructure are designed can either trap or assist in the evacuation of residents during catastrophic events. Many metropolitan areas develop evacuation plans with only passenger cars in mind, forgetting that the public transit system, cycling infrastructure, sidewalks, and other infrastructure supporting alternative modes of transportation may offer safer and faster routes to safety—particularly for low-income families, who often live in the neighborhoods at highest risk of flooding. However, the level of resilience and redundancy of transportation infrastructure can also increase or decrease the relative danger posed by a flooding event. For example, a study in Fort Lauderdale, Florida, USA, a flood- and hurricane-prone coastal city, recommended a variety of infrastructure improvements (e.g., elevating roads, improving drainage, installing pumps, installing alternate route signage) and ongoing maintenance protocols (e.g., expediting road repair at critical intersections and highway exits, tree trimming, equipment for first responders to speed re-opening flooded streets) with the goal of minimizing road blockages during and after flooding events.[508] Evacuation plans that include multiple modes of transportation to move populations out of the most dangerous areas in a community are inherently more resilient than the alternative. For example, an emergency evacuation plan for the Washington, DC, USA, area includes consideration of pedestrian evacuation routes, re-routing city buses, and using the subway system to speed the transfer of people to safe areas—particularly individuals with special needs.[509]

T.7.g.iv Protect Building Systems and Entries from Damage Associated with Water Intrusion

Many sites are flood prone even if they are not technically located within a floodplain. Over the long run, the changes in precipitation patterns and rising sea levels caused by climate change will likely result in new definitions for what constitutes a floodplain. In the short term, cities and regions around the world have started to incorporate flood protection recommendations into their land use and building codes. The Dutch have famously decided to "live with water." In other words, they have built and continue to build a patchwork of canals, waterways, dikes, and green infrastructure to hold excess water and move it away from dry land.[510] Historic buildings in flood-prone areas of the Netherlands and Venice, Italy, also allow for recurrent water entry on the ground floor by installing water resistant finish materials. Historically, these buildings were thoroughly cleaned after each flood event to prevent moisture damage and mold growth.[511] After Hurricane Sandy demonstrated the vulnerability of New York City to flooding from storm surge, the city adopted a set of design guidelines which, among other things, encourage buildings to install flood barriers at grade and to locate mechanical systems, water pumps, emergency generators, and other essential equipment at higher elevations.[512] The US FEMA has developed technical guidance documents for flood-proofing residential[513] and non-residential[514] buildings that provide detailed information about how to design, specify, and install flood barrier systems.

T.7.g.v On-Site Renewable Energy and Microgrids

The extent to which public utilities are decentralized, redundant, and flood-proof helps determine the level of self-reliance or passive survivability that needs to be incorporated into designs at the site scale.[515,516] On-site renewable power or connection to a microgrid can be a valuable resource when the electrical grid is disconnected, as long as they can island (i.e., separate) the property or microgrid from the central grid until power is restored. For example, the desert town of Borrego Springs, California, USA, installed a community microgrid in 2007 after a wildfire destroyed their main transmission line. The system combines rooftop solar and solar farm power production, a thermal water storage facility, and backup diesel generators that can be disconnected from the macro-grid in the event of an emergency. In 2013, when a combination of lightning and flooding cut the same transmission line, the microgrid powered a gas station to allow residents to leave town, a cooling center in the town library to keep those who stayed cool, and the local elder residential community to protect the town's most vulnerable population until the utility regained access to the macro-grid.[517,518] At a larger scale, researchers in Norway predict that the increasing share of on-site photovoltaic installations and zero energy buildings in that country will allow hydropower operators to lower reservoir levels by 20% prior to the annual spring flooding season, thereby reducing flood risk downstream.[519]

T.7.g.vi On-Site Water Capture and Treatment

Many countries allow property owners to collect rainwater to irrigate their gardens. And locations as diverse as Australia, Brazil, China, Taiwan, Thailand, and Texas and Ohio in the US also permit rainwater to be used as drinking water within certain parameters—such as installing a backflow preventer to prevent accidentally contaminating the public water system.[520-522]

On-site drinking water treatment systems are also gaining in acceptance. In rural Tanzania, a photovoltaic-powered reverse osmosis water filtration system has been found to effectively remove contaminants from the local water source.[523] While regulations governing potable water in industrialized countries often stand in the way of distributed water purification systems such as the one used in Tanzania, they may come to be seen as a viable alternative to rebuilding the antiquated central water system in some US cities that have experienced lead contamination, such as Flint, Michigan, and Washington, DC, USA.[524]

Similarly, on-site systems that treat and reuse wastewater are more common in low- and middle-income countries and countries suffering from water scarcity than in industrialized countries as a whole. The systems themselves range from smaller versions of conventional centralized treatment systems (found in the Philippines and Vietnam, for example[525]) to green infrastructure such as constructed wetlands (e.g., China, Colombia, Nicaragua, Peru[525]) to dry/semi-dry treatment systems (e.g., Australia, Germany, Moldova, Philippines, Rwanda, Sierra Leone[526,526]). Constructed wetlands in particular can reduce both flooding risk and the risk of exposure to contaminated water.[528-530] A growing body of research shows that these systems both effectively remove contaminants (sometimes with the help of secondary treatment systems like ultraviolet sterilization) and are less expensive to build and operate than conventional centralized wastewater treatment systems.[525,531] However, the level of adoption varies by jurisdiction, due to different levels of regulatory barriers and comfort among water consumers regarding whether or not they are willing to use treated water as drinking water or only for non-potable uses such as flushing toilets and irrigation.[525,527,532] Several buildings in the US that have been certified under the Living

Building Challenge—including the Arch Nexus SAC office building in central Sacramento, California, USA[533]—are equipped to achieve "net zero" or "net positive" water consumption (i.e., all water consumed on-site is produced and treated on-site) as soon as public health regulations are updated to allow distributed water and wastewater treatment systems.

T.7.g.vii On-Site Food Production

On-site food production offers several advantages in flood-prone areas. First, it can reduce the threat of floodwaters damaging property or putting building occupants in harm's way by collecting rainwater for irrigation and by directly absorbing the precipitation that falls on the plants.[534–536] Combined, the 132 community gardens in New York City, New York, USA, can store over 1 million gallons of rainwater.[534] The daily benefits of on-site food production reducing the risk of under- or mal-nutrition in food deserts are enhanced during the days and weeks following a flooding event if roads are unpassable or the food delivery system has otherwise been temporarily disrupted. For example, a study of disruptions to the food supply in Queensland, Australia, following widespread flooding in late 2010 and early 2011 found that, while deliveries were disrupted to large grocery stores after the flood, local food providers were able to reach customers through small-scale mechanisms like community supported agriculture, farmers markets, and food coops. Furthermore, these smaller food distributors were able to donate excess food to shelters and residents in need of assistance.[537] It is important to harvest food prior to flooding events if the agricultural area is located on the ground level of a site to avoid contaminated floodwaters rendering the plants inedible.[536]

T.7.h Who Is Most Vulnerable?

Vulnerability to flooding is influenced by physiological, social, and contextual characteristics.

T.7.h.i Children and the Elderly

Children and the elderly are more likely to depend on others for transportation. As a result, they are at a higher risk of becoming trapped during a flooding event, potentially in a building that has lost power.[104,105] Children's risk of injury or death is heightened if they become separated from their caregiver during an evacuation.[538–540] Both children and the elderly are also less resilient to the strains that flooding can place on their mental health, particularly if they are displaced from their home and social network.[541(p108)]

T.7.h.ii Pregnant People

Exposure to catastrophic flooding has been associated with increased complications during pregnancy, an increased rate of preterm births, and lower birth weights than pre-disaster.[542,543]

T.7.h.iii Chronic Disease and Pre-existing Conditions

Similar to children and the elderly, patients who are disabled, admitted to hospital, or living in a nursing home or assisted living facility depend on caregivers to safely evacuate them if flooding is severe.[104,544–547] In some cases, this requires healthcare workers to perform heroic acts. For example, three days after Hurricane Katrina flooded New Orleans, Louisiana, USA, in 2007, the emergency generators at Tulane Hospital ran out of fuel. Given that roads remained impassable, hospital staff carried patients down flights of stairs to a makeshift heliport that they had built on the roof of the parking garage, to ensure safe evacuation.[548] Ambulatory patients who depend on routine medical treatment or prescriptions may be at a higher risk of illness after a flooding event if supplies are disrupted or if roads are impassable for long periods of time.[96,97,100,101] Patients who depend on electric powered medical equipment, such as oxygen or ventilators, may be placed at immediate and acute risk if the flood results in a power outage.[104,106,107] Those patients with compromised immune systems (such as cancer patients) are also at heightened risk of infection if they come in contact with contaminated floodwaters.[104,105]

T.7.h.iv Minorities and Minority-Language Speakers

In the US, non-Hispanic African American and Hispanic individuals are at higher risk of flood-related injury and/or death, because a range of social and economic factors increase their level of exposure to dangerous flood conditions.[104,105] Populations who speak minority languages are also at higher risk because they may experience a delay in receiving evacuation orders or other pertinent information relayed by emergency management personnel in the majority language.[104,105]

T.7.h.v Families Living in Poverty and Populations Located in Floodplains

Families living in poverty are more likely to live in unsafe conditions, such as floodplains (where they are directly at risk of flooding-related injuries or death) and substandard housing (where they are at risk after flooding events of indirect health concerns such as mold growth caused by moisture intrusion).[104,105] As a result, these families are more likely to be displaced from their home, place of employment, and social network—three of the most powerful causes of strain on mental health after exposure to a natural disaster.[541(p108)] People experiencing homelessness are arguably the most vulnerable group. Many housing insecure individuals and families live in flood-prone locations such as freeway underpasses, where they could be caught unawares by a flash flood. Their environmental vulnerability is often exacerbated by mental health concerns and/or chronic physical health conditions.[394]

T.7.h.vi Displaced Populations

Displaced populations in shelters (particularly infants and children) may be exposed to infectious disease, either from other shelter residents or from unhygienic surroundings.[104,408] They are also at heightened risk of mental illness, particularly if they have lost loved ones, property, economic security, and/or access to their social network as a result of the flood.[104,406,408,541(p108)]

T.7.h.vii Recovery and Remediation Workers

Mold, bacteria, and their byproducts proliferate after flooding events. If damp materials are not removed within 48 hours of the flood, recovery and remediation workers may be exposed to an unhealthy concentration of contaminants that can trigger or exacerbate respiratory illness, skin rashes, and other symptoms. For this reason, everyone working in flooded buildings should wear personal protective equipment. Rather than using biocides like bleach (which can aggravate respiratory conditions) to kill mold, remediators are encouraged to dry the building as quickly as possible, remove absorptive materials like drywall and carpet, and vacuum dust with a machine equipped with a high efficiency (i.e., HEPA or MERV 13) filter.[429]

T.8 Toolbox—Health Effects of Climate Change: Air Quality

T.8.a Introduction

Poor air quality can result from both natural and human-caused contamination. The three categories of contaminants addressed in this section were selected because site selection, building design, and building operations can reduce their emissions and/or protect occupants from their worst health effects.

The first two groups are emitted by combustion engines—both stationary sources like power plants and generators, as well as mobile sources like the exhaust from cars, trucks, and airplanes.

Ground-level O_3 is generated when VOCs like CO and/or methane (i.e., natural gas) are oxidized in the presence of sunlight and nitrous oxides (NOx). All of these components (except sunlight) are exhausted through the tailpipes of gas- and diesel-powered cars and trucks.[34]

Both gas- and diesel-powered vehicles emit $PM_{2.5}$, whereas PM_{10} is more of a concern for diesel-powered vehicles.[34]

Ozone and its precursors and particulate matter are regulated in many countries in an effort to reduce their impact on the environment and human health. US and WHO thresholds for O_3, NOx, and particulate matter are listed in table T.8.

Ozone and particulate matter ambient air pollution can be reduced in three ways:

1. *Increase the efficiency and filtration of combustion engines, so they burn less fuel and/or exhaust fewer contaminants:* An example of this approach includes US regulations that are slowly increasing minimum vehicle miles per gallon requirements and regulations requiring heavy duty trucks to use filters that reduce emissions of PM_{10} and NOx.[551] The incremental increase in minimum energy efficiency requirements in each subsequent version of the building code is an example from the building sector. The current model international energy conservation code has increased efficiency requirements by 30% over the past decade.[552]

2. *Switch to a non-polluting fuel (such as renewable energy or electric vehicles):* Examples of this approach in the US can be seen at the state level through Renewable Portfolio Standards and Renewable Portfolio Goals, which are policies intended to increase renewable energy as a percentage of a state's energy fuel mix. Thirty-seven out of the 50 states in the US, plus Washington, DC, and three territories have adopted either a Renewable Portfolio Standard or a Renewable Portfolio Goal.[553] At the local level, six cities in the US have fully transitioned to 100% clean, renewable energy sources to power their electric grid and more than 90 cities, 10 counties, and two states (New York and California)—home to 20% of the US population—have committed to achieving 100% renewable energy in their electricity grid by 2050. Internationally, more than 60 countries have committed to reaching net zero emissions by 2050.[554]

3. *Switch to a different approach:* For example, remove cars from the road and replace them with pedestrians and cyclists. In the industrial sector, this switch involves moving away from highly energy intensive production processes to processes that

OZONE
Formed when NOx & VOCs mix in the presence of sunlight. Irritates the respiratory system.

NITROGEN OXIDE
Emitted by fossil fuel combustion. Irritates the respiratory system.

PARTICULATE MATTER
Emitted by fossil fuel combustion. Can trigger or exacerbate cardiovascular disease, respiratory disease, cancer, and cognitive stunting or decline.

AEROALLERGENS
Allergens like grasses, trees, and mold can trigger or exacerbate respiratory disease and allergic conditions.

02 HOW DOES IT AFFECT THE BUILT ENVIRONMENT?

STRESS ON PLANT & ANIMAL LIFE
Pollution can harm plants & animals. It can also lead to higher concentrations of allergens.

URBAN HEAT ISLAND
Heat + air pollution increases the risk of asthma attacks in vulnerable groups.

NON ALLERGENIC LANDSCAPING
Plants that remove pollutants from the air but do not produce allergens.

VEGETATIVE & STRUCTURAL BARRIERS TO EMISSION SOURCES
Reduce exposure to large & heavy air pollutants.

COMPACT, MULTI-USE DEVELOPMENT NEAR TRANSIT & BIKE/PED INFRASTRUCTURE
Reduces the need for car travel, a major cause of air pollution.

LOCATE ON SITE EMISSIONS SOURCES AWAY FROM OPENINGS & AIR SUPPLY
Reduces the risk of pollutants entering the building.

ON-SITE RENEWABLE ENERGY
Use renewables to replace products of combustion on site.

04 WHO IS MOST VULNERABLE...

CHILDREN
More sensitive to exposure because organs & immune system are developing.

ELDERLY
More sensitive & many elderly also have underlying health conditions.

IMMUNO-COMPROMISED
More sensitive because weak immune system.

CHRONIC DISEASE
Increased sensitivity to air pollution.

ALLERGIC SENSITIVITY
Sensitive to exposure to aeroallergens.

POVERTY
Risk of exposure in poorly maintained buildings & polluted neighborhoods.

MINORITIES
Risk of exposure in poorly maintained buildings & polluted neighborhoods.

Toolbox Infographic T.8. Linkages among Air Quality, the Built Environment Determinants of Health, Protective Design and Operations Strategies, the Groups Who Are at Highest Risk, and Related Negative Health Outcomes

01
AIR QUALITY

- Increase in roadway & point source emissions.
- Increase in average temperatures.
- Increase in number & severity of wildfires.

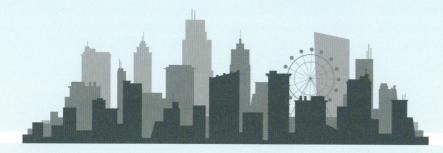

ACCESS TO OUTDOOR ACTIVITIES
It can be dangerous to spend time outdoors in polluted air.

INDOOR AIR QUALITY
Emissions increase indoors when outdoor air is polluted. Paint, adhesives, sealants, interior finishes, & equipment can also emit toxins.

03
HOW CAN DESIGN HELP?

FILTRATION
Filters out pollutants from both outdoor & indoor sources.

VENTILATION
Helpful if most pollution is generated indoors & outdoor air is clean.

LOW EMITTING MATERIALS
Reduces the concentration of pollutants generated indoors.

WELL-MAINTAINED BUILDINGS
Reduces the risk of mold & other allergens; ensures filtration is working.

SUBSTANDARD HOUSING
Risk of exposure to mold, pests, dust, & other allergns.

HEART DISEASE

RESPIRATORY DISEASE

LUNG CANCER

COGNITIVE STUNTING OR DECLINE

ALLERGIC DISEASE

... TO THE HEALTH RISKS? 05

Note: Many of the design and operations strategies in the infographic bring co-benefits to other topics in this toolbox as well. See figure T.4 for a crosswalk of all of the environmental health co-benefits.

can occur at room temperature (e.g., using green chemistry). A number of practices that fall into this category have been piloted in the building sector, such as transit-oriented development, New Urbanism, and complete streets. Many historic districts, tourist towns, and small islands around the world have closed off sections or even an entire territory to car and truck traffic.[555] Additionally, towns like Houten in the Netherlands[556] and Curitiba in Brazil[557] have been designed to make walking, cycling, and transit more convenient than single occupancy cars.

A number of middle- and high-income countries have substantially reduced their population's exposure to $PM_{2.5}$ since 1990 using a mix of these strategies, while O_3 pollution has proven more difficult to address.[220] According to the WHO, over 90% of the world's population are still exposed to air pollution exceeding WHO guidelines, in spite of efforts ramping up starting in the 1990s.[34] In the US, the 1990 revisions to the Clean Air Act resulted in improving ambient air quality in subsequent decades;[558] however, more than 130 million Americans continue to live in metropolitan areas that do not meet national ambient air quality standards for at least one criteria air pollutant.[559]

The third category of air pollution that will be addressed in this section, while produced by plants, is also exacerbated by car-centric land use planning.

Airborne allergens (also called aeroallergens):[436] Numerous studies have shown that allergenic plants like ragweed increase their pollen production along highly trafficked roadways because of increased concentrations of CO_2 from vehicle exhaust.[348,560–563] One study in Maryland found that ragweed at an urban site averaging 2°C higher temperature and 30% higher CO_2 levels than a comparison rural site produced more than double the amount of pollen.[564]

Worldwide, 40% of school-aged children are sensitive to at least one allergen. And the prevalence of allergic diseases such as allergic rhinitis and asthma is growing.[565] A nationally representative survey in the US, the National Health and Nutrition Examination Survey, found that sensitivity to allergens increased two to five times in orders of magnitude from the late 1970s to the early 1990s, depending on the allergen.[566] In 2005–2006, the same survey found that, while sensitization had leveled off or slightly declined across the US as a whole, almost half of the US population six years or older was sensitive to at least one environmental allergen. Interestingly, urban populations were more sensitive to grasses like ragweed and Bermuda grass than rural populations.[567]

T.8.b Health Effects of Air Pollution

Air pollution is the leading environmental risk factor for premature mortality worldwide and fifth overall, after poor diet, high blood pressure, tobacco exposure, and high blood sugar.[220] Exposure to poor air quality can cause or exacerbate respiratory disease, cardiovascular (heart) disease, allergic diseases, cancer, diabetes, chronic kidney disease, immunological, and neurological disease (table T.9).

T.8.b.i Ground-level O_3

Exposure to ground-level O_3 can irritate the respiratory system, triggering asthma, causing difficulty breathing, reducing lung function, and causing lung diseases like COPD.[34] The O_3 precursor NO_2 also irritates the respiratory system, and long-term exposure can lead to reduced growth in lung function.[34] After forming, O_3 can persist in

TABLE T.8.

Air Quality Thresholds: US and World Health Organization (WHO)

Contaminant	US threshold, 1990[560] Annual mean	US threshold, 1990[560] Daily mean	WHO threshold, 2005[561] Annual mean	WHO threshold, 2005[561] Daily mean
Ozone (O_3)	N/A	0.070 ppm, 8-hr mean	N/A	100 µg/m³, 8-hr mean
Nitrogen dioxide (NO_2)	53 ppb	100 ppb, 1-hr mean	40 µg/m³	200 µg/m³, 1-hr mean
Coarse particulate matter (PM_{10}; ≤10 µm)	N/A	150 µg/m³, 24-hr mean	20 µg/m³	50 µg/m³, 24-hr mean
Fine particulate matter ($PM_{2.5}$; ≤2.5 µm)	12.0 µg/m³ (primary) 15.0 µg/m³ (secondary)	35 µg/m³, 24-hr mean	10 µg/m³	25 µg/m³, 24-hr mean

TABLE T.9.

Direct and Indirect Health Effects of Exposure to Air Pollution

Exposure	Health Effects
Direct	• Allergic disease[571,577] • Premature mortality[223,583]
Indirect	• Cognitive stunting or decline[581] • Heart disease or stroke[34,583] • Lung cancer[34,584] • Reduced lung function[34,571,588] • Respiratory disease (especially asthma, COPD)[34,571,577,583]

the environment for days to months, traveling far from its source.[568] The Health Effects Institute estimates that exposure to O_3 accounted for 15% of COPD deaths globally in 2017—roughly 472,000 deaths, 69% of which occurred in China and India. Ozone-attributable deaths have been accelerating worldwide over the past decade, growing 15% from 2010 to 2017.[220] Climate models predict that climate change will slow progress in reducing ground-level ozone in some regions of the US, because increasing temperatures will accelerate the rate of O_3 formation and meteorological changes will increase the risk of stagnant air masses in some areas.[436] Climate models predict an annual increase of hundreds to thousands of O_3-related cases of acute respiratory illnesses, hospital admissions, and premature deaths in the US by 2030.[436]

T.8.b.ii Particulate Matter

The term "particulate matter" refers to a range of small particles and liquid droplets, including relatively benign substances like dirt as well as toxic chemicals like polycyclic aromatic hydrocarbons.[569] It is generally divided into three groupings based on size: PM_{10} (particles £10 µm in diameter), $PM_{2.5}$ (particles £2.5 µm in diameter), and ultrafine particles (UFPM; particles £0.1 µm in diameter). While substances fitting into these size categories could include particles with more or less mass, in general UFPM are considered most harmful to human health within 100 m (330 feet) of major roadways (figure T.3). PM_{10} and $PM_{2.5}$, on the other hand, fall to about 50% of their ambient concentration within 150 m (500 ft) of the roadway. But they can persist at harmful levels well beyond 400 m (0.25 miles),[570] similar to O_3. Exposure to PM_{10}, but particularly $PM_{2.5}$ and UPFM, has been associated with increased rates of premature mortality, cardiovascular disease, and respiratory disease.[571] According to the WHO, 4.2 million deaths glob-

ally in 2016 (over 500 deaths in the US) were attributable to exposure to $PM_{2.5}$—the primary causes of death being heart disease/stroke (58%), respiratory disease (18%), and lung cancer (6%).[34] A number of toxic chemicals found in particulate matter are also suspected or known carcinogens. In fact, the California state office of Environmental Health Hazard Assessment estimates that 70% of cancer risk in the state related to air pollution is caused by exposure to diesel particulate matter.[572] Finally, emerging research has linked long-term exposure to traffic-related particulate matter to reduced cognitive development in children and cognitive decline in the elderly.[569]

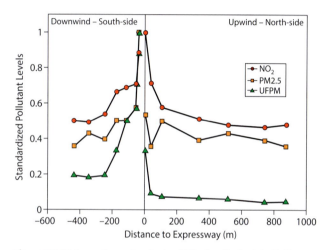

Figure T.3. Distance-Decay Gradients of Ultrafine Particulate Matter Near a Busy Expressway in Toronto, Ontario, Canada, Compared with NO_2 and $PM_{2.5}$. *Source:* Reprinted from Beckerman B et al. 2008[768] with permission from Elsevier

T.8.b.iii Aeroallergens

Environmental aeroallergens like grass pollen, tree pollen, and mold can lead to or exacerbate a variety of diseases in sensitive groups. These include respiratory diseases like asthma, inflammatory diseases like allergic rhinitis, and skin conditions like eczema.[565] It is estimated that up to 30% of populations in Western countries suffer from allergy-related diseases, placing an ongoing burden on the healthcare systems in these countries. For example, 7.5% of US adults (17.6 million)[573] and 9.0% of US children (6.6 million)[574] suffer from hay fever (only one of several allergy-related diseases), and a similar proportion, 8.3%, of US children, have been diagnosed with asthma.[575] In the US, asthma costs an individual, on average, $983 per year in medical costs, and results in 13.8 million days of missed school among school aged children.[575] The prevalence of allergic diseases have increased over the past 30 years worldwide, particularly in urban areas.[565]

T.8.b.iv Relationship with Climate Change

Ambient air pollution and climate change are interconnected in two primary ways. First, they are both caused in large part by the burning of fossil fuels. However, there is also a feedback loop between them: air pollution tends to worsen as temperatures increase. For example, higher temperatures have been found to increase O_3 levels and, separately, to increase the speed and productivity of plants producing aeroallergens.[436] Heat-related deaths have also been found to increase if the extreme heat event corresponds with high levels of O_3 or particulate matter.[577,578] For this reason, future climate projections anticipate worsening air pollution alongside increasing temperatures and other changes to the climate associated with rising GHG emissions.[436]

Climate change may affect particulate matter in a variety of ways. If regulations on gasoline mixes and exhaust controls for combustion engines continue to strengthen as part of climate change mitigation policies, then the ambient concentration of harmful particulate matter may decrease. Changes in humidity, precipitation, and stagnant air events may increase or decrease exposure to traffic-related particulate matter, depending on the circumstance. On the other hand, climate models predict more frequent and lengthy droughts and wildfires. By 2050, wildfires in the western US are predicted to increase emissions of organic carbon by 40% and elemental carbon aerosol concentrations by 20%. The particulate matter from both of these natural hazards can travel long distances, compromising air quality hundreds of miles from the source.[436]

Increased temperatures, increased concentrations of CO_2, and changes in precipitation patterns caused by climate change are predicted to lengthen the allergy season. The quantity, allergenicity, and spatial distribution of pollens are also expected to increase. It is also possible that simultaneous exposure to both allergens and air pollution may magnify the effects of an allergic reaction in some sensitive groups.[436]

According to the IPCC, the built environment is either directly or indirectly responsible for 45% of global GHG emissions: 6% from onsite energy generation and burning fuels for heat or cooking in buildings (including residential cook stoves in low- and middle-income countries), 25% from producing electricity and heat (much of which is used to power and heat buildings), and 14% from transportation (including single-use vehicle trips that are necessary because land use configurations make active modes of transportation and transit impractical).[579] In the US, the percentage of direct emissions from buildings and the transportation sector were both almost twice the global average (11.5% for buildings and 28.9% for transportation)

in 2017. When emissions from electricity use are included in the calculation, the building sector accounts for 31% of total US GHG emissions (16.1% commercial, 14.9% residential). And, almost two-thirds of transportation-related US GHG emissions (58.7%) were generated by passenger cars (41.2%) and SUVs, pickup trucks, and minivans (17.5% combined).[580] In other words, the way land use is configured in the US combined with the way buildings are designed and operated contributes to almost two thirds of the country's annual GHG emissions.

T.8.c How Does Air Pollution Affect the Built Environment?

The built environment and air pollution are interrelated at three scales. Public policy often focuses on the regional scale—regulating fuel and emissions at power plants, industrial installations, and combustion engines in cars and trucks. Once a real estate team selects a site, they have limited influence over those larger scale issues. They may consider whether or not the property is located downwind from a freeway or point source as part of the site selection process. But once a site has been selected, it is usually difficult to address the root cause of pollution. So, design strategies transition to shielding occupants from exposure. The one exception is TRAP. Some developments may have the ability to use traffic calming strategies along perimeter roads or even partner with local government to convert them into part-time or permanent pedestrian roads. The third scale of impact involves reducing exposure to airborne toxins inside the building. At this scale, air pollution may enter from the exterior or be generated inside by high-emitting building materials or operational practices (like cleaning and pest control).

Air pollution can also directly influence design. Outdoor amenities like parks and hike/bike trails may be perceived as less desirable on properties in highly polluted areas. Furthermore, air pollution has been found to increase pollen production among allergenic plants. It can also harm both plants and animals. TRAP is often accompanied by the urban heat island effect, because much of the urban heat island is composed of impervious surfaces for roads and parking lots. In these areas, the combination of air pollution and heat can increase the risk of asthma attacks in vulnerable groups.

T.8.d How Can Design Help?

Starting with the regional scale, public policies and regulations can help lower concentrations of ambient air pollution by accelerating the transition to renewable energy, net zero buildings, and electric vehicles. Land use and zoning requirements that prioritize compact, multi-use development near transit and bike/pedestrian infrastructure can reduce TRAP by reducing demand for and accommodation of single occupancy vehicles. Zoning regulations can also prohibit allergenic plants along roadways and in landscaping on public and private property.

At the property scale, efforts may focus on using vegetative and structural barriers to separate occupants from emissions sources blowing in from off-site. Similarly, project teams can catalog the location of potential on-site emissions (such as combined heat and power installations, emergency generators, and places where vehicles will idle). These sources may be eliminated in equipment by specifying non-emitting models—ideally, connected to on-site renewable power installations. No-idling policies coupled with locating carpool lines, ambulance waiting areas, loading docks, and the like away from doors, windows, and outdoor air intakes can also reduce the risk of introducing pollution into the building.

Inside emissions sources can be reduced by designing a fully electrified building, specifying low emitting finish materials, and establishing green cleaning and integrated pest management policies. Designing the mechanical system to support high levels of ventilation and high-efficiency filtration can further reduce the concentration of airborne pollutants by lowering their indoor concentration and filtering them out of the air.

T.8.e Who Is Most Vulnerable?

The groups who are at most risk of experiencing a negative health effect from exposure to poor air quality are the young, the elderly, people who are immunocompromised, people suffering from chronic disease, people with allergy sensitivities, people living in poverty, minorities, and people living in primitive or substandard housing.

T.8.e.i Children and the Elderly

In many ways, the vulnerabilities of children and the elderly to air pollution mirror each other. For example, exposure to particulate matter can slow cognitive growth in children and speed its decline in the elderly. It can also slow the growth of lung function in children and speed its decline in the elderly.[436,576] As the groups representing the beginning and end of the human life course, both children and the elderly inhabit bodies that are more fragile than healthy adults. The elderly are at high risk of morbidity or mortality after exposure to poor air quality.[576,581] And, children are at heightened risk of developing asthma if they are exposed to allergens.[582] Their developing respiratory and immune systems, coupled with their tendency to spend time outdoors and on the floor, make them highly susceptible to developing sensitivity to aeroallergens.[436]

T.8.e.ii Immunocompromised

People with compromised immune systems, such as people undergoing chemotherapy, are at heightened vulnerability to air pollution because their bodies' defenses are less robust than healthy adults.[583]

T.8.e.iii Chronic Physical and Mental Health Conditions

Exposure to air pollution can trigger severe symptoms in individuals living with chronic conditions like heart disease, asthma, COPD, hypertension, and diabetes.[436,576,584] Exposure to $PM_{2.5}$ in particular has been associated with inflammation and oxidative stress, which—in addition to exacerbating diseases like heart disease, respiratory disease, and diabetes—can exacerbate depression and anxiety symptoms among patients with pre-existing mental health conditions. For example, a population-scale study in Shanghai, China, found that a 10 µg/m³ increase in the 2-day moving average concentrations of sulfur dioxide and particulate matter in ambient air were associated with a 6.9% and 1.3% (respectively) increase in the daily number of psychiatric hospitalizations in the city.[585] A study in the US found that an incremental rise in $PM_{2.5}$ levels increased the risk of anxiety symptoms among patients aged 57 years and older by 60% and increased their risk of depressive symptoms by 16%.[586] Furthermore, a study in South Korea found that patients with underlying diabetes, cardiovascular disease, or COPD were at heightened risk of developing major depressive disorder after exposure to $PM_{2.5}$—possibly via the same physiological pathways (inflammation and oxidative stress).[587]

T.8.e.iv Sensitivities to Allergens

People who are already sensitized to a particular airborne allergen are more likely to respond to exposure to aeroallergens and other types of air pollution with an allergic reaction.[436,565,576] However, the severity of the reaction depends on the number of airborne particles coming in contact with the individual's eyes, nose, and skin; the length of time the individual is exposed; and, the extent to which they can be isolated from the allergen when indoors.[565]

T.8.e.v Families Living in Poverty

Low socioeconomic status increases vulnerability to air pollution for a number of reasons. Lower income neighborhoods are often located closer to the sources of air pollution. Poorly maintained housing can allow higher levels of polluted outside air to infiltrate into the indoors.[436] People living in poverty also often have reduced access to medical services for preventive care and treatment. They are also more likely to live with pre-existing conditions that increase their vulnerability to air pollution.[576] In the US, children living in poverty have been found to be 1.75 times more likely than other children to be hospitalized for asthma-related symptoms.[588,589]

T.8.e.vi Minorities

In the US, racial and ethnic minorities experience higher levels of exposure to both industrial sources of air pollution and mobile sources, due to the history of redlining and other exclusionary regulations that forced non-White families to live and work in neighborhoods that were zoned for industrial use.[590] They also experience higher levels of asthma than the general population. For example, a study in California found that asthma rates among African American and Hispanic children was higher than White children, but they were less likely to use preventative medications to control it. Both groups also reported increased use of the emergency room and rescue medications, regardless of how well they controlled their daily symptoms.[588,589]

T.8.e.vii Primitive and Substandard Housing

Outdoor pollutants make their way indoors through doors, windows, outdoor air intakes, and cracks in the building envelope. Many homes rely on doors and windows to mix the indoor air with "fresh" outdoor air. As a result, contaminants can build up inside unless pushed outside by a fan or similar device. Similarly, if the outdoor air is not healthy, the ritual of opening doors and windows to change out the air inside the house will simply draw more polluted air inside, rather than improving indoor air quality.[591] Even though O_3 concentrations indoors are typically 10%–50% of outdoor concentrations, it is estimated that about half of the health effects felt from O_3 result from indoor exposure, because most people spend the majority of the day inside.[436] Families living in modern housing with central air conditioning can capture many outdoor air pollutants using filtration devices. However, families living in housing with window air conditioning units or in homes that rely on opening the windows to provide cooling and ventilation may be exposed to a higher concentration of contaminants in their homes than immediately outside.[436] In moderate climates that are at risk of wildfire (such as the US Mountain West), residents may be forced to choose between temperature regulation and reducing exposure to potentially toxic air pollution during fire season if they rely exclusively on open windows to cool their home in the summer. In low- and middle-income countries that use coal- or wood-fired cookstoves and in homes in industrialized countries that burn wood in fireplaces or pellet heaters, it is important to switch to a cleaner source of fuel or properly filter the exhaust and ventilate the home to minimize indoor exposure to PM_{10} and CO.[220]

T.9 Toolbox—Health Effects of Climate Change: Disasters

T.9.a Introduction

While severe storms occur less frequently than flooding events, they often lead to significant loss of life, property damage, and economic disruptions. In 2018, 94 storms affected more than 19.5 million people globally, resulting in 1,593 recorded deaths and $69 billion in damages. In comparison, droughts—the second highest cause of economic losses from natural disasters that year—resulted in $9 billion in damages.[351,592] The 42 hurricanes that impacted the US from 1980 through 2018 accounted for only 17% of the total number of billion dollar events during that time but for 55% of the total property losses ($938.2 billion) and 49% of the recorded deaths (6,487 deaths). Severe storms, on the other hand, occurred more frequently (105 recorded from 1980–2018) but were less costly ($13.7 billion total) and resulted in fewer (although still a significant number) of deaths (1,628 deaths).[403]

T.9.b Definition

This section of the toolbox will address tropical cyclones (i.e., hurricanes) and severe storms—meteorological events that combine precipitation with high wind speeds. These are storms that meteorologists have deemed sufficiently dangerous to warrant activating local emergency management personnel by issuing a "watch" or "warning" designation. Severe storms can occur anywhere, whereas tropical cyclones (also known as hurricanes and typhoons) form in a large body of water and move inland from the coast. As a result, in addition to wind damage and street and river flooding, tropical cyclones can cause coastal flooding from the storm surge that develops as they move inland.[593–595] The flooding section of the toolbox addresses heavy precipitation events that do not include the added component of wind.

T.9.c Health Effects of Disasters

The health effects of severe storms, particularly tropical cyclones, are heavily influenced by disparities in location, level of economic development, and the peculiarities of each storm (table T.10). For example, from 1980–2009, Southeast Asia was exposed to only 9% of the total number of tropical cyclones but represented 53% of the global population affected and 80% of deaths. In contrast, the Americas were exposed to 37% of the cyclones that formed during that period and represented 23% of the affected global population but only 8% of the deaths.[596]

Tropical cyclones are also notable because, historically, a handful of storms have been responsible for the vast majority of deaths. For example, globally, Cyclone Gorky (Bangladesh, 1991) and Cyclone Nargis (Myanmar, 2008) accounted for more than two-thirds of all tropical cyclone deaths globally between 1980 and 2009.[596] In the US, Hurricane Katrina accounted for one-third of all hurricane-related deaths (direct and indirect) in the 50-year period from 1963–2012.[28]

Disparities are also marked in information collection. Very little information is available from low- and middle-income countries regarding the causes of death from severe storms, in spite of the high rate of mortality.[596] In the US, on the other hand, detailed records are made public after each extreme weather event occurs. A study of 50 years of hurricane exposure in the US estimated that the number of deaths caused by tropical cyclones in that country is divided roughly evenly between direct and indirect causes.[28] While it is widely acknowledged that low- and middle-income countries suffer a higher number of deaths directly caused by storm surge, rainfall-induced flooding, and high winds, information is lacking regarding the magnitude of indirect injuries and deaths in those countries attributable to tropical cyclones.[596] The reduction in storm-related mortality in high income countries like the US over the past 50 years has been attributed, in large part, to concerted efforts to improve early warning systems, access to emergency shelters, and evacuation plans.[29,597] In fact, prior to implementing these emergency preparedness measures, 90% of deaths from tropical cyclones were caused by drowning in the storm surge.[597]

While drowning is the primary direct cause of injury or death from severe storms, wind often plays a role—particularly in the case of tropical cyclones. For example, almost half (49%) of the 2,544 US hurricane deaths reported from 1963–2012 were caused by storm surge—many of them on the day the levees failed in New Orleans, Louisiana, USA, during Hurricane Katrina (2005). Hurricane Katrina's storm surge along the coast 50 miles northeast of New Orleans reached a record-breaking 28 feet in depth and penetrated 6–12 miles inland on the strength of the waves generated by Category 2–3 wind speeds.[598] The second greatest cause of death from hurricanes in the US from 1963–2012 (27%) was attributed to freshwater flooding/mudslides caused by heavy rainfall. Between 5 and 10% of deaths were attributed to non-tornadic wind exposure, and 3% were attributed to tornadoes.[598] A study of tropical cyclones and severe storms in Australia from 1970–2015 found that drowning deaths also dominated in that country—65% of 192 total. Deaths due to severe storms, on the other hand, were caused primarily by wind gusts. Of the 142 deaths from wind gusts, 30% (42 deaths) were due to drowning, 25% (36 deaths) were caused by vehicle accidents, and 25% (35 deaths) were caused by falling trees/tree limbs.[599]

Exposure to severe storms can exacerbate existing chronic diseases.[541] Death from cardiovascular disease was the number one indirect cause of death from tropical cyclones in the US during the 50 years starting in 1963—roughly equivalent to the number of deaths from drowning in the storm surge. However, that number is influenced by the high number of cardiovascular deaths during Hurricane Katrina—10 times the weekly average in New Orleans.[28] After Hurricanes Gustav and Ike (2008), the American Red Cross field service locations in Louisiana, Mississippi, Tennessee, and Texas, USA reported that 13% of their patients complained of an exacerbated chronic disease; of those, 7% of patients requested help managing hypertension (3.9%) or diabetes (3.1%).[600]

Cases of respiratory disease often increase during and immediately following exposure to a severe storm or tropical cyclone.[29] For example, cases of pneumonia and tuberculosis increased significantly at a hospital in the Philippines during the three months following Typhoon Haiyan (2013).[601] In the three weeks after Hurricane Katrina (2005), 10.5% of illnesses among New Orleans residents were described as acute respiratory infections, second to skin or wound infection (12.8%).[602] Six weeks after the event, acute respiratory infections had increased to become the highest single identifiable set of illnesses—14.8% (538 cases)—while skin or wound infection had decreased to 10% (361 cases).[603] Both severe storms and tropical cyclones have also been found to increase cases of allergic disease, because they tend to increase the concentration of airborne allergens like pollen and fungus in affected areas.[482,617,618] A study of six towns in Australia from 1995 to 1998 found that thunderstorms occurred on more than 30% of the days when asthma visits to the emergency department exceeded four times the expected number.[606]

Many of the other health effects of exposure to storms stem from the damage they can cause to buildings and infrastructure. If damage to the built environment is extensive, the storm could result in health effects that linger for years.

Physical injury is a major cause of death and morbidity before, during, and after the storm. The high wind speeds, maximum gusts of wind, and heavy rains generated by severe storms and tropical cyclones can cause victims to fall or bring them in contact with hazards such as collapsing structures, construction debris, vehicle and machinery debris, downed trees, animals, and severed

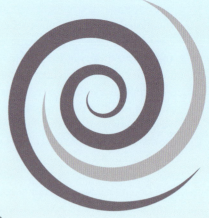

02 HOW DOES IT AFFECT THE BUILT ENVIRONMENT?

STRESS ON PLANT & ANIMAL LIFE
Disasters can damage or destroy ecosystems.

DISEASE-CARRYING VECTORS
Humans can come in contact with vectors through flood water & power outages.

FOOD INSECURITY
Food supply can be disrupted. Risk of spoilage.

WATER QUANTITY & QUALITY
Disasters can compromise centralized water & wastewater systems.

PROVIDE MULTI MODAL EVACUATION ROUTES
Reduces the risk of getting trapped during evacuation if cars are not the only option.

ISLANDABLE SITES & MICROGRIDS
Design on-site energy, water, & food production to allow for multiple days separated from public infrastructure.

04 WHO IS MOST VULNERABLE...

CHILDREN
Dependent on others for safety.

ELDERLY
Many are frail with underlying medical conditions. Dependent on others for safety.

CHRONIC DISEASE
Home medical equipment may rely on electricity.

POVERTY
Risk of exposure in poorly maintained buildings & reduced access to medical care.

MINORITIES
Risk of exposure in poorly maintained buildings & reduced access to medical care.

FLOODPLAINS
Risk of exposure to floodwater; getting trapped or drowning during evacuation.

Toolbox Infographic T.9. Linkages among Disasters, the Built Environment Determinants of Health, Protective Design and Operations Strategies, the Groups Who Are at Highest Risk, and Related Negative Health Outcomes

01 DISASTERS

- Increase in storm intensity.
- Increase in rainfall intensity.
- Storms form more rapidly but travel more slowly after landfall.

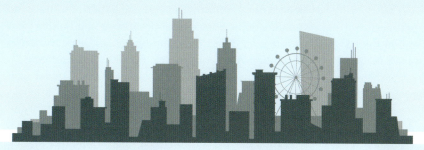

ELECTRICAL GRID INSTABILITY
Excess A/C use during heat events can lead to brown- & blackouts.

INFRASTRUCTURE DAMAGE
Disasters can cause temporary & permanent damage.

STRUCTURAL & MOISTURE DAMAGE
Disasters can cause structural damage & mold growth.

EXPOSURE TO FLOODWATERS
Risk of exposure to chemical and biological contaminants, debris, strong currents.

03 HOW CAN DESIGN HELP?

CONVERTABILITY
Design civic buildings to convert into medical & emergency shelters when needed.

LOW IMPACT DEVELOPMENT
Reduces the risk of injury and property damage by absorbing & slowing stormwater flow across site.

AVOID FLOOD-PRONE LOCATIONS
Avoid flood risk by locating the building outside of floodplains.

... TO THE HEALTH RISKS? 05

DISPLACED
High risk of negative mental and economic health.

RECOVERY WORKERS
Risk of exposure to floodwaters & flood debris.

FLOOD-RELATED INJURY AND DEATH
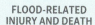

HEART DISEASE

RESPIRATORY DISEASE
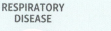

INFECTIOUS DISEASE

TOXIC CHEMICAL EXPOSURE

ALLERGIC DISEASE

MENTAL HEALTH

UNDER- & MALNUTRITION

Note: Many of the design and operations strategies in the infographic bring co-benefits to other topics in this toolbox as well. See figure T.4 for a crosswalk of all of the environmental health co-benefits.

electrical wires. These exposures can cause lacerations, blunt trauma, puncture wounds, stings, and/or electrocution.[29,541] While physical injury is a major cause of tropical cyclone-related mortality,[598] most of the injuries that present at emergency departments after the storm are minor.[607] For example, a database of tropical cyclone-related illness in Hong Kong found that only 2.8% of the 460 injuries reported from 2004–2009 were triaged as high priority.[608]

The majority of deaths from drowning that occurred during Hurricanes Katrina and Camille (1969) in the US were caused by the storm surge trapping residents in their houses.[598] Residents who shelter in place also run the risk of power outages, which can expose them to unsanitary and sometimes dangerous conditions. A 50-year study of US tropical cyclones attributed 12.8% of indirect deaths (182 deaths) to electrical fires (68 deaths), residential fires ignited by candles (45 deaths), or CO poisoning (69 deaths) caused by indoor generator use during a power outage.[28] A study of Hurricane Sandy (USA, 2012) found that the reported number of CO poisonings during and immediately following the storm were three times the same period in 2011 and over five times the same period in 2010.[609]

Evacuation presents its own sets of risk. Hurricanes Harvey (USA, 2017) and Florence (USA, 2018) demonstrate that climate change is making evacuation more difficult and dangerous. The speed at which both storms intensified tested the lead time that evacuation plans need to be successfully implemented. Furthermore, evacuees were forced to retreat from both the historical hazard along the coast—storm surge—and a new inland hazard—freshwater flooding caused by slowly moving storms.[610] The 50-year study of US tropical cyclones found that 14% of indirect fatalities (199 deaths) occurred during evacuation.[28] Studies in Japan have also identified flood victims who drowned as they walked to a shelter.[485] While walking in floodwaters is dangerous, vehicular accidents are also a major cause of indirect deaths from tropical cyclones.[405] Of the indirect tropical cyclone deaths in the 50-year study of US tropical cyclones (264 deaths), 18,6% were caused by vehicular accidents, 63 of which occurred during evacuation.[28]

In addition to drowning, evacuees could be exposed to floodwaters that are contaminated with sewage, toxic chemicals, and/or pathogens, as well as animals and debris.[104,404,406–408,413(p160)] (For a more in-depth review of the health effects associated with exposure to floodwaters, please consult section 7 of this toolbox: "Flooding.") Even after they reach an emergency shelter, evacuees are at a higher risk of infectious disease than the general population due to the large volume of people housed in a communal setting and the heightened risk of disease transmission in unsanitary conditions.[104,408] For example, a widespread norovirus outbreak impacted residents as well as staff and volunteers at a mega-shelter in Houston, Texas, USA that opened to house 24,000 Hurricane Katrina (2005) evacuees from the New Orleans area.[611] Populations in low- and middle-income countries may be particularly vulnerable to the spread of infectious disease in shelters, due to low immunization rates.[29]

Flooding from storm surge and heavy rainfall can compromise the potable water system, leading to increased risk among the general population of waterborne and infectious diseases that proliferate in unsanitary environments.[428(pp161–63)] A number of studies have found associations between tropical cyclones and dramatic increases in the rates of waterborne infectious diseases such as diarrheal and other gastrointestinal diseases in countries as diverse as China,[612] India,[613] South Korea,[614] and the US.[615] Hurricane Mitch (1998) compromised water and sanitation networks throughout Central America to such an extent that cholera outbreaks were reported in Guatemala, Nicaragua, and Belize; Nicaragua also reported an outbreak of leptospirosis; and Honduras reported an outbreak of gastrointestinal disease. The Pan American Health Organization concluded that overcrowded shelters, widespread population displacement, and disruption to health services likely exacerbated the outbreaks.[616]

Strong winds and flooding can disrupt the electrical grid, sometimes for weeks or months. Hurricane Maria (2017) devastated the Caribbean island of Puerto Rico, initially disrupting the electrical supply for the entire island. Only 50% of the island had access to power three months after the event.[617] And, in some rural and low-income urban areas,[618] populations remained without access to the central electrical grid for over 10 months after the storm.[619] In a world that is increasingly dependent on building systems and electronics to function, a long-term disruption to the electrical grid can have cascading consequences to the economy and human health.[104,610]

Tropical cyclones are warm weather occurrences. As a result, a prolonged loss of power can increase the risk of heat-related illness among vulnerable groups who lose access to air conditioning.[620] Fresh food spoils quickly in the absence of refrigeration, leading to an increased risk of foodborne illness and food insecurity when the power remains disrupted for multiple days or longer.[621] For example, New York City experienced a 70% increase in emergency department visits from diarrheal disease in 2003 after a prolonged power outage prompted some residents to eat spoiled food out of non-functioning refrigerators.[622] Furthermore, when roads and other transportation networks are disrupted by flooding or physical obstacles (such as uprooted trees), food and water delivery networks may be disrupted for long periods of time,[623,624] which can increase the risk of food insecurity and malnutrition.[625] For example, a major storm in the US Pacific Northwest in

January 2009 caused flooding, avalanches, and mudslides that were so widespread and severe that freight trains and trucks were not able to access the major port of Seattle.[623]

The strain on mental health of relocating and/or rebuilding a storm-damaged home has been found to increase the risk of depression, anxiety, post-traumatic stress, aggression, and suicidal thoughts.[104,404,408] In the days and weeks immediately following Hurricane Katrina, adults who were exposed to the storm were 4% more likely to report poor mental health than adults who were not directly exposed to the storm.[626] Similarly, in the weeks following Hurricanes Gustav and Ike, 5.4% of the patients treated at American Red Cross field service units in Louisiana, Mississippi, Tennessee, and Texas, USA, requested treatment for agitation, depression, suicidal thoughts, or other mental illnesses.[600] And a study in India 4.5 years after the 2004 Asian tsunami found that more than three-quarters of victims continued to suffer from mental health concerns, including 71% with post-traumatic stress, 33% with depression, and 23% with anxiety.[627] The long-term mental health effects of exposure to devastating storms can lead to tragic outcomes. For example, the rate of homicide-suicides in Miami-Dade County doubled from one per month to two per month during the six months following Hurricane Andrew (1992).[628] Also, women who were living in temporary housing in Louisiana and Mississippi 18 months after Hurricanes Katrina and Rita were 78.6 times more likely to attempt suicide and 14.7 times more likely to follow through to completion than the regional average.[629]

Individuals involved in the rebuilding effort could be exposed to toxic chemical contamination of building finishes that were exposed to floodwaters.[429] Starting within three days of the event, mold growth becomes a major (and sometimes lasting) concern—both for the people refurbishing flooded buildings and for occupants once they move back in.[476,480,481] Respiratory disease dominated the illnesses reported by Hurricane Katrina relief workers both immediately after the hurricane—22.5% (119 cases)[602]—and 6 weeks post-hurricane—25.5% (179 cases).[603]

Cases of insect bites and animal bites often increase during storm and cyclone events, because humans are more likely to come in contact with desperate animals in the floodwaters.[29,541] Unless all of the storm debris is removed during the first two to three weeks after the event, the population of disease-carrying vectors such as mosquitoes, cockroaches, and rodents spikes, which increases the risk of storm victims contracting vector-borne diseases.[444,445] The Philippines saw a sharp increase in dengue cases several months after Typhoon Haiyan (2013) made landfall,[601] and Nicaragua and Guatemala reported a sharp increase in cases of malaria two to three weeks after

TABLE T.10.

Direct and Indirect Health Effects of Exposure to Disasters

Exposure	Health effects
Direct	• Animal bites and stings[29,612] • Drowning[28,610,611] • Mental health concerns[218,649,650] • Physical injury[28,29,610–612] • Vehicle accidents[28,611]
Indirect	• Allergic disease[492,617,618] • Carbon monoxide poisoning[28] • Cardiovascular disease[28,612] • Electrical and residential fires[28] • Exposure to toxic chemicals[644] • Foodborne disease[635] • Heat- or cold-related illness[218,623] • Hypertension, diabetes[613] • Infectious disease[218,649] • Malnutrition[639] • Respiratory disease[29,612,651,652] • Vector-borne disease[452,654] • Waterborne disease[218,649,650,653]

Hurricane Mitch (1998).[626] These timelines align with the amount of time needed for mosquitoes carrying the diseases to proliferate. It also coincides with a period of time when standing water was readily available for eggs and larvae and mosquito control measures were temporarily disrupted. Furthermore, human populations might be more vulnerable to contracting the disease immediately following a disaster, because many people had lost their homes and were living exposed to the elements.[626]

Finally, severe storms and tropical cyclones often trigger or exacerbate compound events (i.e., multiple hazards occurring simultaneously or sequentially), which can lead to cascading disruptions of human and natural systems.[630] When wind damage and flooding disrupt critical infrastructure,[631] they can result in simultaneous or cascading exposures, such as extreme heat during hurricane season, waterborne diseases if the potable water supply is compromised, or disruption in medical care.[343,541] The COVID-19 pandemic added yet another stress to population health and public health infrastructure worldwide when it coincided with the 2020 and 2021 tropical cyclone seasons, extreme heat events, and massive wildfires in many parts of the world. All-cause mortality in France jumped 18.2% during heat waves in 2020 compared with the previous five years (2015–2019). Since less than 100 deaths were attributed to COVID-19 during this time, researchers concluded that the pandemic lockdowns and other pandemic-related conditions (such as difficulty receiving medical attention) were likely responsible for the dramatic uptick in mortality rates.[632] Compound events can have long-term consequences on economic development and social cohesion, particularly in low-income and otherwise vulnerable communities.[630] One study attempting to quantify the economic impact of climate change estimated that every degree Celsius in global warming will result in a 1.2% decrease in the US Gross Domestic Product, and that value over time will migrate north and west in the US, increasing income inequality across regions.[633]

T.9.d Relationship with Climate Change

Both tropical cyclones and severe storms are strongly influenced by climate change.

While it is unclear whether the number of tropical cyclones will increase as the oceans continue to warm, warmer sea surface temperatures are fueling increases in maximum wind speed and rainfall.[630] Historically, the oceans have slowed the effects of human-caused climate change by acting as a carbon sink.[655] Since 1955, they have absorbed more than 90% of the heat that has been added to the atmosphere due to the GHG effect.[656] And, both the upper (0–700 m depth) and lower (700–2000 m depth) ocean have begun to warm as a result.[634] The rate of warming in the upper ocean is particularly concerning, having doubled in the period 1993–2017 compared with 1970–1993.[636] As the oceans warm, the reach of tropical cyclones is moving towards the poles, potentially exposing coastal communities that were not built to withstand their gale-force winds and storm surge to new environmental hazards.[620]

Records from the past few decades show that the proportion of tropical cyclones reaching Category 4 or 5 has increased at a rate of 25%–30% per degree Celsius increase in global average ambient air temperature, with a proportionate reduction in Category 1 and 2 storms.[637] This trend is concerning, because a 10% increase in wind speed has been associated with 30–40% increase in property damage.[638] Cyclones also have begun to intensify more quickly, particularly in the Atlantic Ocean and the western North Pacific Ocean.[630] Both Tropical Cyclone Amos (which impacted the Samoan Islands in 2016)[579] and Hurricanes Harvey and Maria (which impacted several locations in the Gulf of Mexico in 2017)[580] intensified so rapidly that forecasting models struggled to accurately predict both the timing of peak intensity and the maximum wind speeds.[580]

Tropical cyclones are also dropping more rain once they hit the coast and start moving inland, because they are forming in warmer ambient air conditions, which allows them to absorb more water.[342] Climate models predict an average 7% increase in tropical cyclone precipitation rates per degree Celsius increase in sea surface temperature.[630]

As the upper ocean warms, the water molecules expand, exacerbating sea level rise in coastal communities and potentially compounding the effects of storm surge from tropical cyclones.[641–643] Along the East Coast of the US, sea levels are predicted to rise more than 15 cm (6 inches) by 2100 and more than 30 cm (11.8 inches) by 2300 solely as a result of ocean water thermal expansion.[641] That differential is anticipated to increase the devastation caused by storm surges from relatively minor storms to levels experienced historically as a result of major storms like Hurricane Sandy (2012),[643,644] which resulted in more than 250 deaths and $60 billion in property damages.[645] Similarly, a combination of warm ocean surface temperatures, sea level rise from thermal expansion, and storm surge caused by climate change and cyclical meteorological conditions exacerbated the impact of Super Typhoon Haiyan (2013) on the Philippines,[646] where a record-breaking 245 people died and 28,626 people were injured.[630]

Finally, the speed at which cyclones move once they make landfall has slowed 21% in the western North Pacific and 16% in the North Atlantic.[647] Their slowing movement and increased total rainfall have combined to dramatically increase flood hazards.[630] For example, rainfall dramatically increased unexpectedly 400 km southwest of the center of Tropical Cyclone Bilis seven hours after it made landfall in China in 2006, resulting in over 840 deaths and $5 billion in damages.[648] Similarly, the most devastating aspect of Hurricane Harvey in the Houston area, USA, in 2017 was the unprecedented rainfall. Studies have estimated that climate change increased the rainfall intensity of that event by 8%.[630]

Future flood risk models for coastal communities have begun to take into account the compounding effects of higher intensity tropical cyclones coupled with storm surge exacerbated by sea level rise.[630] One such flood index predicts a 4–75 times increase in flood risk under a low GHG emissions scenario and 35–350 times increase under a high-emissions scenario.[649]

Severe thunderstorms are characterized by heavy rain and strong winds. They are also often accompanied by lightening, tornadoes, and/or hail, all of which can pose grave hazards to life and property.[595] The impact of climate change on severe storms is less certain than with tropical cyclones, in part because they are not defined or documented as systematically.[650,651] However, climate modeling predicts severe thunderstorms to occur more frequently in the US, Europe, Australia, and Japan in coming years, particularly in mountainous regions. On the other hand, the frequency of small hail and small tornadoes may decline, replaced with a smaller number of large hail events and severe tornadoes. However, regional variations will play a major role in all of these events, because they are much smaller than tropical cyclones.[650,651]

T.9.e How Do Natural Disasters Affect the Built Environment?

The effects of natural disasters on the built environment could be divided into two rough categories: immediate effects and delayed effects. News coverage often focuses on the immediate effects: flooded or damaged infrastructure, uprooted trees, mudslides, power outages, boil water notices, and locations where residents must be evacuated using boats and helicopters because of dangerous conditions.

The delayed effects of the storm often become apparent a few days or weeks after the event. Residents who are trapped in their neighborhoods may have difficulty accessing clean water and food, leading to food insecurity and an uptick in waterborne and foodborne illnesses. Unless flooded buildings are dried out quickly, they can develop mold, which is hard to remediate—particularly for porous materials—once it has taken up residence in a building. On the outside of the building, standing water can result in a spike in mosquito populations 10 days to 2 weeks after the disaster.

T.9.f How Can Design Help?

Building design and community planning can help reduce the risk of injury and property damage from disasters in two ways. Zoning, siting, and development decisions can dramatically improve neighborhood and site resilience. For example, prohibiting development in flood-prone locations is one of the best ways to protect the population and built environment infrastructure from flooding and storms. Low-impact development—a flood mitigation practice that emphasizes vegetation instead of concrete site design strategies—can slow stormwater flow and reduce the risk of exposure to potentially contaminated floodwaters. Designing a multimodal transportation infrastructure with redundant evacuation routes in mind can save lives during events as well.

The second approach to building resilience to natural disasters considers how a building project can protect occupants during and after disasters. These strategies include designing a building site, campus, or neighborhood to function completely off the grid for a period of time. This approach might include on-site renewable energy or a neighborhood microgrid; on-site rainwater collection, filtration, and storage; and an on-site or neighborhood farm. To support emergency services, civic buildings like schools could be designed to transform into medical and emergency shelters when needed.

The COVID-19 pandemic prompted international organizations like the WHO[652] and non-profit aid organizations like Médecins Sans Frontières[653] to include facility considerations in their guidance on hospital readiness for natural and manmade crises. For example, the question of how to design a brick-and-mortar hospital so that it is flexible enough to allow for surge capacity during mass infection or mass casualty events could dramatically influence facility design into the future. Similarly, COVID-19 forced healthcare facilities to confront the question of how to maintain minimum required infection control standards while simultaneously adapting facility operations to changing needs and avoiding the mistake of sending non-critical patients home to infect their households. Similar to other questions embraced by architectural epidemiology, the question of how to design and operate a hospital that is prepared to respond safely and effectively to the next disaster requires a design and operations response that responds to the social, political, and population health conditions in the surrounding community.

T.9.g Who Is Most Vulnerable?

Vulnerability to severe storms and tropical cyclones is influenced by physiological, social, and contextual characteristics.

T.9.g.i Children and the Elderly

Children and the elderly are both physically and socially vulnerable to the wind and flooding hazards associated with storms.[654,655] Almost half of the people who died during Hurricane Katrina (2005) were over 75 years old,[656] and almost half of the people who died during Hurricane Sandy (2012) were over 65 years old.[104] Similarly, twice as many children (versus adults) were diagnosed with diarrheal disease at a hospital in the Philippines in the months following Typhoon Haiyan (2013).[601] Physically, children and the elderly are more frail than healthy adults and therefore more likely to fall or be harmed after coming into contact with a collapsing structure, a flying object, or something being moved by the current in a storm surge or floodwater.[105] Their immune systems are also more susceptible if they come into contact with pathogens or toxic chemicals in contaminated floodwaters.[392]

If the storm disrupts the systems that make their surroundings comfortable and sanitary—power, water, and transport services—then children and the elderly are more likely to suffer from exposure to the results of that breakdown—temperature extremes, unsanitary water, spoiled food, and disrupted access to medical supplies.[343,655] Children and the elderly often rely on caregivers to keep them safe. They are therefore at a higher risk of harm if they are isolated from help or separated from their caregivers.[104,105,538–540] Finally, both children and the elderly are at higher risk of mental health issues if a storm puts them in harm's way, destroys their home, or separates them from their social network.[551(p108)]

T.9.g.ii Chronic Disease and Pre-existing Mental and Physical Health Conditions

Major storms can disrupt access to medications and to medical devices that require electricity to operate, placing people with chronic disease at risk.[28] For example, The Townsville Hospital in North Queensland, Australia, experienced a 40% increase in emergency department visits immediately following Tropical Cyclone Yasi (2011), including almost double the number of patients who would normally present themselves for help managing chronic health conditions.[657]

The stress of living through or evacuating from a natural disaster has also been found to exacerbate symptoms in some diseases, such as cardiovascular disease;[29] diabetes;[29] hypertension;[29] and mental illnesses like post-traumatic stress, depression, and anxiety.[105,395] The highest number of deaths in Florida, Georgia, and North Carolina, USA, associated with Hurricane Irma (2017), 46 (35.7%) were attributed to exacerbation of existing medical conditions. Of those deaths, 23 (17.8% of the total) were attributed to the effect of stress and anxiety related to the hurricane on individuals with existing cardiovascular disease, and 17 (13.2%) were attributed to the effect of exposure to extreme heat on individuals with underlying medical conditions after the electrical power grid was disrupted.[658] Cancer patients and other immunocompromised people are also at a heightened risk of infection if they come in contact with contaminated water, spoiled food, trash, or disease-carrying vectors like mosquitoes.[392,655]

T.9.g.iii Minorities and Minority-Language Speakers

Racial and ethnic minorities in the US are more likely to be injured or killed by a storm, due to a complex interplay of social and economic conditions that place them in harm's way.[655] For example, the mortality rate for African American adults was 1.7–4 times higher than for White adults as a result of Hurricane Katrina.[656] In the US, a higher percentage of minorities live in areas that are at higher risk of being destroyed during a storm.[655] They are also more likely to have multiple chronic conditions that could be impacted by exposure to the storm.[655] And they have less access to health care, on average, than the White population.[659] They also have lower average incomes than Whites which reduces their resilience to the economic costs of a destructive storm.[660] Finally, populations speaking a minority language are at a disadvantage receiving emergency alerts. They may not respond immediately to an emergency evacuation order, for example, if it is only broadcast in the majority language.[104,105]

T.9.g.iv Families Living in Poverty

Families living in poverty are more likely to live in areas that are more vulnerable to the flooding and wind hazards of storms and in conditions with deteriorated infrastructure.[661] And they may not be able to respond to emergency warnings and evacuation orders in a timely manner, due to a shortage of resources.[661] They are therefore both more likely to experience a disproportionate economic burden and are less likely to have the resources to recover after experiencing a devastating storm.[661,662] The long-term economic impacts of major storms can increase the overall vulnerability of low-income populations by wiping away their savings. If businesses close in the wake of the storm, even temporarily, families without savings may be forced to move away from their social support system to seek a new source of income at the very time when they are most in need of community support.[661,662]

T.9.g.v Populations Located in Coastal Developments or Floodplains

Dense developments in low-lying, coastal areas are particularly vulnerable to storm surges. In developing nations, this vulnerability is exacerbated by poor building construction.[620,654] A global analysis found that the combination of dense, poorly constructed development in low-lying areas and low levels of economic development posed such a significant risk that adaptation efforts in some low- and middle-income countries may not be sufficient to reduce future mortality rates caused by the compounding effect of sea level rise and storm surge.[663]

T.9.g.vi Displaced and Housing Insecure Populations

Storm victims who lose their homes or witness widespread destruction are at risk of post-traumatic stress and other mental illnesses.[395] If they temporarily relocate to an emergency shelter, they may also be exposed to infectious diseases.[104,408] Disruptions to food supplies may increase the risk of malnutrition, particularly for families who lived in poverty prior to the storm, which can increase the risk of infection from a communicable disease.[625] People who become unhoused as a result of the storm are also physically vulnerable to vector-borne diseases, which can spike after tropical cyclones in particular, due to the fact that they take place during mosquito breeding seasons and leave behind them large quantities of standing water.[620]

Roughly 30% of people experiencing homelessness in the US suffer from a mental illness,[664] which adds to both their physical and mental health vulnerability to storms. People with existing mental illnesses are particularly vulnerable to vector-borne diseases that damage the neurological system, such as West Nile virus (WNV; transmitted by mosquitoes) and Lyme disease (transmitted by ticks).[665,666]

T.9.g.vii Recovery and Remediation Workers

In developed nations like the US, the majority of deaths from storms occur after the event, during cleanup (44%), rebuilding (26%), restoring public utilities (8%), and restoring public safety (6%).[104] Recovery workers are often exposed to health and safety risks, in both the physical environment (e.g., unsafe building structures and transportation infrastructure, lack of connectivity, unsanitary conditions, extreme heat or cold) and the social environment (e.g., social unrest and violence).[541,667] A study of Australian first responders who were deployed to Fiji following Tropical Cyclone Winston (2016) found that half reported feeling uncomfortably warm during their work shifts and 30% were not able to find relief from the heat during their leisure time.[668] Finally, the mental strain involved in their work can lead to long term mental health conditions, particularly among local responders. 13%–18% of first responders in a US study reported post-traumatic stress up to four years following their work on large-scale disasters.[669] And local Coast Guard responders to Hurricanes Katrina and Rita reported depression at three times the rate of out-of-town responders.[670]

T.10 Toolbox—Health Effects of Climate Change: Vector-Borne Disease

T.10.a Introduction

Vector-borne diseases are illnesses that are transmitted to humans and other animals via a carrier (or "vector"). Most disease-carrying vectors are bloodsucking insects like mosquitoes, ticks, and fleas. They ingest infectious pathogens during a blood meal of an infected host and then transfer them to another host through a future blood meal.[224,343,671] According to the WHO, 17% of infectious diseases worldwide are transmitted by vectors, resulting in more than 700,000 deaths each year.[671] The overwhelming majority of cases are located in low- and middle-income countries located in tropical and subtropical climates.[672]

The US tracks the number of cases reported each year for 14 vector-borne diseases. Table T.11 displays the average annual number of cases for five of the most well-known, as well as the rate per 100,000 people (a public health method for comparing the risk of a disease between different size groups). This section of the toolbox addresses the health effects, vulnerabilities, and built environment characteristics relevant to these diseases.

T.10.b Common Vector-Borne Diseases

T.10.b.i Lyme Disease

Primary Vector: Ixodes ticks
Vector Habitat: herbaceous forest edge, particularly in fragmented forests
Land Use: suburban, exurban
Animal Hosts: deer, mice

Lyme disease is the most common tick-borne illness globally, resulting in over 30,000 reported cases in the US each year[673] and more than 230,000 cases worldwide.[674] It is notoriously difficult to diagnose, and some estimates place infection rates up to 10 times higher than official counts.[675–677] Lyme disease has been detected throughout the US (particularly in the mountainous regions on the East and West Coasts), Europe, and Asia.[678,679] It is of particular concern in the US, where the number of reported cases has tripled over the past 20 years.[680] *Ixodes* ticks are the primary vector for the bacteria, *Borrelia burgdorferi*, which causes the disease. The tick's two primary hosts are white-footed mice (during the larvae and nymph stage) and white-tailed deer (during the adult stage).[681,682] The ticks are infected through a blood meal from an infected animal host, usually when they are in the immature larvae and nymph phases of their lifecycle. Humans contract Lyme disease when they are bitten by an infected tick—again, usually by nymphs, not adult ticks.[224] *Ixodes* ticks prefer climates with warm, humid summers and mild winters and deciduous and mixed forests with abundant leaf coverage, which give them warm and moist locations to rest in between hosts. Humans are particularly at risk of coming in contact with these ticks in suburban and exurban locations where a forest has been fragmented and deer are therefore likely to intrude on human-occupied land.[681,682]

T.10.b.ii West Nile Virus

Primary Vector: Culex mosquitoes
Vector Habitat: wetlands, agricultural areas, streams, storm sewers
Land Use: suburban, exurban
Animal Host: birds

West Nile virus (WNV) is the most common mosquito-borne disease in the US, averaging over 2,000 cases per year.[673] In comparison, Europe averages roughly 160 cases per year.[683] In 2018, 48 states and the District of Columbia

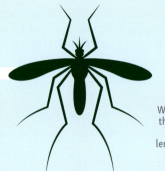

OZONE
Formed when NOx & VOCs mix in the presence of sunlight. Irritates the respiratory system.

PATHOGEN REPLICATION
Warm weather can accelerate the replication rate of many pathogens, increasing transmissibility from vector to host.

VECTOR LIFESPAN
Warm weather can accelerate the rate at which mosquitoes & ticks grow to maturity, lengthening the period of time they can transmit disease.

VECTOR REPRODUCTION
Warm weather & frequent rainfall can accelerate the reproductive lifecycle of mosquitoes & ticks, increasing their numbers.

02 HOW DOES IT AFFECT THE BUILT ENVIRONMENT?

ACCESS TO OUTDOOR ACTIVITIES
Spending time outside in areas with active vector-borne disease transmission can increase the risk of infection.

SPRAWL & HABITAT FRAGMENTATION
Habitat fragmentation places stress on animals, increasing their risk of hosting vectors like ticks. It also brings humans in closer contact with vectors.

STANDING WATER - BREEDING SITES
Mosquitoes use standing water as breeding sites - both impervious surfaces (like plastic & concrete) & marshy vegetation.

COMPACT, MULTI-USE DEVELOPMENT NEAR TRANSIT & BIKE/PED INFRASTRUCTURE
Alternative to sprawl that can help stitch habitat back together, which reduces the risk of disease transmission.

MIX OF VEGETATION ATTRACTING PREDATORS
Native biodiversity in landscaping can attract animals that eat vectors like mosquitoes.

LOW IMPACT DEVELOPMENT
Reduces standing water, which can create breeding grounds for mosquitoes.

04 WHO IS MOST VULNERABLE...

CHILDREN
More sensitive to exposure because developing organs & immune system.

ELDERLY
Many elderly have underlying health conditions and weaker immune systems.

PREGNANT WOMEN
Weaker immune system. Risk of premature birth & birth defects.

IMMUNO-COMPROMISED
Weak immune system reduces protection from exposure.

POVERTY
Risk of exposure in poorly maintained buildings & reduced access to medical care.

MINORITIES
Risk of exposure in poorly maintained buildings & reduced access to medical care.

HOMELESS
Higher risk of exposure if unhoused.

Toolbox Infographic T.10. Linkages among Vector-Borne Disease, the Built Environment Determinants of Health, Protective Design and Operations Strategies, the Groups Who Are at Highest Risk, and Related Negative Health Outcomes

01
VECTOR-BORNE DISEASE

- Increase in average annual temperatures.
- Longer summers.
- Change in seasonal patterns of rainfall.

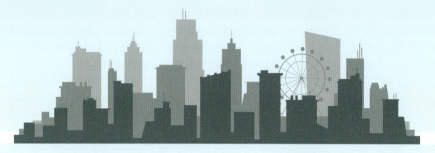

SHELTERING IN PLACE
Vectors like cockroaches, mice, & rats can be attracted to buildings for shelter during heat waves & flooding events.

CHANGE IN GEOGRAPHIC RANGE OF VECTORS
Changes in temperature & rainfall patterns have allowed vectors to move into new regions and infect new hosts.

03
HOW CAN DESIGN HELP?

WELL-MAINTAINED BUILDINGS
Supports IPM. Reduces leaks & opportunities for vectors to enter the building.

SCREENS
Screen windows, doors, porches, chimneys, foundation vents, & outdoor air supplies to prevent vector access when using natural ventilation.

INTEGRATED PEST MANAGEMENT (IPM)
Prevents pests from entering the building & removes their access to shelter, food, & water.

OUTDOOR WORKERS
Risk of occupational exposure.

DEATH OR LONG-TERM DISABILITY

FLU-LIKE SYMPTOMS

SKIN CONDITIONS

HEAD-, MUSCLE ACHES

NEUROLOGICAL CONDITIONS

BIRTH DEFECTS, COMPLICATIONS

... TO THE HEALTH RISKS? 05

Note: Many of the design and operations strategies in the infographic bring co-benefits to other topics in this toolbox as well. See figure T.4 for a crosswalk of all of the environmental health co-benefits.

reported at least one domestically acquired case. 63% of patients were diagnosed with the more serious form of the disease (neuroinvasive), and 6% (167 people) died. Given that many people who are infected with the less severe non-neuroinvasive form of the disease are asymptomatic, the US CDC estimated that the total number of cases was in the range of 52,000 to 118,000.[684]

Culex mosquitoes are infected by taking blood meals from infected birds. Once infected, a mosquito transmits the virus through every future vertebrate blood meal.[685] WNV outbreaks have been found to follow the migratory paths of host birds, appearing in humans several weeks after it is detected in the migratory bird population.[686]

Humans often come in contact with *Culex* mosquitoes in suburban and exurban areas near wetlands, agricultural areas, streams, and other locations with periodic exposure to water, such as storm sewers.[682] *Culex* mosquitoes prefer drier regions where irrigation or intermittent rain events can create the conditions for breeding.[687] In urban areas, on the other hand, larvae may be flushed out of underground breeding spots like storm sewers during heavy rain events.[688]

T.10.b.iii Malaria

Primary Vector: Anopheles mosquitoes
Vector Habitat: agricultural areas, wetlands, streams
Land Use: rural, exurban

Malaria is caused by a type of parasite, *Plasmodium*. It is by far the most devastating mosquito-borne disease globally, averaging 222.8 million cases[81] (5,900 per 100,000[689]) and over 430,000 deaths[689] each year, with sub-Saharan Africa bearing 90% of the burden of disease.[690] The United Nations has set a goal of ending the global malaria epidemic by 2030. However, progress appears to have stalled starting in 2015.[690] One study projected that climate change will increase the number of people at risk of contracting malaria by 200 million from 2030 to 2050.[691]

Anopheles mosquitoes are infected with malaria when they bite an infected human. The parasite undergoes part of its lifecycle inside the mosquito and the remainder in a human host who is infected during a blood meal.[692]

Malaria is most prevalent in rural and agricultural areas, because the *Anopheles* mosquito prefers living in wetlands, fields, and streams. Storm sewers are the most conducive habitat for them in more urban areas.[682]

T.10.b.iv Dengue and Zika

Primary Vector: Aedes mosquitoes
Vector Habitat: trash cans, flowerpots, discarded tires, standing puddles, storm sewers
Land Use: urban, suburban

Dengue and Zika viruses are both spread primarily by *Aedes* mosquitoes, which are also responsible for spreading other serious diseases like chikungunya and yellow fever.[693] Dengue virus is a resurgent disease, having spread from 9 countries in 1970 to over 100 countries today, although 70% of exposures occur in the Asia-Pacific region.[693] According to the WHO, the number of cases of dengue virus worldwide increased sixfold from 2010 (less than 500,000) to 2016 (more than 3.3 million).[693] Close to 4 billion people are at risk of infection, and estimates place infection rates between 284 million and 528 million infections per year and 96 million confirmed cases.[693] In Central and South America, an average of 1.38 million cases (218 per 100,000) are reported each year.[694] In comparison, an average of 675 cases (0.21 per 100,000) are reported each year in the US.[673]

Zika virus is an emerging disease, cases of which increased dramatically in 2016, particularly in the Americas. Transmission rates have since lowered somewhat.[695] The average rate from 2015–2018 in Central and South America was 242,569 cases (31.9 per 100,000).[696] The average rate in the US from 2014–2018 was roughly 1,900 cases per year.[673] Zika virus is currently reported in 87 countries but it is anticipated to spread, because half of the world population lives in areas exposed to *Aedes* mosquitoes.[695]

As the percentage of the world population living in urban areas increases, exposure to the *Aedes* mosquito will likely increase in kind, because their preferred habitat is closely associated with urban and suburban human settlements. They breed in containers that intermittently hold standing water, such as trash cans, flowerpots, and abandoned tires.[682] Storm sewers are a particular concern in dry areas, because they offer safe, moist harborage underground. One study in Australia estimated that up to 78% of the resident *Aedes* mosquito population during the dry season were bred in the storm sewer.[697] Once mature adults, many *Aedes* mosquitoes migrate into buildings, even closer to their human prey.[698]

T.10.c Health Effects of Vector-Borne Disease

T.10.c.i Lyme Disease

Lyme disease is most often contracted during the summer months.[676] It causes a range of symptoms soon after infection, including fever, headache, fatigue, and a characteristic "bulls-eye" rash.[699] It can also lead to pain in the joints, neurological conditions, and other symptoms such as skin lesions.[679] A study in Scotland found that 21.7% of cases presented with symptoms of arthritis, and 7.5% of cases presented with neurological symptoms.[700] The long-term effects of the disease can be debilitating, including permanent damage to the nervous system.[224] Although no vaccine is currently available to prevent infection, antibi-

TABLE T.11.

Vector-Borne Disease: Average Number of Annual Cases, US and Global, Non-US Countries/Regions

Disease	Primary Vector(s)[693]	Vector Habitat, Land Use with High Risk of Exposure, and Animal Host[704]	Average Annual Number of Cases (Rate) US, 2014–2018[695]	Global, Non-US
Tick-Borne				
Lyme Disease	*Ixodes* ticks	*Habitat:* herbaceous forest edge, particularly in fragmented forests *Land use:* suburban, exurban *Host:* deer, mice	36,874 cases (11.46 per 100,000)	Western Europe: ~232,125 cases (56.3 per 100,000)[696]
Mosquito-Borne				
West Nile Virus	*Culex* mosquitoes	*Habitat:* wetlands, agricultural areas, streams, storm sewers *Land use:* suburban, exurban *Host:* birds	2,254 cases (Neuroinvasive: 0.44 per 100,000 Non-neuroinvasive: 0.25 per 100,000)	Europe: 163 cases (90% in Greece, Hungary, Italy, and Romania)[705a] Israel: 62 cases[70a] Russia: 140 cases[705a] Serbia: 80 cases[705a]
Malaria	*Anopheles* mosquitoes	*Habitat:* agricultural areas, wetlands, streams *Land use:* rural, exurban	1,760 cases (0.54 per 100,000)	Global: 222.8 million cases[81b] (5,900 per 100,000)[711]
Dengue	*Aedes* mosquitoes	*Habitat:* trash cans, flowerpots, discarded tires, standing puddles, storm sewers *Land use:* urban, suburban	675 cases (0.21 per 100,000)	Global: 3.34 million cases[715c] Central and South America: 1.38 million cases[716d] (218 per 100,000)
Zika	*Aedes* mosquitoes	*Habitat:* trash cans, flowerpots, abandoned tires, standing puddles, storm sewers *Land use:* urban, suburban	1,921 cases (Non-congenital: 0.59 per 100,000 Congenital: 0.46 per 100,000)[e]	Central and South America: 242,569 cases (31.9 per 100,000)[718f]

[a] 2011–2017 average.
[b] 2010–2017 average.
[c] 2016 globally reported cases, World Health Organization.
[d] 2014–2018 average.
[e] Zika records available in the US from 2016–2018.
[f] 2015–2018 average.

---

otics can be an effective form of treatment, because the disease is caused by a bacterial pathogen. Some patients develop long-term symptoms such as chronic pain and fatigue, which are currently not treatable.[699]

T.10.c.ii West Nile Virus

While WNV is primarily transmitted by mosquitoes, it can also be transmitted through blood transfusions and from mother to baby *in utero*.[701] Most mosquito-borne infections from WNV occur during the summer and early autumn.[684] Between 70% and 80% of people infected with WNV do not show symptoms,[702] which has led to a concern that the actual number of cases is much higher than indicated in official reports. For example, from 1999–2007, it is estimated that more than 1.5 million people in the US were infected with WNV, 300,000 of which were symptomatic.[703] This is a worrying trend, since climate projections estimate that annual cases in the US will more than double by 2050, resulting in up to $1 billion per year in hospitalization costs and premature deaths.[704] Between 20% and 30% of WNV infections develop a serious condition called acute systemic febrile illness, which may manifest through headaches, muscle pains, a rash, or gastrointestinal distress that could linger for several weeks. Less than 1% of infections develop into neuroinvasive WNV, which can lead to inflammation of the brain and/or spinal cord.[703] No vaccines or antivirals are currently available to prevent or treat infection.[702] Environmental and personal protective measures are therefore currently the most effective way to limit the number of WNV cases.

T.10.c.iii Malaria

Malaria symptoms include chills, fever, sweats, headache, nausea and vomiting, and body aches. In countries where malaria is not common, it is often misdiagnosed as cold or flu-like symptoms. In severe cases, patients may experience organ failure or death.[705] Pregnant people can transmit malaria *in utero*, leading at times to premature delivery or low birth weight.[705] Thankfully, malaria is readily treatable with an array of antimalarial medications, particularly during early stages of the disease.[706]

T.10.c.iv Dengue

Dengue virus refers to four strains, or serotypes. Patients who are infected with one serotype develop a long-term immunity to that strain of the disease, but they can become sensitized to more severe forms of the other three serotypes and, possibly, related viruses, like Zika virus.[698] Three-quarters of infections are asymptomatic,[707] meaning that these patients do not realize that they are at a higher risk of contracting a serious form of dengue virus in the future if exposed to a different serotype. Symptoms include fever, nausea and vomiting, rash, and aches and pains (particularly behind the eyes and/or muscle, joint, or bone pain).[707] No vaccines or antivirals are currently available to prevent or treat infection.[708] As a result, similar to WNV, environmental and personal protective measures are currently the most effective way to reduce the spread of dengue virus.

T.10.c.v Zika

Similar to dengue, the majority of people infected with Zika virus either have no symptoms or only mild, non-specific symptoms that are never traced back to the disease.[695] More serious symptoms include swelling of the brain or spinal cord and Guillain-Barré Syndrome—a neurological condition.[709] Pregnant people run the risk of preterm birth, stillborn birth, and babies being born with extremely serious birth defects such as microcephaly.[695] The WHO has expressed concern that the number of reported cases of Zika virus severely undercounts the total number of infections due to the high proportion of patients who are asymptomatic.[695] For example, in Thailand, 45% of the 121 confirmed cases of Zika virus reported among pregnant people in 2016–2017 were asymptomatic.[695] As with the other viruses covered in this section, there is no vaccine or specific medicine available to prevent or treat Zika virus. Environmental and personal protective measures are currently the most effective way to control the disease.

Table T.12 summarizes common direct and indirect health effects associated with Lyme disease, West Nile virus, malaria, dengue, and Zika.

T.10.d Relationship with Climate Change

Vector-borne diseases have a complex relationship with climate change, in part because outbreaks depend on the presence of vectors; pathogens; prospective hosts; and a climatic, physical, and social environment that is conducive to transmission. If one of these factors changes, it has a ripple effect on the overall transmission rate. This is true both in areas that are currently at high risk of exposure to infected vectors and in regions where vector-borne disease is rare or seen as an emerging threat. As a result, it is important to assess local, and even site-specific, conditions to understand its level of risk related to one or more vector-borne diseases, even in areas that are generally considered high risk for those diseases.[224,343]

Changes in temperature and precipitation patterns can influence the gestation and transmission of several diseases, although there is generally a lag time between the climatic event and disease outbreaks. A study in central China found that the average temperature for the previous two months combined with the average rainfall from the current month could be used to predict incidence of malaria.[710]

Warmer temperatures within the mosquito's comfort range accelerate viral replication rates,[711,712] the mosquito life cycle,[711,713] and mosquito biting rates.[711,714] They can also increase a mosquito's lifespan.[715] For example, since the *Aedes* mosquito requires two to three weeks to develop from an egg to adult, the longer season translates to risk of exposure during more mosquito lifecycles each year. Increasing temperatures can cut the development period in half: from 18–19 days to 9–10 days.[715] Similarly, the period of time between an average mosquito's initial exposure to dengue virus and the point at which the virus can be detected in the mosquito's salivary glands decreases from an average of 9 days at 82°F (28°C) to 5 days at 86°F

TABLE T.12.

Direct and Indirect Health Effects of Vector-Borne Diseases

Health Effect	Lyme Disease	West Nile Virus	Malaria	Dengue	Zika
Direct	• Fever • Headache • Fatigue • "Bulls-eye" rash • Joint pain • Neurological conditions • Skin lesions	• Headaches • Muscle pains • Rash • Gastrointestinal distress • Neurological conditions	• Chills • Fever • Sweats • Headache • Nausea and vomiting • Body aches	• Fever • Nausea and vomiting • Rash • Aches and pains (particularly behind the eyes and/or muscle, joint, or bone pain)	*General:* • Non-specific flu-like symptoms • Swelling of the brain or spinal cord • Guillain-Barré syndrome *Babies born to infected mothers:* • Stillbirth • Premature delivery • Low birth weight • Severe birth defects such as microcephaly, neurological conditions, and malformations of the eyes and/or limbs
Indirect	Economic strain, lost days of work or school				

(30°C).[716] And the proportion of mosquitoes that live long enough to transmit dengue virus (10%–39%) increases as the mosquito lifespan lengthens.[711] It is estimated that the global abundance of *Aedes aegypti* mosquitoes has increased 9.5% from 1905–2014 due to a combination of warming temperatures and land use decisions. And that trend is expected to continue, increasing an additional 20%–30% by 2100, with densely populated areas in South Asia, mid-Africa, and South America showing the highest abundance.[717] Extreme heat was found to be the primary climatic driver for an unprecedented outbreak of WNV in Europe, Turkey, and Israel in 2010, possibly because warm temperatures increase the number of mosquitoes and the competence of disease transmission.[718] Warm weather has also been found to speed virus replication.[712]

Warm weather can change or expand a mosquito's geographic range. For example, it may have contributed to the spread and virulence of the Zika epidemic in the Americas from 2014–2016.[353] Climate models predict that the range of mosquito vectors will continue to spread to higher elevations and latitudes[672] and that mosquito season will continue to trend towards beginning earlier and ending later under future climate scenarios. However, it is possible that mosquito populations will fall somewhat during the heat of mid-summer.[719] Human exposure to the *Aedes* mosquito is predicted to increase 30%–60% by 2080, particularly in Australia, Europe, and North America, due to a combination of changes to the climate, demographics, and socioeconomic status.[720]

Warmer weather is also expected to impact the geographic range of *Ixodes* ticks, the length of the Lyme disease season, and the lifecycle of both ticks and the bacteria that causes the disease. Lyme disease is associated with the summer season,[721] when both the *Ixodes* ticks are most active and humans are most likely to spend time in their habitat (possibly wearing fewer protective layers of clothing than in cooler weather). The range of *Ixodes* ticks has expanded north and west from the US Eastern Seaboard starting in the 1970s.[722] And there are some indications that their population expansion is accelerating in some areas. For example, from 2008–2014, the Canadian province of Quebec experienced a fourfold increase in the number of ticks collected, a threefold increase in the percent of ticks infected with Lyme disease, and an increase in the geographic expanse of the ticks' range.[723] One study estimated that, by 2080, the Lyme disease season in the US will start one to two weeks earlier than its average in 2007.[724] Similar to mosquitoes, warmer temperatures increase both the rate of tick development and hatching[725] and the replication rate of the bacteria that causes Lyme disease, *Borrelia burgdorferi*.[726]

Precipitation is another key factor in vector-borne disease transmission. A large-scale study in the US found a one-third to two-thirds increase in WNV infections during a week of a heavy rain, with the increase sustained for an additional two weeks after the rain event.[727] However, the climate-fueled trend of increasingly intense rain events can also work against the spread of WNV. If the rainfall is too heavy, it can flush eggs downstream, temporarily reducing some *Culex* mosquito populations.[728]

On the other end of the spectrum, climate change has also resulted in increased frequency and intensity of seasonal drought in some regions, which can increase rates of WNV transmission up to a year afterwards.[729] A study in southern Florida, USA, found a strong correlation between drought conditions two to six months prior to the study followed by a wet period two to six weeks prior to a marked increase in WNV cases (2 or more cases per month). Researchers hypothesized that the drought brought the *Culex* mosquitoes and sentinel birds needed to transmit WNV together over scarce water supplies, creating hospitable conditions for the virus to amplify in avian hosts. When a wet period a few months later allowed the mosquitoes to breed, the virus was waiting for them in bird hosts.[730] Similarly, in 1993, malaria re-emerged in South Korea, after being eradicated in the 1970s, during a period of extremely hot and dry weather. Subsequent cases increased during similar spells of hot and dry conditions.[731]

Diseases transmitted by the *Aedes* mosquito—such as dengue and Zika—may also increase during drought periods, because mosquito populations have been known to use water storage containers as breeding sites.[732,733] An epidemic of dengue fever in Asia in 2007, where 100,000 people were diagnosed and 1,100 people died in Indonesia alone, was largely attributed to a drought (during which time families stored drinking water in containers that could act as breeding grounds for *Aedes* mosquitoes) followed by a hot and humid summer.[672]

Climate change also affects the relationship between the vector and its hosts—both animal and human. As temperatures have warmed, mosquito and tick habitat have expanded. For example, *Ixodes* ticks have spread more rapidly into regions of Canada that have experienced more moderate winters over the past few years.[734] Climate models predict that up to two-thirds of Canada may be at moderate risk of Lyme disease by 2080 under a high-emission scenario.[735] It is important to note that the density of a vector population can increase without increasing exposure to a vector-borne disease if the vector lives around hosts that are immune or poor carriers for the disease.[224] The impact that climate change will have on the synergy between vector habitats and the habitats of animal hosts (such as mice and deer for ticks and certain species of birds for WNV) is less clear.[224]

Low-lying urban areas are also at a heightened risk of vector-borne disease due to climate change. Many global megacities (population of 10 million or more) with dense, low income neighborhoods that are at high risk of exposure to *Aedes* mosquitoes are also located in coastal areas prone to tropical cyclones and sea level rise.[736] By 2100, the number of people worldwide living in low-elevation coastal zones is estimated to top 1.1 billion.[736] The combined risk of flooding and power outages caused by tropical cyclones and sea level rise heightens the risk of low-income urban populations being exposed to infected mosquitoes several weeks after a severe storm leaves them without adequate housing. For example, studies in Taiwan have identified an association between typhoons, vector populations, and spikes in cases of dengue fever.[737,738]

T.10.e How Does Vector-Borne Disease Affect the Built Environment?

At the regional scale, sprawl development has increased the risk of humans' coming in contact with some ticks and mosquitoes by fragmenting previously wild habitat. This risk increases every year in regions where climate change has led to an expansion of tick and mosquito habitat into areas where landscape and infrastructure are not designed with vectors in mind. Furthermore, the stormwater and road infrastructure that is built to accommodate sprawl developments can harbor mosquitoes that transmit WNV. If vector-borne diseases like Lyme disease and WNV become too prominent in a region, they can reduce local enthusiasm for constructing infrastructure supporting outdoor activities—like hiking, cycling, and fishing.

At the building scale, landscape and hardscape that allows water to stand for more than a week before draining can become mosquito breeding sites. Operable windows and doors without protective screens allow mosquitoes, particularly the *Aedes aegypti*, easy entry to residences where they can hide before biting a human host. Poorly maintained buildings can attract vectors like cockroaches, mice, and rats, particularly when they are looking for shelter from heat waves and floods.

T.10.f How Can Design Help?

Community planning regulations that promote a balance of compact, multi-use development near transit and bike/pedestrian infrastructure separated from large, undisturbed tracts of wildlands can help reduce the risk of human/animal contact (which can lead to exposure to ticks infected with Lyme disease). Similarly, using low-impact development methods instead of traditional (i.e., concrete) stormwater infrastructure reduces the habitat for WNV-carrying *Culex* mosquitoes.

A general landscaping practice of maximizing biodiversity and attracting animals that eat vectors like mosquitoes can be used at the site level hand-in-hand with integrated pest management practices and regular building maintenance audits to reduce access to food, water, and harborage for vectors. Finally, installing and maintaining screens on windows and doors allows for the physical and mental health benefits of natural ventilation and access to nature without allowing vectors like *Aedes aegypti* mosquitoes and cockroaches easy passage inside.

T.10.g Who Is Most Vulnerable?

Vulnerability to vector-borne disease can be caused by physiological characteristics, socioeconomic conditions, or both. Groups who may be vulnerable for physiological reasons include children, the elderly, pregnant people and babies, and the immunocompromised. Socioeconomic circumstances that can increase vulnerability include poverty; minority, Indigenous, or migrant status; insufficient protection from the elements (e.g., housing insecurity, sub-standard or primitive housing); outdoor work or play; and, traveling to countries where vector-borne diseases are endemic.

T.10.g.i Children and the Elderly

Children are disproportionately prone to infection from both tick-borne and mosquito-borne diseases, due to a combination of their immature immune systems[739] and behavioral characteristics, such as playing outside in vegetated areas and being less likely than adults to protect themselves before, during, and after exposure to a vector.[740,741] The highest reporting groups with Lyme disease in the US are children between 5 and 9 years (8.6 cases per 100,000 population) and adults aged 55 to 59 (7.8 cases per 100,000 population).[721] Children under 5 represent 61% of deaths from malaria worldwide.[689] On the positive side, children under 1 year of age may be better protected from milder forms of dengue virus than older children, because the antibodies they receive from their mother *in utero* remain in their bloodstream for several years after birth.[742] But a large international study found that children under 10 years old were at highest risk of mortality if they contract a severe form of the disease.[743]

Studies in the US have found that the risk of contracting a severe form of WNV increases with age. The median age of patients diagnosed with WNV in the US in 2018 was 59, but the median age of patients who died from the disease was 74.[684] A study of the 1999 WNV outbreak in New York City found that people over age 65 were six times more likely to contract a severe form of WNV than younger New Yorkers (one case per 50 infections compared with one case per 300 infections).[744] The elderly may not be at higher risk of contracting other vector-borne diseases, like Lyme disease and mosquito-borne diseases. However, once infected, they are more likely to develop a severe form of the disease and more likely to die from it.[745] A study from 2005–2008 in Singapore found that adults over age 60 were more likely than younger adults to contract both severe dengue (20.3% vs. 14.6%) and the life-threatening dengue hemorrhagic fever (29.2% vs. 21.4%). They also spent more time in the hospital and were more likely to develop secondary infections such as pneumonia and urinary tract infections.[746]

T.10.g.ii Pregnant People and Babies

Pregnant and post-partum people are more susceptible to malaria than the general population.[747] And, while mothers who have developed immunity to one or more strain of the dengue virus may transfer protective antibodies to their infants (reducing the risk of contracting dengue fever during the first year of life),[742] pregnant people infected with malaria, WNV, Zika, or (to a lesser extent) dengue during the gestation period could transmit those diseases *in utero*, resulting in severe health consequences to the baby. The risks to babies range from abortion and stillbirth to premature delivery; low birth weight; and severe birth defects such as microcephaly, neurological conditions, and malformations of the eyes and/or limbs.[693,695,705,748]

T.10.g.iii Immunocompromised People

Immunocompromised people (such as cancer patients or patients with HIV/AIDS) may be more susceptible to severe forms of vector-borne diseases, because their body's defenses are suppressed.[224,759] For example, immunocompromised patients are at higher risk of secondary infections developing after initial infection by the dengue virus.[225]

T.10.g.iv Families Living in Poverty

Vector-borne diseases are often considered poverty amplifiers. The WHO estimates that the per capita mortality rate from vector-borne diseases is 300 times higher in low-income countries than in high-income countries.[750] Malaria in particular has been seen as a contributor to poverty. In 1946, it was present on every continent except Antarctica. However, as socio-economic conditions improved, it was eradicated from many regions of the world.[751] Today, it is primarily endemic to low-income countries in Sub-Saharan Africa, where it helps perpetuate a cycle of poverty in which families continue to be exposed through the inability to pay for adequate protective measures such as treated mosquito nets and window screens, combined with the government's inability to pay for improvements to water and sewer systems that would reduce the mosquito's habitat.[752]

Lyme disease, on the other hand, has been found to disproportionately affect both the lowest and the highest income quartiles in the US.[753] Given that the average early stage Lyme disease patient in the US spends $800 on treatment and $200 in lost productivity,[754] patients in the lowest income quartile face a disproportionate burden from the disease. A study of the economic effect of dengue virus across eight countries found that the average ambulatory patient lost 14.8 days of work due to the disease resulting in an income loss of $514 US; and, the average hospitalized patient lost 18.9 days of work resulting in a loss of $1,394 US.[755]

Families living in poverty are more vulnerable to exposure to disease-carrying vectors, particularly if their housing and surrounding infrastructure are in poor repair.[682] *Aedes* mosquitoes in particular have been found in high abundance in low-income neighborhoods where empty lots and illegal dumping grounds house discarded tires and containers that can turn into mosquito breeding grounds after rain events.[756] Low-income populations are also less likely to benefit from vector-control measures, and they have reduced access to health care services in many communities.[750]

T.10.g.v Minorities, Indigenous Communities, and Migrant Workers

Minorities, Indigenous communities, and migrant workers are more vulnerable to vector-borne diseases in many regions of the world where they are both more likely to live in poverty and receive lower levels of public health support than the majority population. In the case of the US, different vector-borne diseases are more prevalent among different racial and ethnic groups. Lyme disease—which appears more frequently in suburban and exurban communities—is particularly prevalent among Whites, averaging 7.9 cases per 100,000 population from 2016–2018, compared with 0.7 cases per 100,000 among African Americans and 1.0 cases per 100,000 among Hispanics.[673] Malaria and Zika virus, on the other hand, which are primarily travel-related diseases in the US, are more prevalent among African Americans (2.6 cases per 100,000 on average among African Americans from 2016–2018, compared with 0.1 case per 100,000 among both Whites and Hispanics) and Hispanics (3.62 cases per 100,000 during the 2016 outbreak compared with 1 case per 100,000 among Whites and African Americans), respectively.[673]

Indigenous communities often confront added challenges related to lifestyle, remote living conditions, and political neglect. For example, in Panama, malaria eradication efforts are focused along the Panama Canal and in metropolitan areas in spite of the fact that the less developed region where the Guna Amerindians live represents 45% of all malaria cases in the country. Eradication efforts may be further hampered by the Guna's custom of frequently traveling across their territory.[757] A study in India found that Indigenous communities—which represent 50% of the country's deaths from malaria but only 10% of the population—face cultural and language barriers that can slow or prevent diagnosis and treatment of malaria, as well as implementation of measures to protect the most vulnerable members of the community from exposure.[758]

Migrant workers are more vulnerable to contracting vector-borne diseases both due to their outdoor living and working conditions and because they may not receive public health education about how to protect themselves from exposure or treat themselves once infected. A study of migrant workers from Myanmar and Cambodia who were working in Thailand found that workers who had spent less than six months in Thailand and were less fluent in the majority language were half as likely as long-term migrants to recognize the symptoms of malaria (31% of short-term migrants did not know any symptoms versus 7%–11% of long-term migrants) or to know how to protect themselves from exposure (30% of short-term migrants did not know any protective measures versus 9%–14% of long-term migrants).[759] Migrants also run the risk of being stigmatized if they inadvertently transmit pathogens to new areas as they move from one job to the next.[760]

T.10.g.vi Housing Insecurity and Primitive and Substandard Housing

People experiencing homelessness and families living in primitive or sub-standard housing are at higher risk of exposure to mosquito-borne diseases like dengue and malaria, because they lack access to protective building measures like air conditioning, screens on windows, and repellent-treated bed nets that have been shown to reduce disease transmission.[752] The widespread use of air conditioning and window screens in Laredo, Texas, USA, compared with building conditions across the border in Mexico has been identified as a major factor in its low incidence of dengue fever (64 cases in Laredo from 1980 to 1999, compared with 62,000 cases across the border) in spite of much higher counts of infected mosquitoes.[761] In Cuba, chronic disruptions in the drinking water supply has led many families to store water in containers that could become breeding grounds for *Aedes* mosquitoes. This practice is at least partially responsible for the persistence of dengue fever in urban areas of the country. For example, an epidemic in 1997 in Santiago de Cuba resulted in 17,114 cases of dengue fever, 205 cases of dengue hemorrhagic fever, and 12 deaths. In 2001–2002, Havana experienced an outbreak of 12,000 cases of dengue fever.[762]

T.10.g.vii Outdoor Activities

People who work or recreate outdoors in areas with a high concentration of infected vectors are at higher risk of exposure to vector-borne disease (e.g., landscapers, construction workers, agricultural workers, hikers, and children playing outdoors). For Lyme disease, in particular, outdoor activities in suburban and exurban areas that have been built into or along the edge of fragmented forest ecosystems can bring humans into close contact with tick populations.[721] A study in Scotland found that people who lived near the edge of a forest were at 50%–74% higher risk of infection than their neighbors living farther away.[763] Also, an outbreak of Lyme disease in New Jersey in the early 1980s found a higher incidence of Lyme disease among outdoor workers than among adults who worked indoors.[764]

T.10.g.viii Travelers

Vector-borne diseases can readily spread with the help of human travelers.[752] The most famous case of a disease outbreak caused by travel was the black death (bubonic plague), which was transported from Asia to 14th century Europe by rats aboard Norwegian trade ships.[672] Modern international travel and trade have similarly facilitated the international spread of vector-borne diseases. For example, in 2010, the top two illnesses presented by European travelers after returning from a trip abroad were malaria and dengue.[765] Similarly, the majority of recent cases of dengue virus and Zika virus in the continental US were acquired abroad.[766] However, if local *Aedes* mosquitoes bite infected travelers at home, thereby ingesting the virus, they may ultimately transmit it to a local host. While locally acquired cases of dengue virus and Zika virus remain rare,[701] WNV spread across the country within a few years after its introduction as a travel-acquired disease in New York City in 1999.[767] By 2003, it had spread to the West Coast of the US. By 2005, it had spread all the way to Argentina.[703]

Toolbox Crosswalk

Many of the evidence-based design and operations strategies presented in this toolbox create co-benefits for more than one environmental health topic. Figure T.4 facilitates the co-benefit design process (figure T.1) by displaying all of the strategies in a single crosswalk. Project teams can use the figure to build their design around the subset of strategies that could contribute to the greatest number of environmental health priorities identified in the neighborhood assessment (see chapter 2).

Figure T.4 supports design decisions at the building, campus/neighborhood, and community scales. It also explains how the design strategy benefits each relevant environmental health topic in the toolbox. Project teams can use this additional information to design for maximum positive impact—for future occupants, the surrounding neighborhood, and the global supply chain.

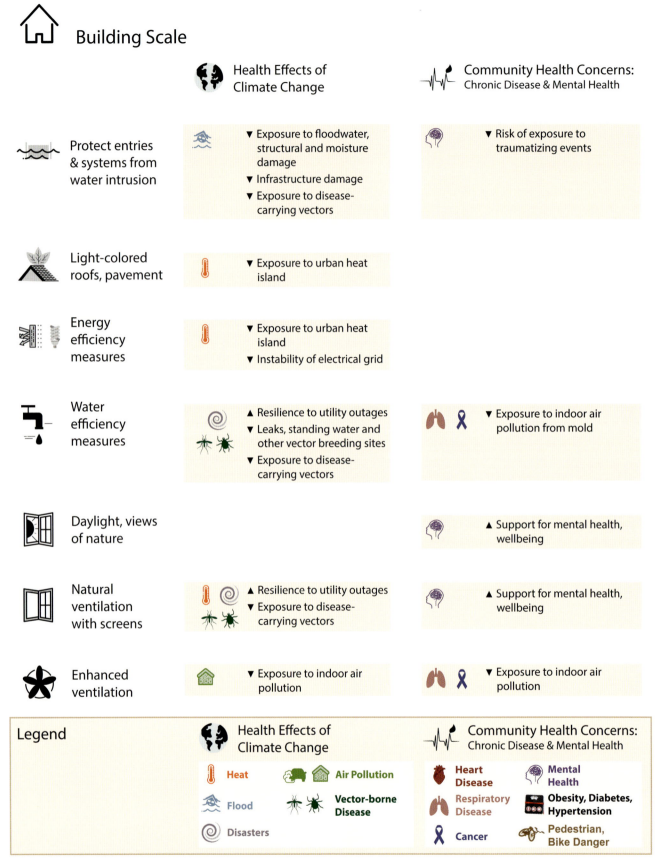

Figure T.4. Health-Promoting Green and Healthy Building Strategies Cross-Tabulated by Climate Change and Community Health Categories.

Note: Environmental determinants of health are listed under health topics.

168 ARCHITECHTURAL EPIDEMIOLOGY

Building Scale (*cont.*)

		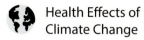 Health Effects of Climate Change	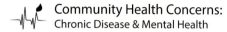 Community Health Concerns: Chronic Disease & Mental Health
	Enhanced air filtration	▼ Exposure to indoor air pollution	▼ Exposure to environmental tobacco smoke ▼ Exposure to indoor air pollution
	Low-emitting, non-toxic materials, finishes	▼ Exposure to indoor air pollution, particularly during heat events	 ▼ Exposure to indoor air pollution
	On-site renewable energy Rainwater capture, filtration, storage	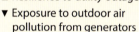 ▼ Exposure to urban heat island ▲ Resilience to utility outages ▼ Exposure to outdoor air pollution from generators ▼ Exposure to indoor air pollution ▼ Infrastructure damage ▼ Structural, moisture damage	▼ Exposure to indoor air pollution ▼ Risk of exposure to traumatizing events
	Well-maintained buildings and integrated pest management (IPM)	▼ Exposure to urban heat island ▼ Flooding, leaks, mold ▼ Exposure to indoor air pollution ▲ Resilience to utility outages ▼ Leaks, standing water and other vector breeding sites ▼ Habitat for vectors and animal hosts ▼ Exposure to disease-carrying vectors	▼ Exposure to indoor air pollution ▼ Risk of exposure to traumatizing events

Figure T.4. (*cont.*)

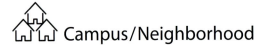 Campus/Neighborhood

 Health Effects of Climate Change

 Community Health Concerns: Chronic Disease & Mental Health

 Avoid flood-prone locations

- ▼ Stress on plant, animal life
- ▲ Water quantity and quality
- ▼ Exposure to floodwater, structural and moisture damage
- ▼ Infrastructure damage
- ▼ Exposure to disease-carrying vectors

- ▲ Resilience of individuals with pre-existing conditions during, after disasters

- ▼ Risk of exposure to traumatizing events

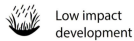 Low impact development

- ▼ Stress on plant, animal life
- ▲ Water quantity and quality
- ▼ Exposure to heat, floodwater, structural and moisture damage
- ▼ Infrastructure damage

- ▲ Access to outdoor activities

- ▲ Access to outdoor activities
- ▼ Fragmentation of preditor habitat
- ▼ Standing water, vector breeding sites
- ▼ Exposure to disease-carrying vectors

- ▼ Risk of exposure to traumatizing events

 Vegetative and structural barriers to emission sources

- ▲ Access to outdoor activities
- ▼ Stress on plant, animal life
- ▼ Exposure to outdoor air pollution
- ▼ Exposure to indoor air pollution
- ▼ Exposure to urban heat island

- ▼ Exposure to environmental tobacco smoke
- ▼ Exposure to outdoor air pollution
- ▼ Exposure to indoor air quality

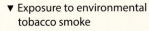

Legend

 Health Effects of Climate Change

 Heat 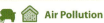 Air Pollution

 Flood   Vector-borne Disease

Disasters

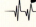 Community Health Concerns: Chronic Disease & Mental Health

 Heart Disease   Mental Health

Respiratory Disease   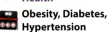 Obesity, Diabetes, Hypertension

Cancer   Pedestrian, Bike Danger

Figure T.4. (cont.)

170 ARCHITECHTURAL EPIDEMIOLOGY

Campus/Neighborhood (*cont.*)

	Health Effects of Climate Change	Community Health Concerns: Chronic Disease & Mental Health
Native, non-allergenic landscaping	▼ Stress on plant, animal life ▼ Exposure to urban heat island ▼ Exposure to outdoor air pollution ▼ Exposure to floodwater ▼ Infrastructure damage ▼ Exposure to disease-carrying vectors	▼ Unsafe bike/pedestrian infrastructure ▲ Access to outdoor activities ▼ Exposure to allergy-triggering plants
Mix of vegetation attracting predators	▼ Stress on plant, animal life ▼ Habitat fragmentation ▼ Standing water, vector breeding sites ▼ Exposure to disease-carrying vectors	▲ Access to outdoor activities
On-site food production/grocery	▼ Stress on plant, animal life ▼ Food insecurity ▼ Exposure to urban heat island ▼ Exposure to floodwater	▲ Access to outdoor activities ▼ Food desert ▼ Exposure to urban heat island ▼ Exposure to flood water
Locate on-site emissions sources away from openings and air supply	▼ Exposure to outdoor air pollution ▼ Exposure to indoor air pollution ▼ Exposure to urban heat island	▼ Exposure to environmental tobacco smoke ▼ Exposure to outdoor air pollution ▼ Exposure to indoor air pollution
Islandable sites and microgrids	▼ Electrical grid instability ▼ Infrastructure damage ▼ Exposure to urban heat island ▼ Exposure to floodwater	▲ Ability to charge electrical medical devices during utility outages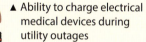 ▼ Risk of exposure to traumatizing events

Figure T.4. (*cont.*)

Community

		Health Effects of Climate Change		Community Health Concerns: Chronic Disease & Mental Health
Compact, multi-use development near transit & bike/pedestrian infrastructure		▼ Exposure to urban heat island ▼ Traffic-related air pollution ▼ Sprawl/single use districts		▼ Barriers to physical activity related to sprawl/single use districts ▼ Unsafe bike/pedestrian infrastructure ▼ Exposure to outdoor air pollution
Provide multi-modal evacuation routes		▲ Access to outdoor activities ▼ Exposure to floodwater ▼ Infrastructure damage		▲ Resilience of individuals with pre-existing conditions during, after disasters
Function as cooling center, resilience hub		▼ Exposure to urban heat island ▼ Exposure to floodwater ▼ Exposure to air pollution from generators ▲ Population resilience during, after disasters		▲ Resilience of individuals with pre-existing conditions during, after disasters ▼ Risk of exposure to traumatizing events

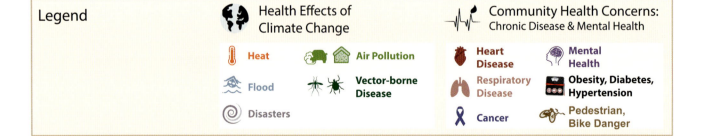

Figure T.4. (*cont.*)

CHAPTER 3

Architectural Epidemiology at Each Phase of the Project Delivery Process

KEY MESSAGES

1. Architectural epidemiology brings value to every phase of the building project delivery process and is particularly useful during the programming/visioning phase because it can help with site selection.

2. The health situation analysis sets the foundation for identifying the most significant environmental health risks to a project based on its environmental and population health context.

3. Health metrics are key to successful implementation of the ArchEPI methodology throughout the full project delivery process. In the earlier phases of the project, they are used to help the team scope the environmental health challenges to be addressed by design strategies or operations protocols. Later on, they are used to track implementation and quality control/quality improvement.

3.1 Introduction

While projects at various scales—including regions, districts, neighborhoods, and master plans—can benefit from a process that focuses on improving health outcomes through design interventions, the main focus of this book is to outline specifically how these methods can improve projects at the building scale and smaller (such as renovations, additions, and interiors projects). Our goal is to help these smaller scale projects contribute to larger scale efforts to address climate, health, and equity. See "The Value Proposition for Architectural Epidemiology" in chapter 1 for a more detailed discussion of the last mile gap between neighborhood/community plans and the tendency of building design projects to limit their focus to inside the boundaries of the project site.

3.1.a What is the Project Delivery Process?

*The process of performing design and construction services on a capital development project is called **project delivery**.* It starts when an owner, operator, or developer identifies the need for a new or expanded space and continues through design and construction. Traditionally, the relationship between the owner and the design and construction team would end when the new space is handed over to the owner for occupancy. However, project delivery is increasingly expanding to spill over into the occupancy phase of the building through activities such as measurement and verification (i.e., tracking energy and water use) and post-occupancy evaluation (i.e., canvassing occupants on their level of satisfaction with their new space).

While the project delivery process can vary from project to project—depending on the contractual relationship between the owner, the design team, and the general contractor—the overall process falls into six major phases: (1) programming/visioning; (2) schematic design; (3) design development; (4) construction documents; (5) construction and construction administration; and (6) occupancy. See figure 1.2 in chapter 1 for a visual crosswalk of ArchEPI decision points at different phases of the project delivery process for 15 design topics.

This chapter lays out the ways in which Architectural Epidemiology (ArchEPI) can contribute to each phase of the project delivery process.

3.1.b Integrating Architectural Epidemiology into the Project Delivery Process

The role of ArchEPI will vary from one project delivery phase to the next. This chapter follows the traditional Design-Bid-Build project delivery process for the sake of convenience. However, the ArchEPI activities outlined below are applicable to any project delivery model. See chapter 4 for more detail about how ArchEPI can be applied to different contractual arrangements.[SR3.1]

3.2 Phase 1—Programming/Visioning

3.2.a Overview

The very first step in any project is to develop a vision of the desired outcome through a conceptualization process.[CC3.1] Here are some of the questions that need to be answered for capital development projects:[1]

- Why is the project needed and what are the specific needs to be met?
- Who should be involved in the visioning process to increase the likelihood that the project will be a success?
- What metrics should be developed to define success?
- What schedule and budget are realistic, given the priorities set out by the owner?
- How will the current project fit into the development's master plan to accommodate future needs?

The phase ends after the project requirements and site considerations are condensed into a *"program"*: *a list of the space functions, square footage, budget, and schedule required to meet the project's vision*. Identifying health goals during this phase of the project delivery process allows them to be considered and planned for from the beginning.

3.2.b Health Situation Analysis

A health situation analysis (HSA)[D3.1] is an essential first step of six in the ArchEPI approach outlined in chapter 2. It sets up any real estate project to create conditions for a positive ripple effect on the health of future building occupants and the community as a whole.[CC3.2,SR3.2] An HSA helps project teams develop goals and prioritize strategies that impact environmental health goals for the project. For project teams with limited time and energy, conducting an HSA is the most efficient method for integrating health priorities at the initial stages of project development.

Site analysis is a key step in the visioning process. It establishes the parameters within which the project will be developed. And it can be pivotal to the site selection process if an owner or developer is evaluating more than one option. Site analysis begins with an inventory of candidate sites and their immediate surroundings. The inventory catalogs the physical, regulatory, and social context

---

> **STAKEHOLDER ROLES 3.1**
>
>
>
> Opportunity for the development team to demonstrate leadership in community benefit design

> **CORE COMPETENCY 3.1**
>
> **Facility Design, Construction, Operations**
> Programming and Analysis
>
> **Sustainability**
> Integrative Services
>
> **Philanthropy**
> Vision Setting

> **DEFINITION 3.1**
>
> **Health Situation Analysis**
> "Study of a situation that may require improvement. This begins with a definition of the problem and an assessment or measurement of its extent, severity, causes, and impacts upon the community; it is followed by appraisal of interactions between the system and its environment and evaluations of performance"
>
> Porta, M. *A Dictionary of Epidemiology*. Sixth Edition, Oxford University Press; 2014.

> **CORE COMPETENCY 3.2**
>
> **Epidemiology**
> Assessment and Analysis; Community Dimension of Practice
>
> **Sustainability**
> Project Surroundings; Public Outreach

> **STAKEHOLDER ROLES 3.2**
>
>
>
> Opportunity for local public health practitioners to perform this task, coach others, and/or provide quality control

into which the project will be embedded. By comparing the project vision and scope with the site analysis for various properties, the developer can determine which site would be most advantageous for the project. This process offers the first opportunity for the project team to brainstorm the ways in which the project vision might result in different design choices, depending on which site is chosen for development.[SR3.3]

An HSA of properties under consideration can inform the site analysis and site selection process. As described in more detail in chapter 2, HSAs identify the priority health concerns in the community where the project is located and their relevance to the physical, regulatory, and social context of the site. After a property has been secured, HSA recommendations can support architects, landscape architects, and civil engineers in determining where the building will be located on the property and its orientation in relation to the sun, topography, nearby streets, and public infrastructure.

The HSA results should be organized into a set of conceptual diagrams and associated environmental public health indicators (EPHIs). The following sections share examples of some of the ways in which an HSA can enhance a traditional site analysis.

3.2.c Physical Context

The climate, topography, soil characteristics, and biodiversity of a site play a fundamental role in shaping ecologically sensitive building designs. These characteristics also influence the health status of the populations living and working in the neighborhood surrounding the site.[CC3.3]

An HSA might also consider the relationship between the utilities serving the site and the health and resilience of future occupants and the surrounding neighborhood.[CC3.4] For example, exposure to combined sewer overflows (CSOs) can lead to waterborne disease.[11,12] It is estimated that waterborne disease accounts for 40,000 hospitalizations each year in the US, representing $970 million in medical expenses.[13] Worldwide, only 56 countries report that 50% or more of their domestic wastewater is safely treated. (Sustainable Development Indicator 6.3.1).[14] Since over half of the waterborne outbreaks in the US occur immediately following heavy rain events,[15] it is particularly important to include on-site storm water prevention and retention capabilities in regions with combined sewers.

> **STAKEHOLDER ROLES 3.3**
>
>
>
> Opportunity for developers, local government, and community groups to work with all stakeholder groups to establish trust, credibility, and accountability to the community

> **CORE COMPETENCY 3.3**
>
> **Facility Design, Construction, Operations**
> Physical Analysis
>
> **Sustainability**
> Energy and Atmosphere; Sustainable Sites

> **CORE COMPETENCY 3.4**
>
> **Epidemiology**
> Assessment and Analysis
>
> **Facility Design, Construction, Operations**
> Technical Capabilities

BOX 3.1.

Example—Environmental Exposures Shift from One Neighborhood to the Next in Phoenix, Arizona, USA

A study of heat vulnerability in Phoenix, Arizona, USA, found that the urban heat island varied greatly from neighborhood to neighborhood. The mean air temperature was more strongly associated with density and vegetation than with distance from the urban core. The warmest and coolest neighborhoods were both located near the center of town, roughly 3 km (2 miles) from each other. In spite of their close proximity, the mean temperature in the warmest neighborhood increased more than twice as much as the coolest neighborhood (6.4°C vs. 2.9°C) during heat waves.[2]

Add to these physical vulnerabilities a population that is more likely to require medical care after exposure to a heat wave—the elderly, children, and/or individuals suffering from chronic respiratory or heart disease[3]—and a health situation analysis of a future long-term elder care facility in the warmest neighborhood in Phoenix might emphasize design strategies that reduce exposure to extreme heat—both inside the building and through shading and vegetation outside.

BOX 3.2.

Example—Kaiser Permanente Community Health Initiative, USA

The Community Health Initiative at Kaiser Permanente uses mapping technology to perform health situation analyses—proactively targeting location-based, population health interventions. When they see high concentrations of populations with diabetes and hypertension, for example, in a specific area, they combine traditional clinical care and public health interventions with programs that modify the built environment—such as improving public parks and redesigning the layout and display of healthy food at stores and in school cafeterias. Over the long term, they can evaluate the program's relative success by tracking the extent to which key behavioral or health indicators change in their member population.[4] For example, the program funded a playground redesign at the intermediate public school in Leadville, Colorado, USA, serving 5th and 6th graders, over 70% of whom identify as Hispanic and 77% of whom receive a free or reduced-price lunch. One year after completion of construction, 67% of students participated in moderate or vigorous exercise during their 25-minute daily recess, compared with only 50% prior to the playground renovation.[5] Kaiser Permanente has integrated environmental stewardship into the Community Health Initiative program, so that green building practices can be integrated into their larger focus of promoting community health—both in their facilities and in the community.[6]

BOX 3.3.

Example—Traffic-Related Air Pollution, Hong Kong, China

A study in Hong Kong raises interesting questions about how to protect vulnerable groups from exposure to traffic-related air pollution (TRAP) in dense cities with large numbers of so-called "street canyons": streets that are lined with tall buildings on both sides. Street canyons are often found in central business districts and in mega-cities where high-density residential towers have proliferated. The concentration of traffic in these semi-enclosed outdoor spaces can lead to high levels of TRAP both at street level and inside the buildings lining the street. The study measured outdoor and indoor concentrations of fine particulate matter ($PM_{2.5}$) and black carbon at six residential towers in TRAP hotspots in Kowloon and northern Hong Kong Island.[7,8]

While the study found that the overall average exposure to $PM_{2.5}$ and black carbon among residents was 20% lower inside than immediately outside, the median infiltration efficiency increased to 91% for both $PM_{2.5}$ and black carbon during the cool season, which also corresponds with the highest ambient concentrations of $PM_{2.5}$ pollution in the city. During summer months, the median infiltration efficiency fell slightly for black carbon (88%) and a bit more for $PM_{2.5}$ (81%). Students and working age adults were exposed to higher levels of TRAP annually, because they spent more time outdoors commuting than the elderly and people who neither worked nor studied outside the home. In contrast, the infiltration efficiency for mechanically ventilated office buildings was much lower: 45% during the cool season and 40% during the warm season. Overall, increased exposure correlated with higher risk of all-cause, cardiovascular, and respiratory disease mortality.[8] An additional social consideration is the relative scarcity of air conditioning in homes[9] (leaving windows and doors as the only access point for ventilation) and the fact that many of the TRAP hotspots in the study correspond to pockets of concentrated poverty.[10]

The design questions raised by a health situation analysis using these findings might focus on design strategies that address the combined challenges of Hong Kong's hot, humid climate; the regional air flow that brings industrial pollution from factories in mainland China northwest of the city down towards Hong Kong; the orientation, footprint, and massing of Hong Kong's street canyons; and cost considerations associated with installing air filters and/or mechanical systems to reduce indoor exposure to ambient air pollution.

BOX 3.4.

Example—Green Alley Program, Chicago, Illinois, USA

The city of Chicago's Green Alley Program is an example of a built environment intervention that reduces exposure to two climate-related health risks: extreme heat and exposure to combined sewer overflows (CSOs) due to flooding. It encourages replacing impervious surfaces in the 2,000 miles of public alleys throughout the city with vegetation and pervious surfaces. From 2006 to 2014, more than 200 Green Alley projects were installed in Chicago, diverting 17 million gallons of storm water away from the combined sanitary and storm sewer system each year. Chicago has also aggressively promoted the use of vegetated (e.g. garden) roofs. As of 2014, 5.5 million square feet of vegetative roofs had been installed in the city, detaining 70 million gallons of stormwater annually.[16] Other green infrastructure best management practices encouraged by the city include rain gardens, rain barrels, converting turf to native grasses, and on-site storm water management measures. Given the dual health risks of extreme heat and CSOs in Chicago and the availability of municipal resources such as the Green Alley Program, a health situation analysis for a site located in high-risk Chicago neighborhoods would likely identify heat and street flooding as primary health concerns that should be prioritized by the project.

BOX 3.5.

Example—Sanitation Options for Sustainable Housing Tool, South Africa

The Sanitation Options for Sustainable Housing (SOSH) tool is designed to help projects in South Africa select the most appropriate wastewater conveyance system for their needs, based on an understanding of the project scope, budget, and characteristics of the surrounding infrastructure.[17] Wastewater infrastructure is a major concern in the country, because 18.5% of the population live in residences with substandard sanitary systems[18(p96)] and 9.8% do not have access to clean drinking water.[18(p95)] The SOSH tool was developed in response to the combination of drought (exacerbated by climate change), ageing and poorly maintained infrastructure, and concerns in South Africa that widely used technologies like pit latrines might increase the risk of waterborne disease. It guides users through a series of questions about the building project's expected lifespan (e.g., temporary or permanent); building density; risk of flooding; existing access to a potable water system; and access to funding/local capacity to construct, operate, and maintain a wastewater system. The sanitation options recommended for different types of settlements range from flush toilets connected to municipal wastewater conveyance systems to septic systems, pit latrines, and composting toilets.

Two case studies—an informal settlement and a student residence—demonstrate how the SOSH tool could inform the utility infrastructure section of a health situation analysis for a potential building site in South Africa. The tool returned a recommendation for providing composting toilets in the informal settlement and flush toilets with a neighborhood treatment plant for the student housing project. The recommendation for neighborhood treatment rather than connecting to an existing municipal wastewater conveyance system was based on user input regarding the relative capacity of the university to operate and maintain a sanitary sewer system on campus compared with the municipality, which was reportedly under strain with its current capacity. Furthermore, user input suggested that the university might be able to reuse the treated wastewater to irrigate landscaping.[17]

> **CORE COMPETENCY 3.5**
>
> **Epidemiology**
> Policy Development
>
> **Real Estate Development**
> Market Research
>
> **Facility Design, Construction, Operations**
> Programming and Analysis
>
> **Philanthropy**
> Collaboration/Partnership

> **STAKEHOLDER ROLES 3.4**
>
>
>
> Opportunity for local regulators to tailor requirements and incentive programs to address neighborhood needs

> **STAKEHOLDER ROLES 3.5**
>
>
>
> Opportunity to center questions of equity and social justice in the project

> **CORE COMPETENCY 3.6**
>
> **Epidemiology**
> Community Dimension of Practice; Cultural Competency
>
> **Facility Design, Construction, Operations**
> Research, Technical and Analytical
>
> **Sustainability**
> Project Surroundings and Public Outreach
>
> **Philanthropy**
> Collaboration/Partnership

3.2.d Regulatory Context

The codes and regulations governing land use development[CC3.5] often determine key features of the project, such as its size, density, setback from the street, and parking requirements. While the data gathered by an HSA may not override regulations that inadvertently exacerbate disease (such as single-use zoning),[19] it can be used to request variances.[SR3.4]

Many building and zoning codes in the US encourage single occupancy car use by accommodating large volumes of traffic and requiring that all developments set aside space for a minimum number of parking spots. These same codes may ignore or not permit the construction of sidewalks, bike paths, bus stops, and other infrastructures that encourage less polluting and more active modes of transportation. They also may reduce density, which discourages active transportation. Other regulations, such as codes affecting open space, energy and water efficiency, and storm water management, often offer a range of options for compliance. Overlaying population health data onto these regulatory requirements can help project teams prioritize design strategies that both protect health and meet the goals of the regulation.

An HSA for a development located in a community with a high rate of chronic heart and respiratory disease might flag TRAP as a health priority for the project, particularly because the concentration of air pollution from cars and trucks has been found to be many times worse inside urban homes than in suburban homes in the US. A study comparing the homes of asthmatic children in inner city Baltimore, Maryland, USA, with homes in the surrounding suburbs found that the average concentration of PM_{10} in inner city homes was 47 µg/m³ (compared with 18 µg/m³ in the suburbs), 34 µg/m³ for $PM_{2.5}$ (compared with 8.7 µg/m³), 19 ppb for NO_2 (compared with "below detection"), and 1.9 ppb for O_3 (compared with 0.015 ppb).[20]

However, it can be difficult for a single building project to reduce ambient air pollution on its own. The examples below from the South Bronx neighborhood of New York City, New York, USA, and the Hackney borough in East London, UK, demonstrate that community groups, real estate developers/landowners, and land use regulators may need to collaborate over a period of years or even decades to push through the policy changes that are needed to streamline the process of seeking variances to building and zoning codes in order to protect population health.

3.2.e Social Context

The social and economic context of the site is arguably the closest a conventional site analysis comes to addressing public health considerations—specifically, the social determinants of health.[SR3.5] For example, a brownfield site can expose the entire neighborhood surrounding it to environmental toxins through air pollution, contaminated dust, and/or compromised stormwater or groundwater. If a concentration of low-income and/or minority groups live and work in neighborhood, an HSA can be used both to build public support for the project and to identify supplemental funding sources to pay for a high level of remediation.[CC3.6]

The HSA may also include a health equity assessment to position the site-specific demographic, socioeconomic, and health data within an historical context. The result can be leveraged to support community members in revitalization efforts with an eye to minimizing population displacement (i.e., gentrification) and future proofing the long-term real estate value of the new development.

178 ARCHITECHTURAL EPIDEMIOLOGY

BOX 3.6.

Architectural Epidemiology in Action
South Bronx, New York City, New York, USA

The South Bronx Neighborhood is one of the most acutely affected environmental justice neighborhoods in the US. It is home to four natural gas power plants,[21] a wastewater treatment plant that represents 11% of the city's treatment capacity,[22] a major food distribution hub that is responsible for 12% of all food sales and 22% of regional wholesale produce sales in New York City (NYC),[23] and nine solid waste transfer stations. Every day, 750 diesel truck trips pass through the neighborhood, hauling an average of 2,500 tons of commercial waste.[24] Roughly one-quarter of the residents in South Bronx are African American, and three-quarters are Hispanic (compared with 22% African American and 29% Hispanic in NYC as a whole). Twenty-nine percent of residents live below the poverty line (compared with 20% in NYC), 58% of households pay more than 30% of their income for housing (compared with 51% in NYC), and 12% are unemployed (compared with 9% in NYC). They are almost twice as likely to be diagnosed with obesity (42%) and diabetes (20%) as the citywide average (24% and 11%, respectively). Pediatric asthma-related emergency department visits in the eastern half of South Bronx (Hunts Point/Longwood) are almost twice the rate of NYC (432 per 10,000 compared with 223 per 10,000 in NYC). Rates in the western half (Mott Haven/Melrose) are even higher: 647 per 10,000. Residents under age 65 also experience a higher death rate from heart disease than NYC as a whole: more than 50 deaths per 100,000 compared with 33 deaths per 100,000 in NYC.[25,26]

Arbor House, a 124-unit, LEED Platinum certified affordable housing apartment building, took the most inward-looking approach of the three projects in this case study. Rather than attempting to change the rights-of-way or zoning requirements adjacent to the site to reduce traffic and improve outdoor air quality, the project installed an advanced airtight envelope system, a whole building continuous background direct exhaust vent with air regulators, trickle vents in each unit, and building materials with low levels of volatile organic compounds. The building is also designated as no-smoking—another public health step that could be taken with minimal input from code reviewers.[27]

The Eltona, a 63-unit, LEED Platinum affordable housing apartment building, was developed by the same developer as Arbor House, Blue Sea Development Company, and pursued many of the same green building strategies to improve indoor air quality.[28] However, The Eltona also benefitted from the 15 years of regulatory and code negotiations associated with the LEED Silver Certified 30 block Melrose Commons urban infill renewal area where it is located. The community plan for Melrose Commons complements the efforts at indoor environmental quality within housing units by emphasizing pedestrian-oriented streets and pocket parks inside the development—two strategies that can reduce the concentration of traffic-related air pollution.[29]

Finally, the Peninsula (figure 3.1) is a major renovation project, converting a decommissioned juvenile detention facility into a mixed-use project with 740 units of affordable housing, a health and wellness center, a supermarket, a daycare center, 15,000 square feet of commercial space, 50,000 square feet of light industrial space, and a jobs center, among other programmatic elements.[30] The Peninsula project aligns with a number of objectives in the Hunts Point Vision Plan (figure 3.2), which calls for changes to land use, greater regulation of diesel trucks, and

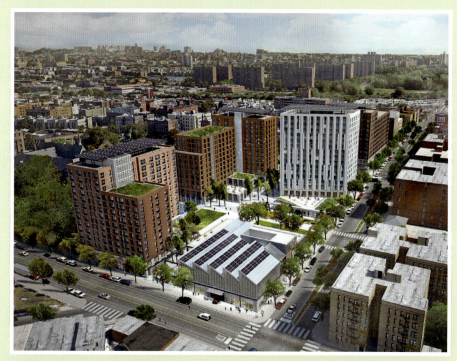

Figure 3.1. Rendering of the Peninsula Redevelopment, South Bronx, New York City, New York, USA.
Source: The Peninsula https://www.thepeninsulabx.com/

BOX 3.6. (cont.)

redesigning 10 miles of streets. Its three main goals are economic development, improving neighborhood air quality, and improving access to parks and green space.[32] Together with the renovation of a neighborhood playground and library, the installation of rooftop solar and energy storage on neighborhood schools, and the construction of new employment opportunities in the neighborhood, The Peninsula contributes to the Vision Plan's goal of improving the neighborhood's quality of life without displacing its residents. Such a bold and expansive vision required close coordination with many city departments to overcome a wide array of regulatory hurdles, which can be a slow process.[32] While the Vision Plan was published in 2004,[32] construction on The Peninsula project did not break ground until late 2019.[33]

Health Situation Analysis Snapshot

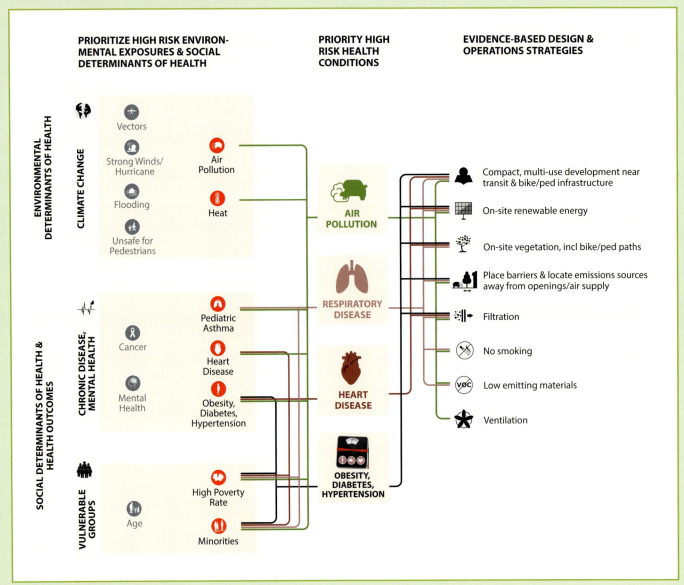

HSA 3.1. South Bronx

Note: This snapshot reflects the information in the case study. Additional research and data collection might uncover additional environmental risk factors, population health risk factors, priority health concerns, and/or evidence-based design strategies. For more examples, see figure T.4 in the toolbox to explore a crosswalk of climate change and community health co-benefits associated with common design and operations strategies.

Stakeholder Roles: South Bronx

 Development team

Provided affordable and middle-income housing units and small-scale retail and light industrial space in a neighborhood in need of both types of real estate asset

 Local government

Took a leadership role in convening a community-centered vision for urban renewal, including confronting the barriers caused by antiquated building code and zoning regulations

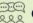 **Community groups**

Active community groups advocated on behalf of existing residents, increased visibility of environmental exposures, and the economic and health effects associated with decades of underinvestment in the neighborhood

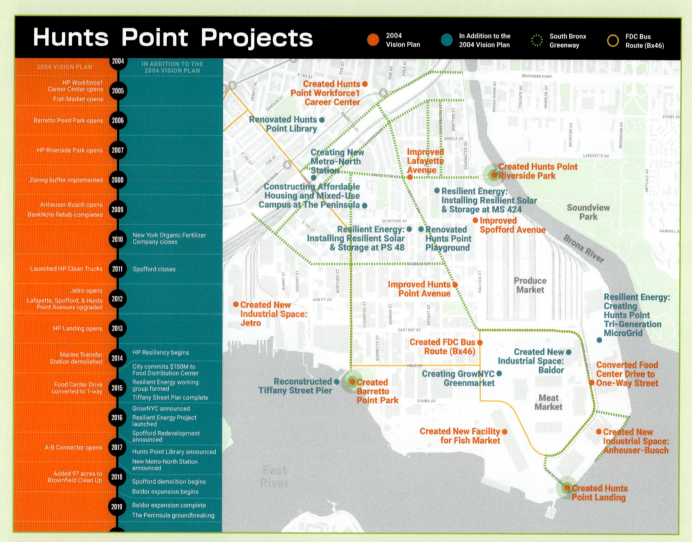

Figure 3.2. Hunts Point Redevelopment Project Map, South Bronx, New York City, New York, USA. *Source:* New York City Economic Development Corporation 2020[32]

EACH PHASE OF THE PROJECT DELIVERY PROCESS **181**

BOX 3.7.

Architectural Epidemiology in Action
Gillett Square, London, UK

Gillett Square in the Hackney borough in East London, UK, is an interior pedestrian plaza that provides access to opportunities for physical activity at a distance from the traffic-related air pollution, dangerous pedestrian environment, and absence of parks or open space characterizing the surrounding neighborhood.[34] The project began in the 1980s and has developed over the course of 40 years into an ongoing three-pronged initiative aimed at (1) reducing crime, (2) acting as a catalyst for economic development among neighborhood women- and minority-owned small businesses, and (3) resisting gentrification.[35] The project is spearheaded by Hackney Co-operative Developments, a community interest company, which leads a public-private partnership that funded the renovation of the square and surrounding building using United Kingdom and European Union urban renewal funding sources.[36,37]

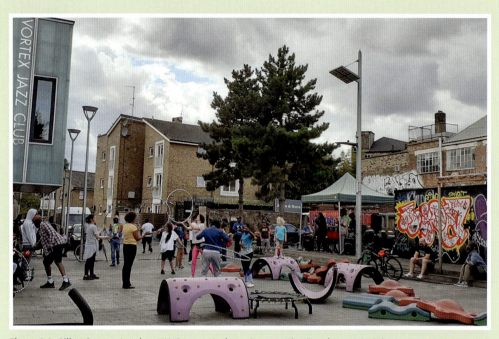

Figure 3.3. Gillett Square, London, UK. *Source:* Hackney Co-operative Developments CIC

Hackney was originally developed in the 18th century as an industrial zone interspersed with worker housing. However, between 1921 and 1981, most of the warehouses and factories were abandoned, and the residential population fell by 50%. The borough began to repopulate in the 1990s. By 2016, its population had increased by 37%, and it had become the 3rd most populated and the 6th most diverse borough in London, with a mix of 50% White, 23% Black, and 10.5% Asian residents.[38] By this time, community members had begun to worry about gentrification: a process by which low-income families are forced to relocate due to rapidly rising property values. Seventy-five percent of Hackney residents are renters, which increases their vulnerability to changes in housing costs. And many residents are low income, particularly among the elderly and the young. The borough reports the second highest poverty rate in England among the elderly and the fourth highest poverty rate among children in London.[38]

Rezoning was central to the success of the project, starting with a multi-step conversion of a parking lot in the middle of a block into the project's namesake—a pedestrian plaza and play area known as Gillett Square (figure 3.3). A row of Victorian flats were converted into 30 workspaces and 10 new retail spaces facing the interior of the block, while retaining the existing street-facing ground-floor retail. The renovated building, rechristened Bradbury Works, replaces the original interior stairs with outdoor stairs and galleries facing Gillett Square to increase connection with activity in the plaza. The entire project prioritizes tenants from neighborhood start-ups and cultural organizations. Existing tenants either stayed in the building throughout the renovation or were accommodated by the development team in temporary space off-site to help them continue operations during the construction process.

The renovation also enhanced the historic building's resilience to extreme heat and cold by improving its thermal performance (e.g., adding insulation and installing double-paned windows), increasing energy efficiency, installing operable windows and designing the building to take advantage of cross-ventilation, and preparing the project for a future solar array on the south-facing roof.[36,37,39] A clothing factory along the west side of the square was converted into a jazz club. And an empty factory on the north side of the square was converted into a mixed-use development with office space and social housing.[36]

Health Situation Analysis Snapshot

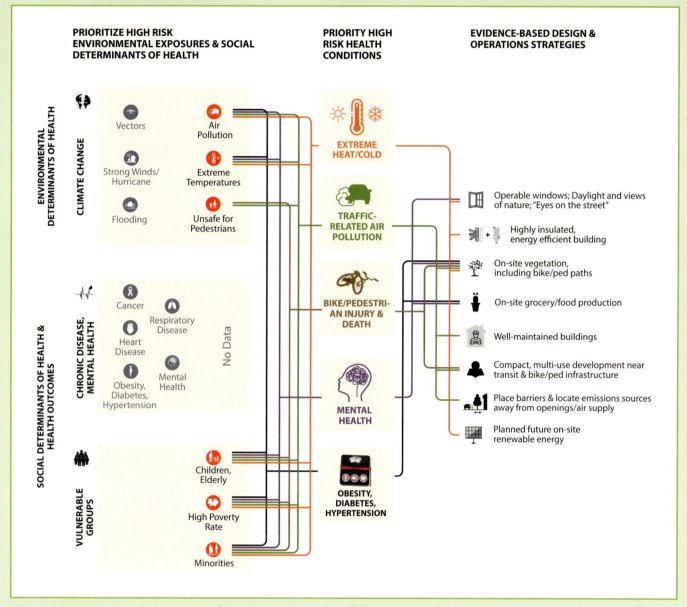

HSA 3.2. Gillett Square

Note: This snapshot reflects the information in the case study. Additional research and data collection might uncover additional environmental risk factors, population health risk factors, priority health concerns, and/or evidence-based design strategies. For more examples, see figure T.4 in the toolbox to explore a crosswalk of climate change and community health co-benefits associated with common design and operations strategies.

BOX 3.7. (*cont.*)

Stakeholder Roles: Gillett Square

Development team	Local government	Community groups
Organized as a community-interest company to manage a public-private partnership that centered existing residents' interests in the project	Supported a rezoning effort that converted a parking lot into a pedestrian plaza, allowed building use rezoning, and permitted the construction of kiosks	Active engagement over more than four decades ensured that the existing residents' goals of reducing crime, supporting economic development opportunities for women- and minority-owned businesses, and resisting gentrification were reflected in the final project

BOX 3.8.

Architectural Epidemiology in Action
High Point, Seattle, Washington, USA

The 120-acre High Point redevelopment in Seattle, Washington, USA, is a 1,600 unit mixed-income development[40] located in a working-class area that, from 1990 to 2000, transformed from majority White to majority minority. During that same period, the rate of educational and professional attainment in the neighborhood fell in comparison with the citywide average. And the median home price fell to $100,000 lower than the Seattle average in 2000. While the risk of exposure to toxic air pollution decreased 96% across Seattle from 1990–2007, the remaining industrial facilities are clustered in West Seattle, where the High Point neighborhood is located.[41] The High Point site itself was a public housing development with buildings dating from the 1940s. Due to income-eligibility requirements for residents, prior to the redevelopment, 85% of households lived at or below 30% of the mean income for King County.[42] Furthermore, more than 10% of the population suffered from asthma.

The new development responded to the historical context of the site and the needs of the existing population by actively involving residents in the design process. The resulting design moved beyond a typical "green" development. In addition to building energy- and water-efficient homes and installing landscaping that purifies and retains storm water onsite, the development includes 35 so-called "Breathe-Easy" homes (figure 3.4) for families suffering from asthma.[43] The site design was also tailored to encourage walking and other forms of physical activity (figure 3.5), including working in the community garden.[40] Post-occupancy studies have also been performed since completion of construction to quantify the health benefits associated with the project. A study comparing asthmatic children who moved into Breathe-Easy homes with similar children living in other public housing residences found that one year after move-in, the children in Breathe-Easy home experienced improvements in symptom-free days, lung capacity, and caretakers' quality of life, as well as a reduction in hospital visits.[44] Another study looking at the combined impact of design elements to encourage physical activity and supportive programs like walking groups reported similarly positive results. Study participants increased the number of minutes they walked each day (from 64.6 to 108.8) and reported feeling healthier, both physically and mentally.[40] The development has also managed to maintain its reputation as a mixed-income neighborhood with a high quality of life even as it experiences 11% churn among renters each year and the continued build-out of market rate housing.[45]

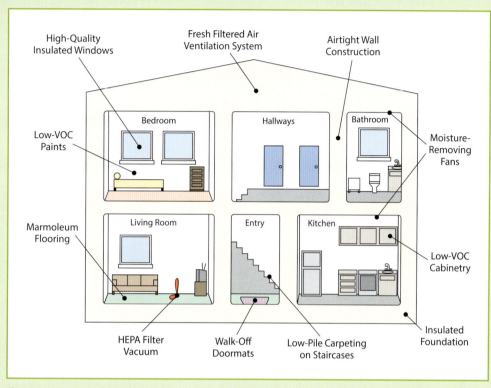

Figure 3.4. Diagram of Breathe-Easy Home. *Source:* Illustration courtesy of Seattle Housing Authority and Mithun

EACH PHASE OF THE PROJECT DELIVERY PROCESS **185**

BOX 3.8. (cont.)

Health Situation Analysis Snapshot

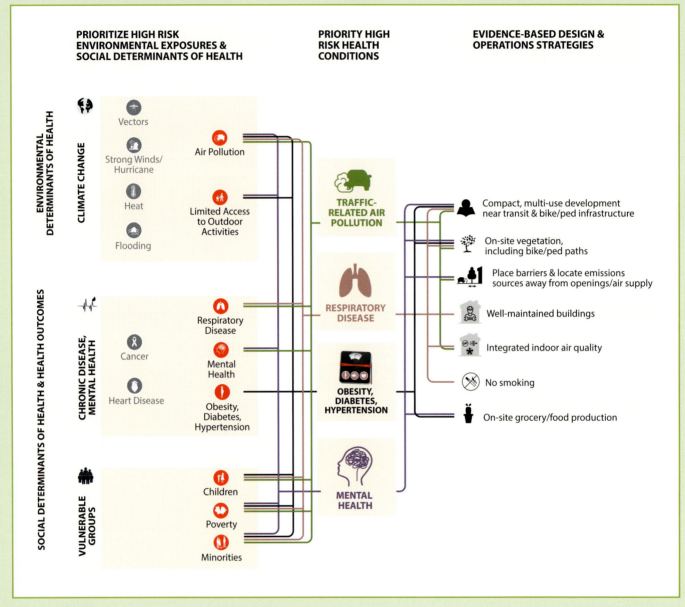

HSA 3.3. High Point

Note: This snapshot reflects the information in the case study. Additional research and data collection might uncover additional environmental risk factors, population health risk factors, priority health concerns, and/or evidence-based design strategies. For more examples, see figure T.4 in the toolbox to explore a crosswalk of climate change and community health co-benefits associated with common design and operations strategies.

Stakeholder Roles: High Point

Development team	Local government	 Community groups
Committed to maintaining the development as mixed income over time	Converted a public housing site into a mixed-income development that includes opportunities for home ownership	Active involvement in the design process led to a dual emphasis on home with healthy indoor air quality and access to opportunities for recreational physical activity

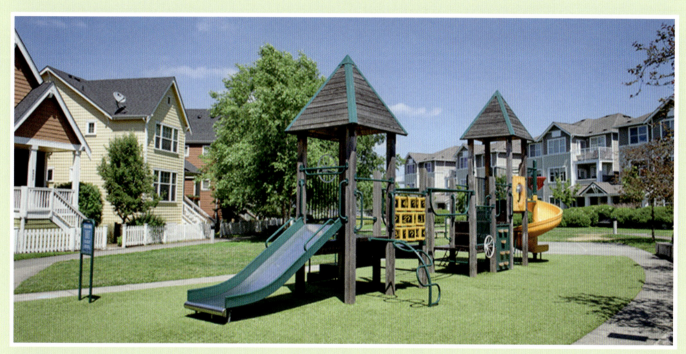

Figure 3.5. Pocket Park in High Point Neighborhood, Seattle, Washington, USA. *Source:* Barnett 2017.[45] *Image credit:* John Vicory.

BOX 3.9.

Architectural Epidemiology in Action
Bon Pastor, Barcelona, Spain

The low-income neighborhood of Bon Pastor in Barcelona, Spain was originally developed by the Municipal Institute of Housing and Rehabilitation of Barcelona in 1929 primarily to house families who were displaced from slums on the mountain of Monjuic in southwestern Barcelona as part of urban renewal efforts to prepare for the International Exhibition held that year. By 2002, the 784 one-story, low-income houses in the original development—nicknamed "cheap houses" (Casas Baratas)—were in poor condition, and, the City proposed replacing them with apartment buildings. In the end, one block of the original houses was retained as a cultural heritage museum. The remainder of the development was demolished and is in the process of being replaced with apartment buildings interspersed with pocket parks and pedestrian plazas (figure 3.6).

Barcelona has historically suffered from flash flooding, due to its semi-arid climate, dense urban fabric, and steep topography. In recent years, heavy precipitation events have occasionally overwhelmed the centralized network of storm sewers, which is designed to drain rainwater into the Mediterranean as fast as possible. As a result, in 2006, the city began to supplement the central system with smaller scale sustainable urban drainage systems (SUDS), which have the opposite goal. By building smaller scale stormwater controls in multiple locations, SUDS slow down and purify stormwater using green infrastructure methods such as infiltration and detention. In addition to reducing the risk of flooding, the water SUDS capture and store can be used for landscape irrigation or drinking water (if properly filtered).

The city-wide stormwater management plan identified Bon Pastor as a good candidate for a SUDS installation, because it is both adjacent to the Besòs River and low in elevation. Because the SUDS installation was limited to the boundaries of the new apartment complex, the neighborhood association was able to exert a strong level of influence over the final design. They were included in a consensus-building design process that included representatives from the SUDS design team and the municipal government.

In the final design, SUDS have been integrated into the vegetated areas that were made available by increasing density in the development. They vary in design, including gravel infiltration wells located under rain gardens in the green areas surrounding the apartment buildings, a bio-retention material located between the street and the sidewalks, and pervious pavement on the streets and sidewalks (figure 3.7). The local parks department is currently maintaining the SUDS, but the neighborhood association is considering taking a more active role to increase the participation of residents in the success of the flood-control system.

The project has brought multiple benefits to the neighborhood. It is credited with preventing street flooding and humidity entering the new apartment buildings during multiple flash flooding events in 2018. The increased vegetation surrounding the apartment buildings has lowered the urban heat island effect in the neighborhood—which previously did not have access to any green space. It has also increased interest in green building technologies among residents. For example, Bon Pastor volunteered to become a pilot project for a citywide Zero Waste project, which is designed to virtually eliminate municipal waste through waste reduction, reuse, and recycling practices.[46]

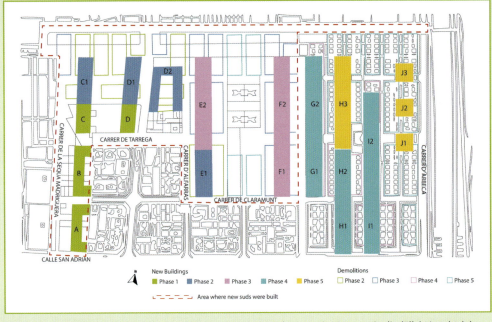

Figure 3.6. Bon Pastor Redevelopment and SUDS Network, Barcelona, Spain. *Source:* Xiaolin (Elle) Li and Adele Houghton. *Reference:* Carriquiry et al. 2020.[46]

188 ARCHITECHTURAL EPIDEMIOLOGY

Health Situation Analysis Snapshot

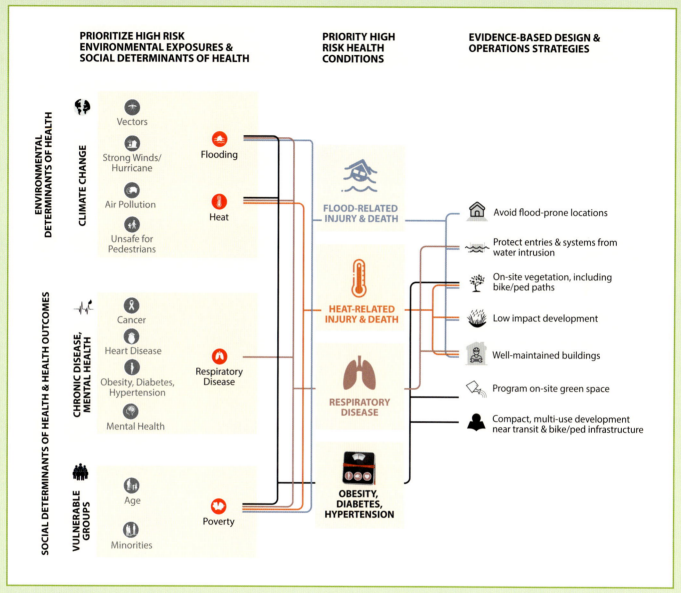

HSA 3.4. Bon Pastor

Note: This snapshot reflects the information in the case study. Additional research and data collection might uncover additional environmental risk factors, population health risk factors, priority health concerns, and/or evidence-based design strategies. For more examples, see figure T.4 in the toolbox to explore a crosswalk of climate change and community health co-benefits associated with common design and operations strategies.

BOX 3.9. (cont.)

Stakeholder Roles: Bon Pastor

 Development team

 Local government

 Community groups

Coordinated the negotiations between the City and the neighborhood association

Revised the apartment design to accommodate the sustainable urban drainage systems (SUDS) and the neighborhood association's proposals

Combined a health and safety goal of improving the quality of low-income housing in the Bon Pastor neighborhood with a city-wide goal of reducing the risk of flash flooding

Exerted influence over the final design of the apartment buildings and stormwater management system, so that the SUDS double as resident green space and are designed to reduce the risk of water infiltration into the buildings after rain events

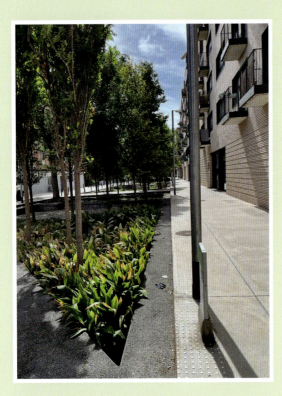
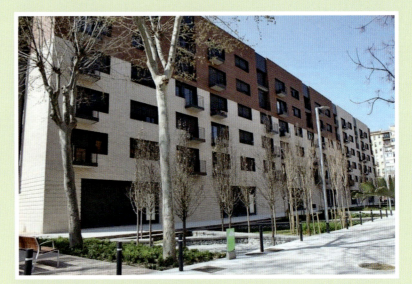

Figure 3.7. New Apartment Buildings and SUDS Installation in Bon Pastor Neighborhood, Barcelona, Spain. *Source:* Jaume Canela Soler

3.2.f Health Mission Statement

The ArchEPI process can also contribute to the programming/visioning phase by translating the results of the HSA into a health mission statement for the project. A **health mission statement** is a short declaration of the project team's objectives promoting health and wellbeing.[47(p137)] Writing a health mission statement offers an opportunity for the entire project team to process the results of the health situation analysis and lay out in clear terms[SR3.6]

- the set of values that are guiding the project,
- the environmental health risks that are most relevant to the project,
- vulnerable groups on-site or located in the surrounding community, and
- the EPHIs that the project intends to track to measure progress towards reducing risk and enhancing health and wellbeing.[CC3.7]

The health care sector is a leader in the adoption of health mission statements for both capital investments and ongoing facilities operations. In the early 2000s, the *Green Guide for Health Care*[48] was the first green building rating system to require that all registered projects develop a health mission statement and program as part of the project's design intent document. In 2010, the LEED for Healthcare[49] rating system adopted health mission statement language similar to the *Green Guide for Health Care*. Some health systems have developed system-wide health mission statements. For example, Kaiser Permanente announced a set of environmental stewardship goals in 2016 that the organization is working toward achieving by 2025:

- Become "carbon net positive" by buying enough clean energy and carbon offsets to remove more greenhouse gases from the atmosphere than we emit.
- Buy all our food locally or from farms and producers that use sustainable practices, including using antibiotics responsibly.
- Recycle, reuse, or compost 100% of our non-hazardous waste.
- Reduce the amount of water we use by 25% per square foot of buildings.
- Increase our purchase of products and materials meeting environmental standards to 50%.
- Meet international standards for environmental management at all of our hospitals.
- Pursue new collaborations to reduce environmental risks to foodsheds, watersheds and air basins supplying our communities.[49]

These goals directly link the organization's environmental commitment to its obligation to advance health and wellness among the people they serve. Similarly, real estate and health care institutions like Anthem and Alexandria Real Estate Equities, Inc. have established goals for their real estate portfolios centered on health for the building occupants by certifying them with healthy building certification systems like Fitwel and WELL.

On an even larger scale, the National Health Service (NHS) in the UK, which owns or manages 8,253 sites covering 5,560 hectares of land in England alone,[50] adopted a "vision of sustainable health and care" in 2014 with the following declaration: "A sustainable health and care system works within the available environmental and social resources protecting and improving health now and for future generations. This means working to reduce carbon emissions, minimizing waste & pollution, making the best use of scarce resources, building resilience to a changing climate and nurturing community strengths and assets."[51] Table 3.1 details recent progress the NHS has made related to specific environmental goals.

STAKEHOLDER ROLES 3.6

Opportunity for the development team to demonstrate how the design supports community goals

CORE COMPETENCY 3.7

Epidemiology
Policy Development

Real Estate Development
CRE Asset Management

Facility Design, Construction, Operations
Project Planning and Design

Sustainability
Integrative Strategies

Philanthropy
Vision Setting

TABLE 3.1.
National Health Service England Health Check Scorecard 2018

Table 3.1.a. NHS Scorecard Goal 1: A Healthier Environment

ID	Indicator	2017	Trend	2018	Context
1.01	Progressive of Health and Social Care to achieve 34% 2020 carbon reduction target	*	▬	*	Making progress
1.02	% NHS providers reporting on track to meet 34% carbon reduction target by 2020	41%	▼	39%	Improvement needed
1.03	NHS provider building energy use carbon emissions (2013–2014 baseline)	−0.5%	▼	−9%–4%	Making progress
1.04	Implementation of SDMPs by NHS providers	71%	▬	71%	Making progress
1.05	Implementation of SDMPs by Commissioners (CCGs)	34%	▼	26%	Improvement needed
1.06	% of health bodies' Greening Government Commitments on target (2020 targets)	Some		88%	Very good
1.07	Implementation of healthy travel plans by NHS providers	60%	▼	57%	Making progress
1.08	NHS Staff commuting active travel modal share by distance	Undefined	New	5.7%	Making progress
1.09	Air pollution costs to health by NHS travel and transport	£324m	▼	£311m	Improvement needed
1.10	NHS staff valuing health and wellbeing benefits from green spaces access	Undefined	New	95.4%	Very good
1.11	Sustainability as a core to qualify care and leadership throughout the system	Undefined		Undefined	Definition needed
1.12	Waste weight generated by NHS providers		New	224 Mt	Making progress
1.13	% Waste avoiding landfill by NHS providers		New	85.5%	Very good
1.14	Change in water volume use by NHS providers (2013–2014 baseline)	3.5%	▼	1.80%	Improvement needed
1.15	NHS providers and CCGs with an annual sustainability report	69%	▲	85%	Very good
1.16	NHS providers and CCGs with "good" or "excellent" reporting	36%	▲	45%	Making progress
1.17	% NHS organisations with a Good Corporate Citizen assessment in 2016–2017	15%	▼	13%	Improvement needed
1.18	Good Corporate Citizen assessment - average score in 2016–2017	50%	▬	50%	Making progress

Note: NHS = National Health Service; CCGs = clinical commissioning groups; SDMP = sustainable development management plan.

Table 3.1.b. NHS Scorecard Goal 2: Communities and Services Are Ready and Resilient for Changing Times and Climates

ID	Indicator	2017	Trend	2018	Context
2.01	NHS staff who value environmental sustainability in the workplace	Undefined	New	93%	Very good
2.02	NHS Staff perception of their employer actively supporting the environment		New	71%	Making progress
2.03	NHS Staff feeling encouraged by their employer to support the environment outside of work		New	50%	Making progress
2.04	NHS providers reporting includes employment practices (e.g., living wage)	29%	—	66%	Very good
2.05	JSNAs including good assessment of sustainability	23%	—	23%	Making progress
2.06	Housing and fuel poverty included in the JSNA assessment	37%	—	37%	Making progress
2.07	Percentage of households in England that experience fuel poverty (low income; high cost)	10.69%	▲	11.0%	Improvement needed
2.08	Partnership working for adaptation plans referenced in JSNAs	11%	—	11%	Making progress
2.09	Implementation of adaptation plans by NHS providers	38%	▼	32%	Improvement needed
2.10	NHS providers reporting on adaptation in annual report	55%	▲	71%	Very good
2.11	Number of overheating events in NHS provider clinical areas		New	2,980	Improvement needed
2.12	Percentage of NHS provider clinical space monitored for temperatures		New	48.2%	Improvement needed
2.13	Local areas (e.g., STP counties) with a sustainability ambassador		New	64%	Making progress
2.14	% Local sustainability ambassadors with a live local sustainability project		New	22%	Improvement needed

Note: JSNA = joint strategic needs assessment; STP = sustainability and transformation plan.

(*cont.*)

Table 3.1.c. NHS Scorecard Goal 3: Every Opportunity Contributes to Healthy Lives, Healthy Communities, and Healthy Environments

ID	Indicator	2017	Trend	2018	Context
3.01	Commissioners CCGs using sustainability in managing demand for services	46%	▼	44%	Making progress
3.02	Use of guidance and tools to assess environmental impacts of patient pathways	Low	—	Low	Improvement needed
3.03	Use of a Sustainability Impact Assessment in NHS commissioning	Low	—	Low	Improvement needed
3.04	Commissioners (CCGs) encouraging providers in sustainability	12%	▲	13%	Improvement needed
3.05	NHS providers encouraging supply chain in sustainability	9%	▲	21%	Improvement needed
3.06	Measures of sustainable procurement: Ethical, SME & third sector spend	Undefined	New	Low	Improvement needed
3.07	Proportion of people with long term conditions feeling supported to manage their condition	64.3%	▼	64.0%	Making progress
3.08	Emergency admissions for acute conditions that should not usually require hospital admission (per 100,000 population)	1,314	▲	1,357	Improvement needed
3.09	Fraction mortality attributable to particulate air pollution	5.1%	▼	4.7%	Making progress
3.10	Utilisation of outdoor space for exercise/health reasons	17.9%	—	17.9%	Making progress
3.11	% of non-propellant inhalers dispensed in the community	27%	▼	26%	Improvement needed
3.12	Reduction in anaesthetic gases emissions	Undefined		Undefined	Definition needed

Source: Adapted from NHS England, Sustainable Development in the Health and Care System: Health Check 2018, 2018.

STAKEHOLDER ROLES 3.7

Opportunity for local public health practitioners to perform this task, coach others, and/or provide quality control

CORE COMPETENCY 3.8

Epidemiology
Assessment and Analysis; Cultural Competency

The key to developing a health mission statement with measurable objectives is to include public health experts on the project team.[SR3.7] As discussed in more detail in chapter 2, section 2.4, chances are that readily available population health data could be used to develop a health mission statement supporting the overall vision for the project. This same data could be converted into baseline health indicators for tracking the design's level of compliance with the health mission statement.[CC3.8]

3.2.g ArchEPI Activities (Phase 1)

- The programming/visioning phase is the ideal time to perform a health situation analysis, because all topics are still on the table. This is particularly true if the owner is considering more than one location for the project. The earlier the team begins to think about the potential for the project to improve environmental health conditions in the surrounding neighborhood, the more likely those considerations will become central to the ultimate design.[CC3.9]

- Health metrics alongside economic, environmental, and other data that are gathered through the HSA should be collected during this stage for use in developing the schematic design in the next phase of the project.[CC3.10]

3.3 Phase 2—Schematic Design

3.3.a Overview

During the schematic design phase, several preliminary design options are developed, each of which emphasizes a different aspect of the project vision or the unique characteristics of the site. This phase is characterized by research, experimentation, and an iterative design process.[57] Health goals established during visioning are supported through the use of design strategies and high-level decision-making.

The major design disciplines (architecture, engineering, landscape, etc.) engage in intensive collaboration during this phase with the goal of integrating as many systems as possible.[CC3.11] The higher a building's performance goals, the more integrated building systems must become. For example, the Living Building Challenge requires that all certified projects generate on-site the quantity of energy and water required to run the facility. The Bullitt Center in Seattle, Washington, USA, achieved this requirement by designing the structural, energy, water, daylighting, and landscaping systems all in relation to each other, rather than running parallel design processes for each building system—which is the conventional design approach. (For more detailed information, see the Bullitt Center's website: http://bullittcenter.org.)

3.3.b Health Impact Assessments

Many ArchEPI projects will use the Health Impact Assessment (HIA) framework to translate the EPHIs developed through the HSA into design and operations recommendations tailored to the project site and program.[SR3.8] The most effective time to perform an HIA for a building project is the schematic design phase, because the project vision has been set but the design is still in flux. An HIA can be used to synthesize the health, environmental, regulatory, and cultural data gathered during the programming/visioning phase into design recommendations about the location, footprint, massing, layout, orientation, materials, and technologies included in the final design. See section 2.6 in chapter 2 and appendix N for an in-depth discussion of HIAs and health equity impact assessments.

3.3.c ArchEPI Activities (Phase 2)

- Translate the environmental health data gathered in the Programming phase into evidence-based design recommendations using tools like HIA.[SR3.9] Green and healthy building certification systems, such as LEED, Fitwel, WELL, Enterprise Green Communities, and Living Building Challenge, are useful at this stage as sources of evidence-based design strategies depending on the environmental health goals of the project. These recommendations can be presented through the HIA, as an addendum to the HSA, or as a separate report linked to design and community engagement workshops.[CC3.12]

CORE COMPETENCY 3.9

Epidemiology
Assessment and Analysis

Sustainability
Integrative Strategies

CORE COMPETENCY 3.10

Facility Design, Construction, Operations
Site Inventory; Contextual Analysis

CORE COMPETENCY 3.11

Facility Design, Construction, Operations
Project Development and Documentation

Sustainability
Integrative Strategies

STAKEHOLDER ROLES 3.8

Opportunity for developers, local government, and community groups to align project goals with community climate, health, and equity goals

STAKEHOLDER ROLES 3.9

Opportunity for local public health practitioners to perform this task, coach others, and/or provide quality control

CORE COMPETENCY 3.12

Epidemiology
Assessment and Analysis

Sustainability
Integrative Strategies, Green and Healthy Building Certification Process

BOX 3.10.

Architectural Epidemiology in Action
The Family Health Center on Virginia, McKinney, Texas, USA

The idea for developing this Federally Qualified Health Clinic (figure 3.8) in a rapidly growing community near Dallas, Texas, USA, originated at a local bank, Independent Financial, whose CEO was committed to giving back to his community. The project attracted support from regional health systems, foundations, non-profits, and private companies, who partnered to create the North Texas Family Health Foundation, which oversees the health center's operations.[52–55]

Mission and Health Impact Statement:[56]

Our mission is to research, partner and advocate for projects that promote stronger, healthier communities.

Working Together to Build Up Community, Health & Hope

The North Texas Family Health Foundation believes that by working together, local communities can make tremendous progress on health equity and improve health outcomes and opportunity for everyone. Our focus is on supporting cross-sector collaborations and strategic public-private partnerships to create sustainable solutions.

The Foundation's first project, Family Health Center on Virginia (FHC) is the result of a seven+ year commitment to expand primary care resources in McKinney and North Texas. To date, the clinic has established a medical home for more than 4,000 individuals and families, and with the recent completion of the new home for FHC, we look forward to growing that impact further.

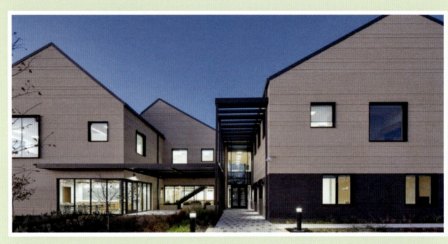

Figure 3.8. The Family Health Center on Virginia, McKinney, Texas, USA. *Image Credit:* Iwan Baan

The development team strategically located the Family Health Center in East McKinney, a low-income neighborhood where fewer households report access to health insurance or dental insurance than the city as a whole. Given the high rate of chronic diseases such as diabetes in the neighborhood, the health center provides both traditional primary care services as well as behavioral health services and a food pantry. In an effort to present the project as a community center that supports health (rather than as a traditional institutional medical facility), the design reflects local residential architecture in terms of scale and aesthetics and intersperses community spaces with spaces for clinical care.

Stakeholder Roles: The Family Health Center on Virginia

Development team	Local government	Community groups
Non-profit partnership was created to envision, finance, and operate a federally qualified health center in a neighborhood that did not previously have access primary care	Awarded a permit to a health center with unconventional programming	Community-based organizations like the local food bank partnered with the project team to provide wraparound services complimenting baseline primary care services

196 ARCHITECHTURAL EPIDEMIOLOGY

Health Situation Analysis Snapshot

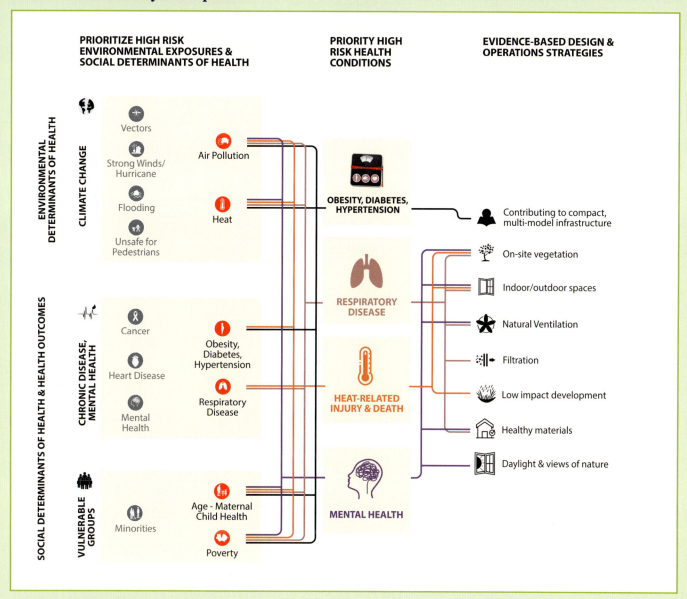

HSA 3.5. The Family Health Center on Virginia

Note: This snapshot reflects the information in the case study. Additional research and data collection might uncover additional environmental risk factors, population health risk factors, priority health concerns, and/or evidence-based design strategies. For more examples, see figure T.4 in the toolbox to explore a crosswalk of climate change and community health co-benefits associated with common design and operations strategies.

BOX 3.11.

Architectural Epidemiology in Action
Jack London Gateway, West Oakland, California, USA

The Jack London Gateway project (figure 3.9), a 61-unit low-income senior housing development in West Oakland, California, USA, commissioned an HIA to identify opportunities to mitigate health impacts associated with the site's proximity to two freeways and the port. The HIA identified four factors associated with negative determinants of health: poor air quality, noise levels, pedestrian safety, and access to health-promoting retail options.

The report's recommendations were shared with the developer early enough in the design process to influence the final project's ventilation and filtration system, the location of resident balconies, and the location of building entrances to enhance perceived safety and connection with the surrounding community.[58] The HIA further recommended attracting an outlet to the retail space on the ground floor to provide affordable, fresh food.[59]

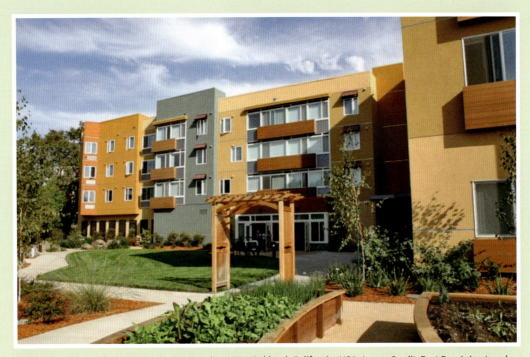

Figure 3.9. Jack London Gateway Senior Housing, West Oakland, California, USA. *Image Credit:* East Bay Asian Local Development Corporation

Stakeholder Roles: Jack London Gateway

 Development team | **Local government** | **Community groups**

The non-profit developer centered both the neighborhood's environmental justice legacy and the specific vulnerabilities of future occupants (low-income seniors) in the design discussions from the beginning	Awarded a permit to convert a shopping center parking lot into a senior living facility	Active community-based organizations have raised the profile of health disparities in West Oakland related to a history of industrial pollution and environmental exposures associated with the Port of Oakland

Health Situation Analysis Snapshot

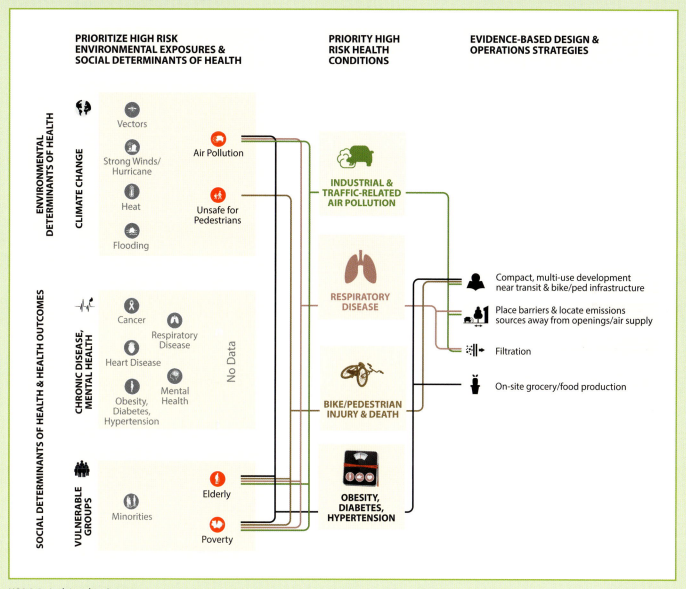

HSA 3.6. Jack London Gateway

Note: This snapshot reflects the information in the case study. Additional research and data collection might uncover additional environmental risk factors, population health risk factors, priority health concerns, and/or evidence-based design strategies. For more examples, see figure T.4 in the toolbox to explore a crosswalk of climate change and community health co-benefits associated with common design and operations strategies.

BOX 3.12.

Architectural Epidemiology in Action
Aerotropolis Atlanta, Atlanta, Georgia, USA

Aerotropolis Atlanta—a development located on the former Hapeville Ford Assembly Plant site next to the Hartsfield-Jackson Atlanta International Airport in Atlanta, Georgia, USA—had already undergone brownfield remediation prior to performing a Health Impact Assessment (HIA) of the project. The new development represents over 3 million square feet of office space, retail, hospitality, and parking (figure 3.10). The HIA combined an empirical assessment of demographic, health status, and environmental data with anecdotal information gathered from an Advisory Council representing the existing neighborhoods surrounding the site. The site is surrounded by a mix of industrial areas, the airport, and low-income neighborhoods, some of which are majority minority. Residents living in the neighborhoods surrounding the site have historically experienced disproportionately high disability rates; visits to the emergency room; and death rates from cardiovascular disease, stroke, HIV, homicide, diabetes, and septicemia compared with the state average. Additionally, the hospital discharge rate for asthma was about 30% higher than the average rate in Georgia.

The resulting recommendations identified a variety of ways the new development could better integrate into the surrounding community, thereby increasing potential revenues for the property owner and converting the development into an amenity for the surrounding neighborhood. For example, the HIA recommended moving high-speed traffic corridors (such as freeways) to the edge of the development, laying out the interior of the development as small blocks with frequent intersections and easy access to multiple modes of transportation, zoning for a mix of uses that would attract nearby residents in addition to the intended occupants of the site, and building public spaces such as parks throughout the development. The HIA also recommended zoning language that accommodates small-scale industry with the goal of providing employment opportunities for existing residents.[60] Furthermore, by linking the amenities offered by the new development with the health effects associated with current gaps in the social and economic fabric of the community, the HIA offers an opportunity for the new development to negotiate financial benefits from the public sector—such as variances, expedited plan review, reductions in property taxes, and direct investment.

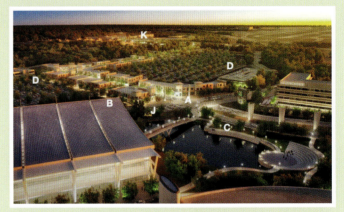

Figure 3.10. Aerotropolis Atlanta, Atlanta, Georgia, USA. *Image Credit:* Aerotropolis Atlanta Alliance

Stakeholder Roles: Aerotropolis Atlanta

Development team	Local government	Community groups
Public-private partnership whose goal is to use the Aerotropolis site to catalyze economic development and promote community health, particularly in existing neighborhoods adjacent to the site whose residents experience disproportionately higher rates of poor health outcomes compared with the rest of the metropolitan region	Public-private partnership explicitly raises community benefit as one of the project's overarching goals	The health impact assessment recommends improving integration between the Aerotropolis master plan and existing surrounding communities, so that it can be used as an opportunity both to catalyze economic development in low-income and underserved neighborhoods and increasing residents' access to parks, community amenities, and other benefits of the development

Health Situation Analysis Snapshot

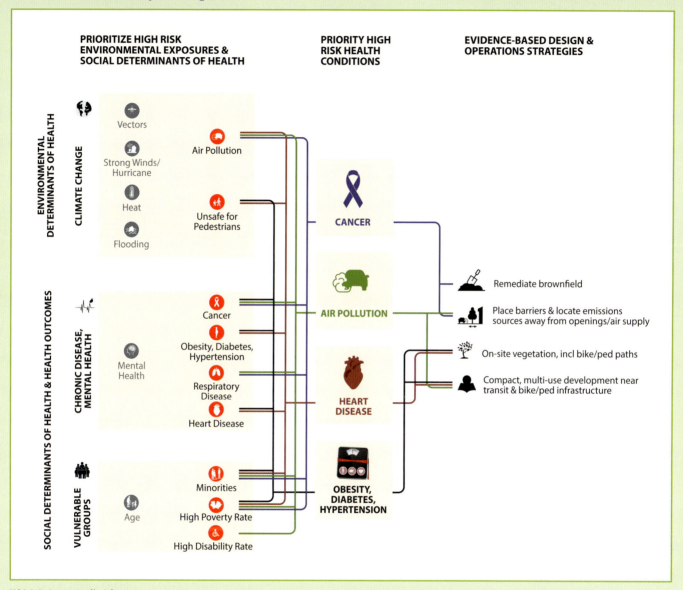

HSA 3.7. Aerotropolis Atlanta

Note: This snapshot reflects the information in the case study. Additional research and data collection might uncover additional environmental risk factors, population health risk factors, priority health concerns, and/or evidence-based design strategies. For more examples, see figure T.4 in the toolbox to explore a crosswalk of climate change and community health co-benefits associated with common design and operations strategies.

3.4 Phase 3—Design Development

3.4.a Overview

During the design development phase, the most promising design concepts from the schematic design phase are developed in more detail.[SR3.10] The shape of the building can change a great deal during this phase, because the design moves from an abstract idea to a set of interconnected buildings systems that will be constructed using materials with specific sizing, structural, and performance characteristics. Space must also be allocated for the mechanical, electrical, plumbing, and telecommunications systems. Finally, the design is checked against municipal building codes (e.g., fire code, flood control and water quality regulations, seismic codes, green building requirements, aesthetic requirements), which can have a dramatic impact on the final design.[57,CC3.13]

The role of ArchEPI during the design development phase is to help the project team flesh out the health promoting strategies incorporated in the schematic design, so that they are tailored to the unique circumstances of the project site, program, budget, and regulatory obligations. This is also the phase in which the team creates a mechanism for tracking the EPHIs that were developed through the health situation analysis.[CC3.14]

3.4.b Maximizing the Value of Computer Software Programs to Promote Health

Both real estate development and public health practice have undergone digital revolutions over the past 30 years. For designers, this shift has changed the focus of day-to-day work from generating technical drawings and specifications to developing a computer model that can be shared among design specialties and—in some cases—with the contractor and facility operators after completion of construction. During the design development phase, project teams begin to utilize digital tools to describe their designs. These tools can also link a wealth of health information into the project models and construction methods for the remainder of the project delivery process.

The National Institute of Building Sciences defines building information modeling (BIM) as a product, a collaborative process, and a facility lifecycle management tool.[61] BIM software allows project teams to develop an "intelligent digital representation of data about a capital facility."[61] By integrating building systems data from all project team members—architects, engineers, other design consultants, and contractors—into a single digital model, BIM enables increased collaboration throughout the design and construction process. Once the facility has been successfully constructed, the "as-built" model can be handed over to the facility manager, where it can be used to optimize building performance.[61] The data embedded in the BIM model can also be used to support green building goals, such as energy performance, water conservation, and materials selection.[62] When optimized, BIM can also support integrated project delivery, because all team members base their design on the same computer model. This setup is particularly useful for refining the engineering design, which traditionally developed calculations using assumptions extrapolated down from the building scale.[62] The savings in terms of enhanced productivity and coordination are projected to have been substantial. For example, in 2002, inadequate interoperability was estimated to cost the industry $15.8 billion in the US alone.[63]

Public health researchers, policymakers, and practitioners have turned to a similar software package to perform spatial analysis. Geographic Information Systems (GIS) are information systems that link data with geospatial attributes.[64]

STAKEHOLDER ROLES 3.10

Opportunity for the development team to demonstrate how the design supports community goals

CORE COMPETENCY 3.13

Facility Design, Construction, Operations
Project Development and Documentation

Sustainability
Integrative Strategies; Green and Healthy Building Certification Process

CORE COMPETENCY 3.14

Epidemiology
Assessment and Analysis; Communication

BOX 3.13.

Example—NASA Sustainability Base, Moffet Field, California, USA

As shown in figure 3.11, the NASA Sustainability Base project at the Ames Research Center in Moffet Field, California, USA, was able to tune the design to optimize energy performance by transferring relevant data from the BIM computer model to an energy modeling program as the design was fleshed out.[70]

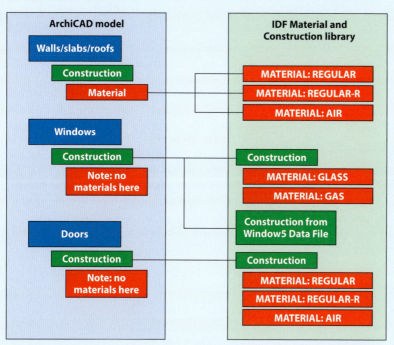

Figure 3.11. Data Mapping between BIM (ArchiCAD Software) and Energy (Energy Plus Software) Models for the NASA Sustainability Base Project at the Ames Research Center, Moffet Field, California, USA. *Source:* Adapted from O'Donnell et al. 2013[70]

GIS is often used in public health to map the spatial distribution of a disease or a factor that could lead to disease (such as toxic air pollutants). It is also used to identify clusters of disease and to perform spatial statistical analysis, which establishes spatial autocorrelation between a location and the event of interest (such as the relationship between lung cancer and distance from a high traffic roadway). Most powerfully, perhaps, it can be used to develop maps displaying spatial relationships in a visually compelling way.[65,66] See section 2.4.d in chapter 2 and appendices I–L for additional details about how to use GIS in an ArchEPI assessment.

While BIM software is optimized to model individual real estate developments in great detail and GIS software is designed to develop maps at larger spatial scales, both software packages essentially offer the same product: a visual representation (i.e., a computer model) linked to a database of relevant information. In the case of BIM, a line representing a wall in the computer model might link back to information in the database such as the wall materials (i.e., tilt up concrete, a steel stud cavity wall with brick veneer, or an aluminum and glass curtain wall), its height and thickness, what kind of insulation and waterproofing system will be built into it, and what green building characteristics are inherent in the wall (such as the percentage of recycled content and its insulation value). The computer model could use the information about insulation and the location, size, and types of windows to estimate building energy use and the level of daylighting in each room. All of this information is stored in a database that is dynamically edited and amplified as the computer model becomes more detailed.

While it can be tedious to extract the information embedded in a building model manually, a number of plugins have been developed that automatically benchmark BIM models against a wide array of sustainability goals, including green building standards, life cycle assessment frameworks, energy modeling goals, carbon footprinting targets, low-impact development goals, and stormwater management regulations.[67,68] In some cases, the plugin only extracts the data, which is then analyzed using a separate software program. In other cases, the plugin performs the analysis inside the BIM software program.[69]

BOX 3.14.

Example—Bulgari Manufacturing Plant, Valenza, Italy

A manufacturing plant for jewelry maker Bulgari located in Italy used a BIM model to calculate whether or not the HVAC system had been designed to comply with LEED minimum outdoor air ventilation rates. The team developed an external spreadsheet (figure 3.12, bottom right) that communicated with the BIM model (figure 3.12, top left) using an export/import script (figure 3.12, bottom left and top right). The spreadsheet collected data from the BIM model on room area, room volume, and maximum occupancy. After calculating the required minimum outdoor airflow, the script imported the results back into the BIM model so that the design team could compare them with the HVAC design. If the design did not supply sufficient outdoor air, the HVAC engineers revised the design until the entire project met LEED thresholds (figure 3.12).[71]

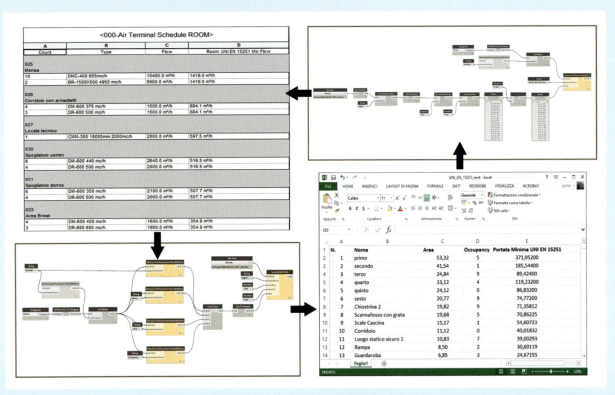

Figure 3.12. Data Flow for Automatic Calculation of LEED Indoor Air Quality—Ventilation Prerequisite and Credit, Bulgari Factory, Valenza, Italy. *Source:* Bergonzoni et al. 2016.[71] Reproduced by arrangement with Taylor & Francis Group.

204 ARCHITECHTURAL EPIDEMIOLOGY

BIM models routinely import information generated using GIS software, such as the location of utility lines adjacent to the site. Civil and plumbing engineers use this information to locate drinking water intakes and sewer and stormwater outlets at the site boundary.

The process of adding health and vulnerability data to a BIM model would follow the same lines. However, instead of reviewing environmental data exclusively (such as the location of regional watersheds and flood maps), a synthesized map might be imported that also displays the density of impervious surface within 100-year and 500-year flood plains, the location of combined sanitary and storm sewers, the neighborhoods with the highest rate of complaints about CSO, and the density of populations who are vulnerable to waterborne disease.[CC3.15]

Furthermore, if the BIM model is tracking information such as LEED, WELL, or Fitwel credits,[72] the credits that are most likely to reduce the risk of exposure to public health concerns (such as combined sewer overflows) could be flagged within the software as priority credits. As the design continues to develop, users can generate reports identifying areas of the model that comply with the designated green and healthy building credits and areas that require more attention.[CC3.16]

CORE COMPETENCY 3.15

Facility Design, Construction, Operations
Research, Technical and Analytical; Technical Capabilities

CORE COMPETENCY 3.16

Facility Design, Construction, Operations
Green and Healthy Building Certification Process

3.4.c Complying with Building Codes

The design development phase is when many of the details are worked out regarding how the project will comply with multiple layers of (sometimes conflicting) regulations.[CC3.17] Tracking EPHI metrics through the ArchEPI process can help projects apply for building code variances to incorporate innovative features. For example, some homeowner associations in Texas, USA, have attempted to prohibit rainwater catchment systems and solar photovoltaic displays in master-planned communities in spite of laws allowing their use (Texas Property Code §202.007 and §202.010, respectively).[73] The conceptual frameworks developed through the health situation analysis can be used to build support for the project by laying the foundation for an evidence-based communications pamphlet speaking to the environmental health vulnerabilities of the neighborhood and the ways in which the project's controversial technologies or design strategies will benefit its neighbors.

The ArchEPI lead can also help the full project team navigate conversations with the local health department if innovative design features conflict with public health regulations.[SR3.11] For example, the Bullitt Center in Seattle, Washington, USA, took advantage of the City of Seattle's Living Building Challenge Pilot Program (Seattle Municipal Code § 23.40.060)[74] to facilitate the permitting process for 10 micro-foam-flush composting toilets and a solar array on the roof that extends over the property line—neither of which was allowed by code.[75,76] The composting toilets, in particular, conflicted with the King County plumbing code (King County Code § 13.24.035)[77] requirement that buildings within the urban growth boundary connect to the sanitary sewer. As a result, the project was required to install an overflow connection to the sewer system to guard against a failure of the composting toilet system.[75] The solar array, on the other hand, was granted an exception to the land use code (Seattle Municipal Code; Title 23 LAND USE CODE; Subtitle III Land Use Regulations; Chapter 23.40: Compliance with Regulations Required-Exceptions)[78] and permitted as a sky bridge project.[76]

CORE COMPETENCY 3.17

Facility Design, Construction, Operations
Project Planning and Design

STAKEHOLDER ROLES 3.11

Opportunity for local regulators to tailor requirements and incentive programs to address neighborhood needs

> **STAKEHOLDER ROLES 3.12**
>
>
>
> Opportunity for community to help refine the design based on knowledge from lived experience

> **CORE COMPETENCY 3.18**
>
> **Epidemiology**
> Community Dimension of Practice
>
> **Facility Design, Construction, Operations**
> Project Development and Documentation
>
> **Sustainability**
> Project Surroundings and Public Outreach
>
> **Philanthropy**
> Collaboration/Partnership

> **CORE COMPETENCY 3.19**
>
> **Facility Design, Construction, Operations**
> Research, Technical and Analytical; Technical Capabilities

> **CORE COMPETENCY 3.20, 3.21**
>
> **Epidemiology**
> Assessment and Analysis
>
> **Facility Design, Construction, Operations**
> Research, Technical and Analytical; Technical Capabilities
>
> **Sustainability**
> Green and Healthy Building Certification Process

> **CORE COMPETENCY 3.22**
>
> **Epidemiology**
> Community Dimension of Practice
>
> **Facility Design, Construction, Operations**
> Project Development and Documentation
>
> **Sustainability**
> Project Surroundings and Public Outreach
>
> **Philanthropy**
> Collaboration/Partnership

> **CORE COMPETENCY 3.23**
>
> **Facility Design, Construction, Operations**
> Project Management

> **STAKEHOLDER ROLES 3.13**
>
>
>
> Opportunity for the development team to demonstrate how the design supports community goals

3.4.d Community Engagement

The ArchEPI lead may also spearhead the effort to check in regularly with community stakeholders and track dynamic community health indicators over the course of the design development phase.[SR3.12] Continuously monitoring the proposed design's level of success meeting environmental health and equity goals is particularly important for projects that serve the public or are otherwise high profile. The design development phase is an ideal time to communicate the project health goals and supportive design strategies with the community as a way of reinforcing the public's understanding of the project's commitment to the health of community residents. See section 2.6 in chapter 2 and appendix N for an in-depth discussion of HIAs and health equity impact assessments.[CC3.18]

In summary, design development is a crucial inflection point during the project delivery process in terms of embedding health considerations into the design and communicating that commitment to the team and the public. If appropriate EPHI metrics are included in the checklists that the design team uses to keep the project on course as the design is fleshed out, then progress towards meeting environmental health goals can be routinely tracked alongside ongoing updates to other technical aspects of the project, such as the energy model, daylighting model, and the LEED scorecard.

3.4.e ArchEPI Activities (Phase 3)

- Insert the EPHIs from the contextual health assessment into the project documents.[CC3.19]
- Create a combined green building/carbon footprint/environmental public health checklist for the project. Use this document to track compliance with all three goals, including best practice rating systems like LEED, Fitwel, WELL, Enterprise Green Communities, and Living Building Challenge.[CC3.20]
- Integrate EPHIs into BIM and other design software.[CC3.21]
- Perform community health spot-check assessments as the design is further refined.[CC3.22]

3.5 Phase 4—Construction Documents

3.5.a Overview

The construction documents phase focuses on developing the technical requirements for translating the building design into a three-dimensional building.[CC3.23] Drawings and technical specifications are finalized during this phase, including construction details and explicit instructions regarding required performance criteria for every product and system installed on the project.[56] Green and healthy design strategies that are included during this phase are one step closer to protecting occupants and community members as the project is completed.[SR3.13]

The contractor and/or a professional cost estimating company develops a definitive estimate of construction costs during this phase, leading to a cost-cutting exercise called "Value Engineering" (VE). Unless design strategies to enhance environmental health are deeply embedded in the architectural design, the VE process can result in stripping them out of the project. See the example below for a successful approach to embedding active living principles in the design of an affordable housing development in the South Bronx neighborhood of New York City, New York, USA, so that they survived the VE process.

BOX 3.15.

Architectural Epidemiology in Action
St. Antony's School, Gudalur, India

The design of St. Antony's School in Gudalur, a town in southern India, prioritized thermal comfort, indoor air quality, and the mental health benefits of daylighting as the primary health goals for the project. Gudalur, situated in the Nilgiris hills in Tamil Nadu, has a mild and humid climate year-round, due to its 3,000 ft (900 m) elevation above sea level.

The school design focused on providing as much daylighting and thermal comfort as possible using natural sources, such as the wind and the sun. The building was designed with a narrow footprint (figures 3.13 and 3.14), in order to maximize cross ventilation in the classrooms. Classrooms alternated across a covered outdoor passageway. In between classrooms, covered spaces were designed to act as semi-outdoor extensions of the classroom and covered play areas.

Local regulations required a higher density of students than recommended by international standards. As a result, the design tailored window size and location to increase ventilation rates to dissipate the carbon dioxide and heat generated from the increased number of pupils in the classroom.

Computer modeling tools such as computational fluid dynamics and daylighting analysis were used to support design development and determine the window/floor area configuration that would maximize both ventilation rates and daylighting during the academic year. The analysis found that the ratio of window to floor area needed to be 20% to achieve sufficient ventilation and 30% to achieve optimal daylighting. The final design incorporated the larger window configuration, because excessive heat loss during winter months is unlikely in such a mild climate.[79]

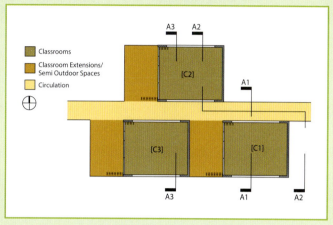

Figure 3.13. Plan of a Classroom Cluster Maximizing Natural Ventilation and Daylighting, St. Antony's School, Gudalur, Tamil Nadu, India. *Source:* Kohli 2006.[79] Used with permission.

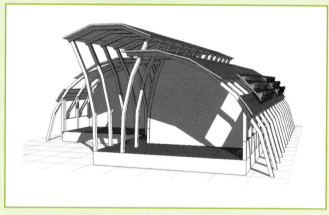

Figure 3.14. Perspective View of Classroom Cluster, St. Antony's School, Gudalur, Tamil Nadu, India. *Source:* Kohli 2006.[79] Used with permission.

Stakeholder Roles: St. Antony's School

Development team	Local government	 Community groups
This project was developed by an owner-occupier: a school	The local requirement to accommodate a higher density of students than recommended by international standards prompted the design team to focus on opportunities to maximize natural ventilation	No information

BOX 3.15. (cont.)

Health Situation Analysis Snapshot

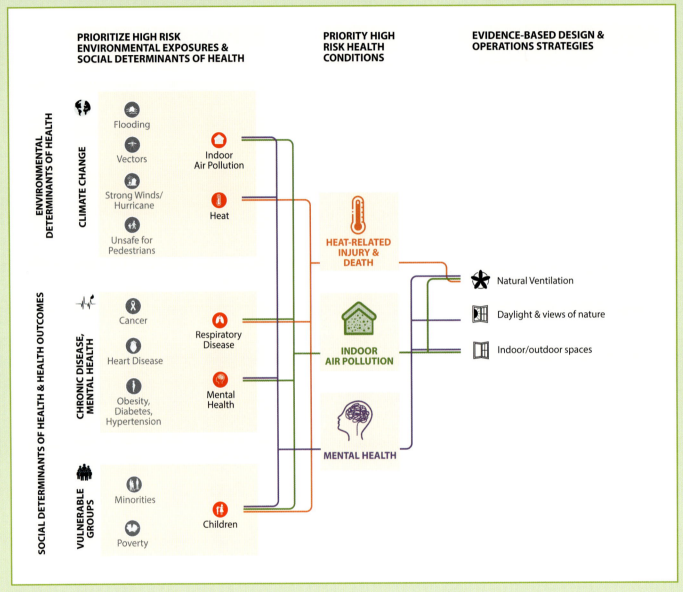

HSA 3.8. St. Antony's School

Note: This snapshot reflects the information in the case study. Additional research and data collection might uncover additional environmental risk factors, population health risk factors, priority health concerns, and/or evidence-based design strategies. For more examples, see figure T.4 in the toolbox to explore a crosswalk of climate change and community health co-benefits associated with common design and operations strategies.

3.5.b Quality Control/Quality Improvement

The role of ArchEPI during the construction documents phase is to perform quality control/quality assurance on the health promoting aspects of the design, to ensure that they are not removed during the VE process and to establish a tracking protocol that will facilitate quality-control activities during the construction administration phase.[CC3.24]

The construction documents phase concludes when the authority having jurisdiction accepts the project documents (e.g., drawings and specifications) and issues a construction permit.

3.5.c ArchEPI Activities (Phase 4)

- Collect baseline EPHI data sets (or proxies) from the health situation assessment conducted during the programming/visioning phase.[CC3.25]
- Establish a framework and milestones for tracking performance during construction administration to ensure that the project remains on track to meet the health goals set out in the ArchEPI assessment.[CC3.26]

3.6 Phase 5—Construction Administration

3.6.a Overview

Construction administration refers to the process of maintaining quality control during the construction process.[CC3.27] Occasionally, the owner may lead this process; however, the architect often coordinates construction administration as a natural extension of the construction documents phase. The design team's role during this phase (including ArchEPI team members) is to verify that the project is constructed in compliance with the permitted drawings and specifications.[57,SR3.14] ArchEPI leads should remind team members who are checking shop drawings or reviewing material substitution requests of the importance of delivering the building that was designed, including environmental health objectives.[CC3.28]

3.6.b Quality Control/Quality Improvement

Similar to the construction documents phase, environmental health data sets should be collected and periodically evaluated during this phase.[CC3.29] This is particularly important when the health outcomes identified by an HIA include the risk of exposure to environmental toxic chemicals. The example below describes the monitoring activities that were enacted during the demolition of a bridge in Cincinnati, Ohio, USA. While not all projects will be confronted with remediation of environmental toxins, ArchEPI projects should develop a protocol for tracking relevant EPHIs during the construction phase of the project.

3.6.c ArchEPI Activities (Phase 5)

- Follow the data collection framework developed during the construction documents phase.[CC3.30]
- Incorporate routine spot-check assessments into the site visit and project coordination schedule.[CC3.31]
- Track performance based on goals set at the beginning of the project.[CC3.32]

CORE COMPETENCY 3.24

Facility Design, Construction, Operations
Quality Control and Quality Assurance

Sustainability
Green and Healthy Building Certification Process

CORE COMPETENCY 3.25

Epidemiology
Assessment and Analysis

Facility Design, Construction, Operations
Research, Technical and Analytical

Sustainability
Green and Healthy Building Certification Process

CORE COMPETENCY 3.26, 3.30

Facility Design, Construction, Operations
Project Management; Quality Control/Quality Assurance

Sustainability
Green and Healthy Building Certification Process

CORE COMPETENCY 3.27

Facility Design, Construction, Operations
Construction and Evaluation

STAKEHOLDER ROLES 3.14

Opportunity for local public health practitioners to perform this task, coach others, and/or provide quality control

CORE COMPETENCY 3.28

Facility Design, Construction, Operations
Construction and Evaluation; Quality Control/Quality Assurance

Sustainability
Green and Healthy Building Certification Process

CORE COMPETENCY 3.29

Epidemiology
Assessment and Analysis

CORE COMPETENCY 3.31

Facility Design, Construction, Operations
Construction and Evaluation; Quality Control/Quality Assurance

CORE COMPETENCY 3.32

Facility Design, Construction, Operations
Project Management

Sustainability
Green and Healthy Building Certification Process

BOX 3.16.

Architectural Epidemiology in Action
Via Verde, New York City, New York, USA

If an office building design encourages physical activity through minor alterations to the stairs (such as upgrading the decor and finishes) but situates them behind closed metal doors at the end of a series of corridors, it is easy for the value engineering (VE) process to convert them into fire stairs that sound an alarm when someone tries to use them. The entire massing of the Via Verde (http://viaverdenyc.com/) mixed-income housing complex in the South Bronx (LEED Gold certified), on the other hand, was designed to encourage residents to climb up the outside of the structure (figure 3.15). Indoor stairwells are conveniently located, colorfully painted, and daylit. The plantings on the stepped roofs also serve multiple purposes. They are both integral to the design concept and increase access to fresh, healthy food by growing fruits and vegetables on-site. The accessible roof gardens also create an opportunity to highlight the project's attempt to reduce its reliance on the centralized energy grid by installing a portion of the building's rooftop solar array as a shade structure. By knitting these design features together, the design team reduced the likelihood that one of the strategies would be eliminated during the VE process to reduce capital costs at the expense of healthy occupant outcomes.

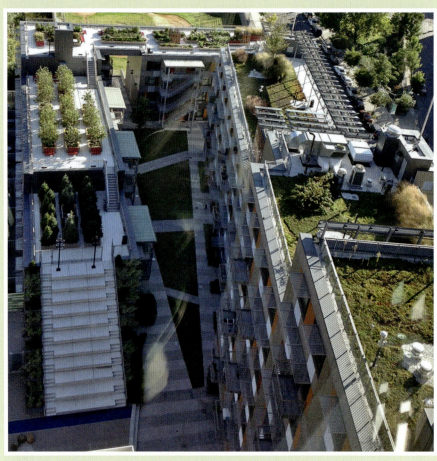

Figure 3.15. View of Exterior Stairs at Via Verde, South Bronx, New York City, New York, USA. *Photo Credit:* Adele Houghton

Stakeholder Roles: Via Verde

Development team	Local government	 Community groups
A for-profit and a non-profit development company teamed together to win the public request for proposal (RFP) for this site, which served to center community benefit as a core project goal	The City of New York used the RFP process to set minimum community benefit thresholds for the winning development team, including a minimum number of low-income rental units	The project houses non-profit social services and contracts out to a local non-profit to help manage the on-site community garden and social programming

Health Situation Analysis Snapshot

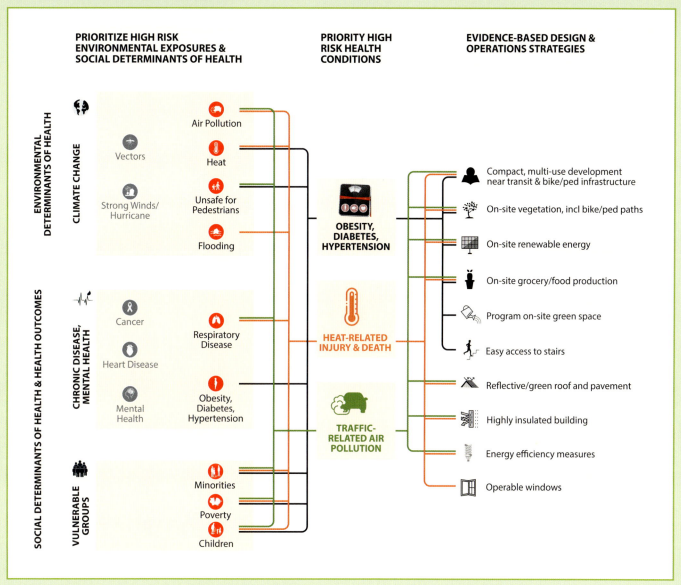

HSA 3.9. Via Verde

Note: This snapshot reflects the information in the case study. Additional research and data collection might uncover additional environmental risk factors, population health risk factors, priority health concerns, and/or evidence-based design strategies. For more examples, see figure T.4 in the toolbox to explore a crosswalk of climate change and community health co-benefits associated with common design and operations strategies.

BOX 3.17.

Architectural Epidemiology in Action
The Technological and Higher Education Institute Chai Wan Campus, Hong Kong, China

The design goals of the Chai Wan campus of the Technological and Higher Education Institute (THEi) in Hong Kong were to create a connection between the school and the surrounding neighborhood; integrate the site with existing outdoor spaces and the public realm; provide natural daylight, views, and ventilation to occupants; and reduce exposure to noise pollution.

The campus adopts a twin tower design, forming definitive visual corridors between the city and the harbor. A pedestrian pathway, fully open to the public, goes through the campus, encouraging the community to commute through the school and creating connections between the amenities and spaces in the immediate neighborhood. The pathway and a plaza between the towers also connect a park and a public housing development on the south side of the site to the previously inaccessible waterfront.

Vegetation on balconies, cantilevered planters facing the plaza and multi-level greening on the buildings' terraces mirror the adjacent public park and extend upwards throughout the THEi campus. The balconies open sideways to provide daylighting and natural ventilation and double as external shading devices for the commuting corridors, while the towers are oriented to take advantage of prevailing winds and light from the north. The geometry of the façade is designed to reduce noise pollution, enhance natural ventilation, and help daylight penetrate deeper into the interior of the classrooms (figure 3.16).

While a comparison of design renderings with Google Earth imagery demonstrates a loss of original urban greenery on the ground, the re-vegetated outdoor spaces and the greening on sky decks mitigate this loss by providing high site permeability, a green breezeway, and a connection to nature for this vertical campus (figure 3.17). The result is a low-carbon campus with excellent energy performance and a high greenery coverage.[80,81]

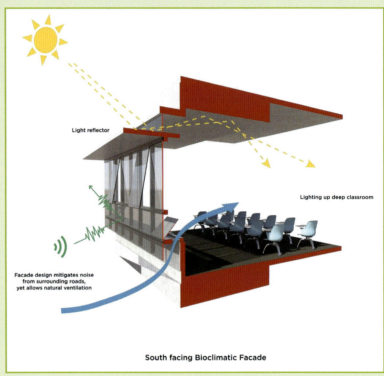

Figure 3.16. The Technological and Higher Education Institute Chai Wan Campus, Hong Kong, China, South-Facing Façade Showing Daylighting, Natural Ventilation, and Noise Pollution Design Elements. *Source:* Ronald Lu & Partners 2015.[81] Used with permission.

Stakeholder Roles: The Technological and Higher Education Institute

Development team	Local government	Community groups
This project was developed by an owner-occupier: a university that offers technical education, including courses that could benefit residents in the neighboring public housing development	The local government allowed the project to span a public right of way to make access from the public housing development easier and safer	The design makes explicit efforts to make community members feel welcome, including opening up access to the waterfront, which was previously inaccessible to neighborhood residents, and making rooms available to the general public on the ground floor

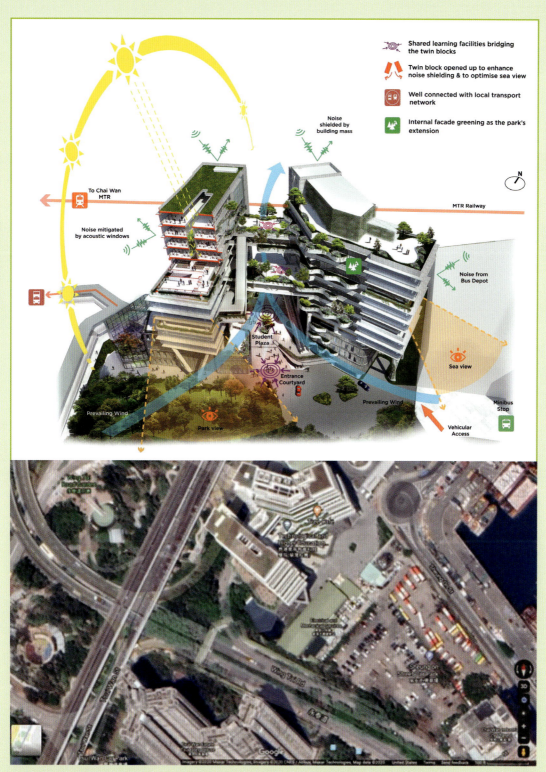

Figure 3.17. Project Rendering of The Technological and Higher Education Institute Chai Wan Campus, Hong Kong, China and Aerial Photo of the Completed Project. *Source:* Ronald Lu & Partners 2015.[81] Used with permission.

EACH PHASE OF THE PROJECT DELIVERY PROCESS **213**

Health Situation Analysis Snapshot

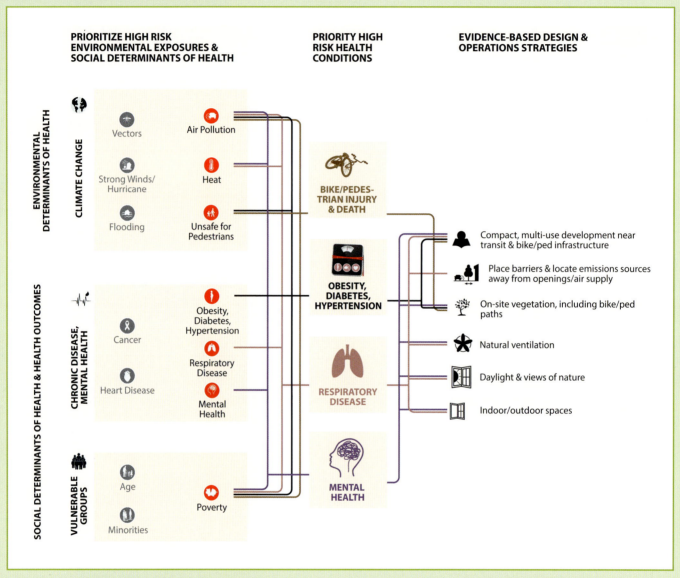

HSA 3.10. The Technological and Higher Education Institute

Note: This snapshot reflects the information in the case study. Additional research and data collection might uncover additional environmental risk factors, population health risk factors, priority health concerns, and/or evidence-based design strategies. For more examples, see figure T.4 in the toolbox to explore a crosswalk of climate change and community health co-benefits associated with common design and operations strategies.

> **BOX 3.18.**
>
> ## Example—Health Impact Assessment of Bridge Demolition, Cincinnati, Ohio, USA
>
> An HIA in Cincinnati, Ohio, USA, assessed the potential health co-benefits and co-harms associated with the demolition of a bridge coated in lead-based paint that was located next to a residential neighborhood in Cincinnati. In this case, the HIA included a plan for monitoring ambient levels of lead and particulate matter ($PM_{2.5}$ and PM_{10}) throughout the demolition process. The report also includes recommendations to reduce the risk of exposure. For example, neighborhood sidewalks and streets should be washed on a daily basis during the demolition project. Since the demolition was scheduled to take place during the school year, the neighborhood school's air filters should be changed frequently, entryway systems should be installed to trap dust tracked into the school through foot traffic, school vacuums should use HEPA filters, windowsills should be wet wiped frequently, and outdoor activities should be limited during the demolition process. Monitoring activities should also include school children with asthma and children enrolled in neighborhood daycares. Finally, a community education campaign should be launched to encourage residents to remove their shoes before entering their homes and to wash their hands more frequently during the demolition process—particularly when preparing or consuming food.[82]

> **BOX 3.19.**
>
> ## Example—Construction Air Pollution Study, Montreal, Quebec, Canada
>
> The global construction sector is estimated to contribute 23% of direct carbon dioxide (CO_2) emissions,[83] mainly due to their use of diesel-powered off-road equipment. In Canada, off-road vehicles account for 21.8% of carbon monoxide (CO), 9.4% of nitrogen oxides (NOx), and 1% of fine particulate matter emissions.[84] However, these emissions are generally not monitored during the construction process. A demonstration project in Montreal, Quebec, Canada, installed air sensors at two construction sites as a test case for using air monitoring as a construction management tool. The sensors collected data every 30 minutes for a number of air pollutants, including CO, NO_2, CO_2, noise levels, ultraviolet radiation (UV), temperature, humidity, and dust. An online portal allowed users to view on-site concentrations real time, as well as an estimate of pollutant concentrations 5 km (3 mi) downwind from the construction site. If the concentration of a certain pollutant exceeded the programmed threshold, the sensor sent an alert to the email account monitoring air quality at the construction site.
>
> The first site was a 15-story condominium development under construction in the Griffintown District of Montreal, Quebec, Canada. In this case, the air quality sensors issued alerts of unhealthy NO_2 concentrations during the earthmoving process, due to the diesel emissions from heavy-duty earthmoving equipment. The second site was a wastewater infrastructure project in downtown Montreal. In this case, the system sent alerts of unhealthy concentrations of both NO_2 and CO_2. Again, diesel-fired construction equipment was suspected to be the cause of the unhealthy conditions.[85]

3.7 Phase 6—Occupancy

3.7.a Overview

The occupancy phase begins when the project receives a "certificate of occupancy" from the authority having jurisdiction stating that the building meets the minimum regulations required for a building to be safe to occupy.[57,SR3.15] In many development projects, the certificate of occupancy marks the end of the design team's contract. However, this approach is changing somewhat in at least two areas: measurement and verification (M&V) and post-occupancy evaluations (POEs).[CC3.33]

M&V refers to making use of the energy model developed as part of the design process to help facility managers optimize building performance after occupancy. A robust M&V program requires installing sub-meters throughout the facility to tailor ongoing efficiency assessments to appropriate zones within a

STAKEHOLDER ROLES 3.15

Opportunity for the development team to demonstrate leadership in community benefit design

CORE COMPETENCY 3.33

Facility Design, Construction, Operations
Construction and Evaluation

Sustainability
Asset Management; Green and Healthy Building Certification Process

specific building. POEs generally assess more qualitative data, such as comparing the level of satisfaction among building occupants before and after moving into a new space. The example below shares the results from a POE of clinical staff after relocating to a LEED platinum community health clinic.

3.7.b Facilities Management

The role of ArchEPI during the occupancy phase can be limited or far reaching. In a more limited approach, health data can be integrated into facility management data collection and evaluation tools such as M&V and POEs. Building occupants can also participate in the ArchEPI process by self-reporting behavioral and health data that is then compared with the baseline population health metrics defined during the programming/visioning and schematic design phases.[SR3.16]

All data collection should follow the privacy and informed consent guidelines outlined in section 2.3.e in chapter 2 and appendix D. Some projects may include plans for occupancy as early as the programming/visioning phase. For example, a project whose HSA recommends prioritizing protection from extreme heat events may both include in the design a cooling center space equipped with an emergency power supply to enable air conditioning during a blackout and an accompanying operational policy. These conversations are also an opportunity to continue engagement with the surrounding community regarding partnerships to provide mutual support, such as standing up a cooling center or resilience hub when the power goes out or a natural disaster disrupts power, transportation systems, or access to grocery stores for a period of time.[CC3.34]

STAKEHOLDER ROLES 3.16

Opportunity for developers, local government, and community groups to align project goals with community climate, health, and equity goals

CORE COMPETENCY 3.34

Real Estate Development
Facilities Management

Facility Design, Construction, Operations
Quality Control/Quality Assurance

BOX 3.20.

Example—Indoor Air Quality Study, Syracuse, New York, USA

Indoor environmental quality (IEQ) is often a primary health consideration for office building projects, because a large body of research has found that healthy IEQ can increase productivity and reduce absenteeism—both of which benefit the bottom line. Many green and healthy building rating systems devote an environmental category to IEQ with the goal of encouraging the development of facilities that are healthy for both the natural environment and the people who live, work, and play in them.

A small study in Syracuse, New York, USA, tracked IEQ metrics, self-reported health status, and heart rate among 30 participants who worked in either a green building or a conventional building. Twenty-four participants then worked for six days in a LEED Platinum building, four participants remained in their conventional office environment, and two participants remained in their green office environment. During the six-day work stay at the LEED Platinum building, the IEQ conditions were changed to reflect the ventilation levels, carbon dioxide (CO_2) levels, and volatile organic compound (VOC) levels of a conventional building, a LEED-certified building, and a green building with two times the ventilation rate in a typical LEED building.

During the two weeks participants worked in their regular environment, air sensors recorded average CO_2 levels just above 750 ppm in the conventional workspaces and 500 ppm in the green workspaces. Twenty-four percent of participants in conventional buildings reported lack of air movement, and 15% reported that their workspace was too hot (compared with 2% and 3%, respectively among participants working in green buildings). Furthermore, participants working in green buildings reported half the number of health symptoms compared with participants working in conventional buildings. Even more interesting, 38% of the health symptoms reported by participants working in conventional buildings disappeared when they went home over the weekend, compared with 19% of symptoms reported by participants working in green buildings.

During the week participants relocated to the LEED Platinum building where they were exposed to CO_2, VOCs, and ventilation rates typical in a conventional building, a LEED-certified building, and a highly ventilated green building, the number of symptoms reported per participant per day fell by 0.75 on green building days compared with conventional building days. Furthermore, a 1,000 ppm increase in CO_2 levels correlated with a 43% increase in symptom reporting and 2.3 bpm increase in heart rate.[86]

BOX 3.21.

Architectural Epidemiology in Action
Uberlândia, Minas Gerais, Brazil

A post-occupancy evaluation (POE) of a social housing development outside of Uberlândia, Minas Gerais (Brazil) called "Shopping Park" three years after completion of construction uncovered a number of design and construction flaws that increased residents' risk of injury and death from flooding and extreme heat events. The built environment section of the POE covered the following topics: design, construction system and materials, maintenance, services, internal layout, adaptation and refurbishment, adaptation for commerce, comfort, privacy and previous housing. After describing the design characteristics that could increase occupants' vulnerability to flooding and extreme heat, the final report shares recommendations to improve community resilience that were "co-produced" through a collaboration between residents and researchers.

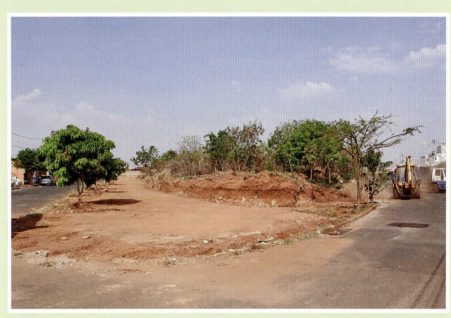

Figure 3.18. Erosion in the "Shopping Park" Social Housing Development, Uberlândia, Brazil.
Source: Prefeitura de Uberlândia, 2020, https://www.uberlandia.mg.gov.br/2020/10/06/praca-do-bairro-shopping-park-passa-por-reestruturacao/

The most critical climatic vulnerability in the development was flooding, because homes were constructed perpendicular to the topography on a hillside with 12% slope—many without containment walls to protect them from landslides. Furthermore, half of the housing units are surrounded by more than 80% impervious cover with bare dirt covering the other 20%. 67.5% of residents complained about the lack of vegetation within their residential lot, and 52.5% complained about the lack of vegetation in the neighborhood. They also reported a lack of knowledge about gardening and a fear of maintenance expense as barriers to investing in private gardens—which would reduce the risk of erosion. Many of the spaces that were set aside for public parks in the community plan had not been maintained. As a result, they had also become bare dirt (figure 3.18). Over time, residents began using them as public dumping grounds. These conditions increase vulnerability to landslides and structural collapse during floods.

The development also suffers from combined sewer overflows (CSOs) during flooding events; because, the rainwater collection systems on each house that were included in the stormwater management design were never built. Flooding from CSOs can expose residents to waterborne disease and increase the risk of mold growth. During a walkthrough conducted as part of the POE, the homes were also found to be at risk of poor indoor air quality caused by capillary water infiltration in exterior walls and recurrent leaks (particularly associated with the poor installation of the solar water heater on the roof).

Co-produced recommendations to reduce the health risks arising from flooding included encouraging residents to increase vegetation on site by planting back gardens and replacing impervious surface on their property with additional vegetation. Larger scale recommendations included proposals for the creation and public maintenance of community parks and street trees within the development as well as a linear park along the river at the bottom of the hillside. Design recommendations included a suggestion that all houses be equipped with rainwater collection systems, which would reduce both water insecurity and reduce flooding risk.

Homes in the Shopping Park development are also vulnerable to extreme heat events, because the area is located in Brazil's Bioclimatic Zone 4, which is characterized by a hot, dry climate. Measurements found that houses averaged 0.7–1.9°C above outdoor temperatures, which could place vulnerable groups at risk of heat-related illness during heat waves. The POE recommendations for mitigating the health risks from heat exposure mirrored its recommendations for mitigating flooding, indicating that planting vegetation around the house and at the neighborhood scale could have co-benefits for both heat and flooding.[87]

BOX 3.21. (cont.)

Health Situation Analysis Snapshot

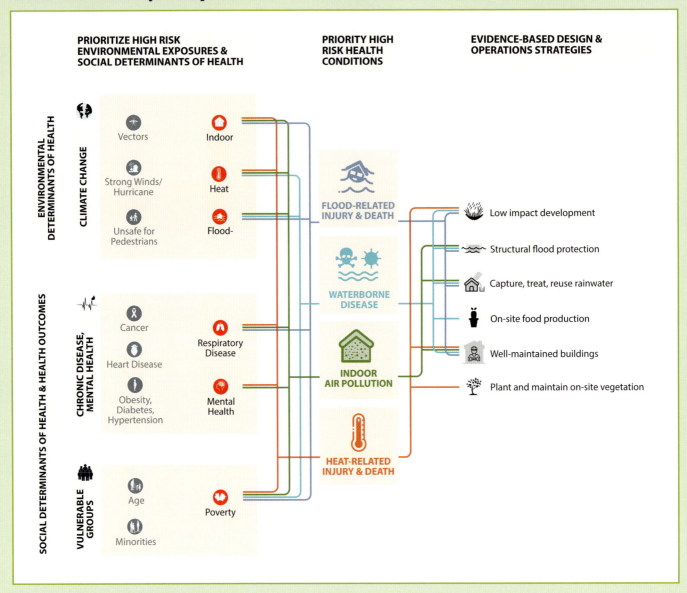

HSA 3.11. Uberlândia Housing Development

Note: This snapshot reflects the information in the case study. Additional research and data collection might uncover additional environmental risk factors, population health risk factors, priority health concerns, and/or evidence-based design strategies. For more examples, see figure T.4 in the toolbox to explore a crosswalk of climate change and community health co-benefits associated with common design and operations strategies.

Stakeholder Roles: Uberlândia Housing Development

Development team	**Local government**	**Community groups**
The report found that the original development was poorly constructed, indicating poor quality control during construction	Many of the conditions in the development that were identified by researchers as compromising health and safety stemmed from an absence of public services such as trash collection and park maintenance	Active participation in a community-based participatory action research project led to a list of recommendations for improvements that were endorsed by residents

3.7.c ArchEPI Activities (Phase 6)

- Include recommendations on health and sustainability operations practices in project hand-off documents provided to the owner upon receipt of the certificate of occupancy.[CC3.35]
- Integrate health data into M&V and POE programs.[CC3.36]
- Compare building operations metrics with baseline metrics gathered during design and construction.
- Coordinate with facility management staff if certain health promoting design features require their active programmatic support in order to be effectively implemented.

3.8 Summary

The role of architectural epidemiology across the project delivery process could be divided into six phases. During the first two phases (programming/visioning and schematic design), the ArchEPI analysis brings added depth and focus to traditional research into the physical, regulatory, and social context of the site. By using an HSA to develop a conceptual framework for project-specific environmental exposures and health needs, projects will be well positioned to streamline implementation of environmental health priorities as the project moves into the final four phases of the process: design development, construction documents, construction administration, and occupancy. Crafting a health mission statement for the project using clear, compelling language can act as a touchstone for the project team as they transition into the implementation phase of the project, where core concepts can sometimes get lost in the details.

The next chapter expands our analysis of ArchEPI's role in project delivery beyond the traditional design-bid-build approach. It considers the roles and responsibilities, advantages, and disadvantages of Design-Build, CM-at-Risk, and Integrated Project Delivery contracts as well as how best to position ArchEPI within each of those frameworks. It also continues the discussion about the value proposition from chapter 1 by framing ArchEPI recommendations within the

---

CORE COMPETENCY 3.35

Real Estate Development
Facilities Management

Facility Design, Construction, Operations
Construction and Evaluation; Project Development and Documentation

Sustainability
Asset Management

CORE COMPETENCY 3.36

Facility Design, Construction, Operations
Construction and Evaluation

Sustainability
Asset Management; Green and Healthy Building Certification Process

context of the developer's goals, the tenant's goals, the project's potential benefit to the community, and the scale of the development.

3.8.a Core Competencies by Discipline
Architectural Epidemiology at Each Phase of the Project Delivery Process: Core Competencies

Field	Core Competencies
Epidemiology	• Assessment and analysis • Communication • Community dimension of practice • Cultural competency • Policy development
Real estate development	• Facilities management • Market research
Facility design, construction, operations	• Construction and evaluation • Contextual analysis • Physical analysis • Programming and analysis • Project management • Project planning and design • Project development and documentation • Quality control and quality assurance • Research, technical and analytical • Site inventory • Technical capabilities
Sustainability	• Asset managements • Energy and atmosphere • Green and healthy building certification process • Integrative strategies • Project surroundings and public outreach • Sustainable sites
Philanthropy	• Collaboration/partnership • Vision setting

DISCUSSION QUESTIONS

1. How does ArchEPI contribute to the six phases of the project delivery process?
2. Describe how health goals can be incorporated into the project programming phase of the process.
3. What is one way that technology tools can improve the efficiency of the contract documents process?
4. What is the significance of the certificate of occupancy? What other points in the project delivery process does the municipality have a role to play in moving the project forward or holding it back, and how can ArchEPI data and communications strategies streamline that process?

CHAPTER 4

Applying Architectural Epidemiology to Different Contract and Financing Structures

KEY MESSAGES

1. Writing ArchEPI process steps and deliverables into the contract can ensure that environmental health priorities are integrated into every step of the project delivery process.

2. While the role of the ArchEPI methodology changes somewhat depending on the contract design (design-bid-build, design-build, CM-at-risk, or integrated project delivery), the health situation analysis (HSA) and associated metrics remain key to both persuading the team to pursue health promoting strategies and demonstrating the value of the approach.

3. Architectural epidemiology can add value to projects that are run by for-profit developers, non-profit developers, public sector agencies, and public-private partnerships as long as the financial and health goals are tailored to the needs and interests of each approach.

4.1 Introduction

This chapter expands the discussion of the value proposition for architectural epidemiology (ArchEPI) in chapter 1. Real estate development is often painted with a broad brushstroke regarding the assumption that all investors require an aggressive return on investment. However, while many of the economic and regulatory drivers remain largely the same across different project types within the same country, the structure of the contract and the way the project is financed can lead to vastly different expectations for the yield and timeline for an internal rate of return on investment.[CC4.1] We included this chapter to help project teams position ArchEPI as a mechanism for advancing the financial and mission-driven goals across all types of project proponents (e.g., private developers, institutions, non-profits, public agencies) and project delivery models.

CORE COMPETENCY 4.1

Real Estate Development
Capital Market Analysis

4.2 Architectural Epidemiology and Project Delivery Models

The way that team members are organized contractually to deliver a building project will largely determine the role of ArchEPI throughout the project delivery process. The term defining that contractual relationship is the project delivery model (PDM).[D4.1]

There are several commonly used PDMs, which focus primarily on the relationship between the three main parties to the contract(s): the owner, the architect, and the contractor. In addition to designing the building(s) in the project, the architect coordinates the entire team of service providers, including the engineers, landscape architects, green and healthy building consultants, and public health/ArchEPI consultants.

DEFINITION 4.1

Project Delivery Model
The way project team members are organized contractually to deliver a building project.

The following paragraphs and table 4.1 explain the differences among PDMs in terms of roles and responsibilities, advantages and disadvantages to each approach, and the unique value that ArchEPI can bring to each model.

4.2.a Design-Bid-Build

The project delivery process described in chapter 3 followed the Design-Bid-Build[1] PDM, which is the dominant approach to structuring real estate contracts worldwide. In the US market, 60% of architects and 37% of contractors report it as the most frequently used PDM on their projects.[2] However, it is slightly less dominant globally, where roughly one-third of owners report Design-Bid-Build as their preferred PDM.[3,CC4.2]

Under this model, the owner signs separate contracts with the architect and the contractor. The contract between the owner and the architect generally starts at the beginning of the conceptualization or schematic design phase. The contractor is usually hired through a competitive bidding process after the completion of construction documents. During the construction phase, the architect holds the contractor accountable for meeting the quality standards set out in the construction documents. All other service consultants (e.g., engineers, landscape architects, green building consultants) are hired as sub-consultants to the architect. The general contractor hires an array of sub-contractors who supply labor and materials for each aspect of the construction process.

CORE COMPETENCY 4.2

Facility Design, Construction, Operations
Project Management

4.2.a.i Advantages

The goal of this approach is to set up the architect and contractor in an adversarial relationship, where the architect looks after the owner's interests in delivering a high-quality product and the contractor attempts to reduce costs. When this model works as designed, the owner receives a building that meets the quality requirements established in the construction documents at the lowest possible construction cost.

4.2.a.ii Disadvantages

The bidding process used to select the contractor encourages construction firms to submit unrealistically low bids, which they then make up during the construction phase through substitution requests and requests for information. When the project is bogged down in this way, it is often delivered to the owner late, over budget, and riddled with building system incompatibilities that can compromise building functionality during the operations phase. Substitutions and design changes must be considered carefully, because they can be of inferior quality or lack health aspects of the original project design.

STAKEHOLDER ROLES 4.1

ArchEPI increases accountability for the final, constructed project to reflect the community's contribution to the design.

4.2.a.iii ArchEPI Added Value

Human health is a powerful motivator for design decisions, particularly among owners who plan to use the health-promoting elements of the new building as a marketing tool. Adding ArchEPI metrics to the construction administration protocol gives the architect and sub-consultants leverage for pressuring the contractor to build according to the construction documents.[SR4.1]

TABLE 4.1.

Role of Architectural Epidemiology (ArchEPI) in the Four Predominant Real Estate Project Delivery Models

Project Delivery Model	Contract Roles and Responsibilities	Advantages	Disadvantages	Role of ArchEPI
Design-Bid-Build	• Separate contracts between owner/architect and owner/contractor. • Architect performs quality control on the contractor's work during construction administration.	• Adversarial relationship between architect and contractor is designed to reduce construction cost without compromising quality.	• Adversarial relationship may reduce collaboration. • Contractor often submits an unrealistically low budget to win the contract, which is recouped during the construction phase through substitution requests and requests for information. • Project is often delayed, over budget, and does not meet the quality requirements in the design documents.	• ArchEPI consultant hired as a subconsultant to the architect. • ArchEPI consultant contributes at each phase of design, similar to other subconsultants. • ArchEPI metrics wrapped into the construction administration quality control process spearheaded by the architect.
Design-Build	• Single contract between owner and design/construction team. • General Contractor is often the lead, because they are bonded companies. The contractor enters into sub-contracts with both service providers and sub-contractors.	• The single contract is simpler for the owner to manage. • The design and construction teams are part of the same team, which may improve coordination, reduce construction delays, and result in cost reductions.	• If the contractor is leading the Design-Build team, the designers may not have as much freedom to innovate. • The contract does not include a third party to perform quality control during construction, which can lead to lower quality construction. • Health goals must be identified in the contract or they may be deleted from the scope during the value engineering process.	• ArchEPI consultant hired as a subconsultant to the Design-Build team. • ArchEPI health situation analysis can be used as a platform for design innovations. • ArchEPI recommendations can be vetted based on cost and constructability during the design phase.

(cont.)

TABLE 4.1. (cont.)

Project Delivery Model	Contract Roles and Responsibilities	Advantages	Disadvantages	Role of ArchEPI
CM-at-Risk	• Contract between owner and architect is similar to Design-Bid-Build. • Two separate contracts between the owner and contractor: (1) pre-construction (contractor consults on constructability of design alternatives); (2) construction (similar to Design-Bid-Build).	• Including the contractor in the design process may improve construction coordination, reduce construction delays, and result in cost reductions. • The architect continues to oversee quality control during construction.	• The contractor reverts to prioritizing self-interest over the owner's interest during the construction phase, which can lead to cost overruns, construction schedule delays, and reduced construction quality.	• ArchEPI consultant hired as a sub-consultant to the architect. • ArchEPI consultant contributes at each phase of design, similar to other sub-consultants. • ArchEPI recommendations can be vetted based on cost and constructability during the design phase. • ArchEPI metrics wrapped into the construction administration quality control process spearheaded by the architect.
Integrated Project Delivery	• A single contract formalizes the relationship between the owner, architect, contractor, facility manager, landscape, sustainability, etc., very early in the design process. • The contract could be divided into two parts, similar to CM-at-Risk, or it could integrate the major parties for the duration of the project.	• Forming a team from the very beginning can improve coordination throughout the project, which can lead to innovations, improve the speed and quality of construction, and help the project stay within its budget.	• Lack of familiarity with this type of project delivery model. • Concern about increased liability among parties who are not used to participating in a contract that promotes cooperation instead of an adversarial relationship.	• ArchEPI consultant included in the single project team contract. • ArchEPI health situation analysis can be used as a platform for design innovations. • ArchEPI recommendations can be vetted based on cost and constructability during the design phase.

4.2.b Design-Build

Design-Build[1] projects use a single contract to define the relationship between the owner and a combined design/construction team. Either party could act as the contract lead. However, in practice, the contractor often acts as the principal party to the contract, because they are more likely than architecture firms to hold bond insurance. The contractor enters into sub-contracts with both service providers and sub-contractors. In the US, 17% of architects and 25% of contractors report this model as the one they use most frequently on their projects.[2] Internationally, more than 40% of owners report a preference for PDMs like Design-Build and Engineer-Procure-Construct that create a single point of contact between the owner and the design/construction team.[3]

4.2.b.i Advantages

The design and construction teams are combined into a single team, which may improve coordination, reduce construction delays, and result in cost reductions.

4.2.b.ii Disadvantages

If the contractor is leading the Design-Build team, designers may not have as much freedom to innovate due to concerns about constructability. Also, by removing the architect's role as a quality control check on the contractor, the project runs the risk of falling short of the owner's expectations for construction quality or healthy design features that are not specifically called out in the agreement and/or contract documents.

4.2.b.iii ArchEPI Added Value

The ArchEPI health situation analysis can be used by the design team to advocate for design innovations that target priority health topics. Design-Build teams that work collaboratively and set clear expectations early have the opportunity to develop innovative, health-promoting design strategies with constructability in mind—including potentially testing out prototypes before scaling up to full construction.[SR4.2]

4.2.c CM-at-Risk

CM-at-Risk[1] is a hybrid model. The contract between the owner and the architect is similar to Design-Bid-Build. On the other hand, the owner's relationship with the contractor is divided into two parts. During conceptualization or just before the start of schematic design, the owner hires the contractor as a service provider to help evaluate design alternatives. In this role, the contractor develops constructability analyses and calculates a "cost to build" estimate. If the owner accepts the contractor's estimate, they sign a second contract with the contractor after completion of the construction document phase. This contract returns the contractor to a similar relationship with the owner and architect as the Design-Bid-Build model. In the US, 14% of architects and 24% of contractors report this model as the most frequently used PDM on their projects.[2] However, this approach is less common internationally, where fewer than 10% of owners report entering into CM-at-Risk or Construction Manager as Advisor contracts.[3]

4.2.c.i Advantages

Including the contractor in the design process can lead to design innovations that take advantage of innovative construction practices and standard dimensions for building products and materials. As a result, these projects may experience cost reductions as well as improvements in the speed and quality of construction. Another benefit of this approach is that the architect performs quality control on behalf of the owner during the construction phase, similar to the Design-Bid-Build model.

4.2.c.ii Disadvantages

The contractor reverts to prioritizing company self-interest over the owner's interest during the construction phase, which can lead to cost overruns, construction schedule delays, and lower quality/health compromised construction.

STAKEHOLDER ROLES 4.2

The efficiencies in Design-Build can increase opportunities to emphasize community benefit.

STAKEHOLDER ROLES 4.3

ArchEPI increases the visibility of community voices, particularly in relation to climate, health, and equity goals.

4.2.c.iii ArchEPI Added Value

The constructability analyses and cost to build estimates developed by the contractor can help price out design scenarios that address priority health topics. As a result, owners can quantify the added expense (if any) associated with introducing health-promoting measures into the design. Those metrics can support funding applications to public agencies, philanthropies, and impact investors.[SR4.3]

4.2.d Integrated Project Delivery

Integrated Project Delivery[1] is a newer PDM, which is used by only 2% of projects in the US[2] and 4% worldwide.[3] Under this model, the owner, design team, and contractor enter into a contractual relationship of shared risk and reward.[4] The contract could be divided into two phases, similar to CM-at-Risk. Or it could completely integrate the major parties by creating a separate LLC for the sole purpose of developing the project.

4.2.d.i Advantages

The goal of Integrated Project Delivery is to remove barriers to collaboration among the design team and contractor, which is often disjointed and compartmentalized under traditional PDMs. Integrated Design uses cross-disciplinary research and inter-disciplinary design teams to transform the traditionally linear design process into a series of iterations, where each phase builds on the results of the previous phase.[5] When successful, Integrated Project Delivery can result in a building that is higher performing and more functional for users at a lower cost to the owner or developer.

4.2.d.ii Disadvantages

Many team members may be unfamiliar with this approach, because it is still rarely used. If team members continue to work in spite of the joint contract, the project may not produce the benefits promised by integration.

STAKEHOLDER ROLES 4.4

Opportunity to formalize community-based participation throughout the development process

4.2.d.iii ArchEPI Added Value

Including the ArchEPI team members in the integrated project team increases the likelihood that the final design will fully embrace the health-promoting strategies recommended by the contextual health assessment. Integrated Project Delivery is more likely to consider the implications of available data sets on the design, because these projects tend to rely heavily on BIM software. And by increasing the level of communication across project team disciplines, projects that follow this model are more likely to weave the recommendations of the health situation analysis throughout the design as a whole, rather than discipline by discipline.[SR4.4]

BOX 4.1.

Architectural Epidemiology in Action
Buckingham County Primary and Elementary Schools, Dillwyn, Virginia, USA

The Buckingham County Primary and Elementary Schools in Dillwyn, Virginia, USA, demonstrates the value of incorporating public health representatives into the integrative design process. This project (completed in 2012) renovated and connected two existing mid-century elementary schools located on adjacent properties. The project team prioritized promoting physical activity and access to fresh and healthy food in response to county-level data indicating a higher prevalence of obesity and physical inactivity among adults living in Buckingham County, Virginia, compared with the state average: 31% obesity rate compared with 28% in Virginia and 29% physical inactivity compared with 23% in Virginia. The county's rural land use configuration stands in the way of most children walking or cycling to school. So, the majority of their daily physical activity during the week is likely to occur after they have arrived on campus. Research also found that many families in the county did not have easy access to fresh and healthy food or otherwise experienced food insecurity. As a result, the design's focus on access to healthy food doubled as a public health intervention bolstering childhood nutrition.[6]

Health researchers from the University of Virginia and the University of Nebraska Medical Center and a furniture manufacturer (VS America) joined educators and design and construction professionals on the integrated design team. The resulting project (figure 4.1) includes a community garden, a teaching kitchen, and a food lab. The school's ergonomic furniture is designed to encourage students to transition between sitting and standing as they move from one lesson to the next. The school facilities are also used for community activities such as farmers markets and yoga classes. And the school curriculum promotes awareness of healthy and sustainable food.[7,8] A post-occupancy study performed a year after opening the new school found that students spent 1.5 fewer hours sedentary each day, took 21 more breaks from sitting down, and spent an additional hour each day engaged in light physical activity compared with baseline students at the same grade level.[9]

Stakeholder Roles: Buckingham County Primary and Elementary Schools

Development team	Local government	Community groups
Project was developed by an owner--occupier: a public school district	School district and designers used public health data collected about students and their families to focus the design on promoting access to healthy food and physical activity	The campus design was complemented with school curricula that promotes awareness of healthy and sustainable food, an approach that indirectly educates the entire community

BOX 4.1. (cont.)

Health Situation Analysis Snapshot

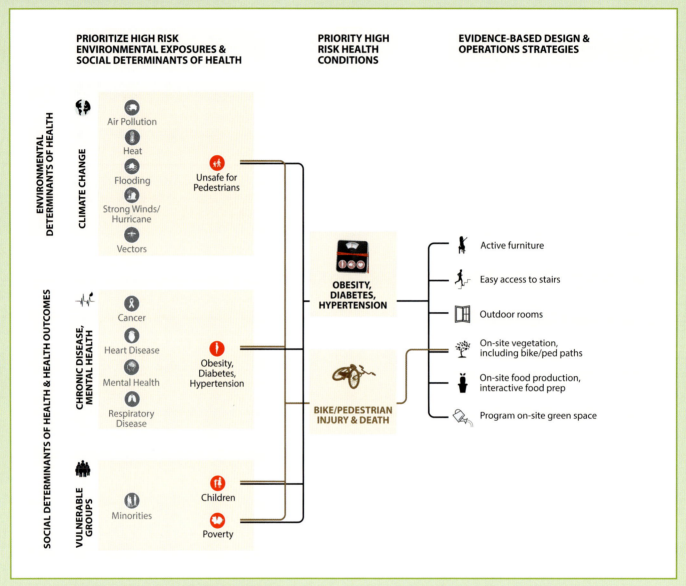

HSA 4.1. Buckingham County Primary and Elementary Schools

Note: This snapshot reflects the information in the case study. Additional research and data collection might uncover additional environmental risk factors, population health risk factors, priority health concerns, and/or evidence-based design strategies. For more examples, see figure T.4 in the toolbox to explore a crosswalk of climate change and community health co-benefits associated with common design and operations strategies.

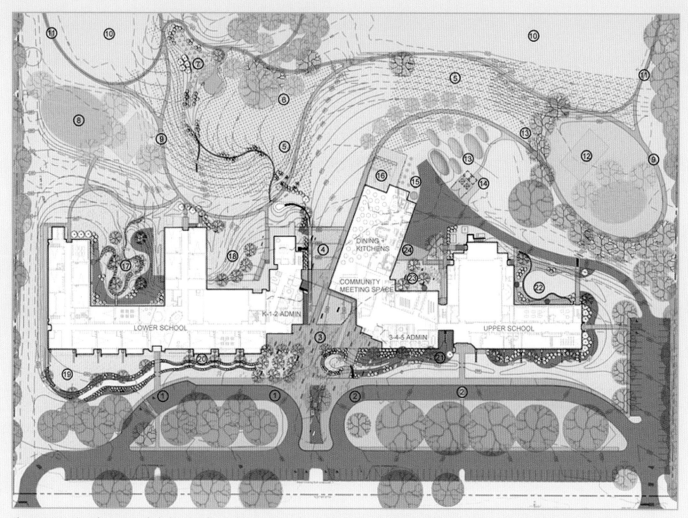

Figure 4.1. Design Elements Included in Woodson Education Complex, Buckingham County, Virginia, USA, that Promote Physical Activity

Key: (1) K-1-2 bus loop and parent pick-up and drop-off; (2) 3-4-5 bus loop and parent pick-up and drop-off; (3) entry courtyard; (4) cafeteria commons; (5) naturalized "no-mow" meadow grass; (6) picnic knoll; (7) frog bog and outdoor classroom/observation deck; (8) K-1-2 play terrace; (9) short-circuit walking paths (physical education circuit); (10) large playfields; (11) long-circuit walking paths (eco-circuit); (12) 3-4-5 play terrace; (13) school gardens (vegetables, frutis, and nuts); (14) composting station and dirt lab; (15) kitchen gardens (permaculture demonstration); (16) outdoor dining and classroom terraces; (17) K-1-2 science garden labs; (18) art terrace and garden; (19) K-tot lot (natural play area); (20) K-pop rain gardens; (21) rain gardens bio-filter; (22) 3-4-5 pollinator garden; (23) sonata garden (outdoor music classroom); (24) loading dock/service.

Source: Huang et al. 2013[60]

4.3 Architectural Epidemiology and Real Estate Investment Models

A general rule of thumb in commercial real estate development is that project budgets should be designed to deliver a three- to five-year return on investment (ROI). The expectation for such a quick turnaround has stifled innovation on many projects for fear of cost overruns. The culture of scarcity introduced by this approach also often makes it difficult to hire specialty sub-consultants—such as green building or ArchEPI consultants—because their fees increase the overall cost of design. Projects following an Integrated Project Delivery model are best positioned to meet short payback period requirements without sacrificing valuable input from specialty consultants, because they frontload project coordination. By integrating systems early in the design process, these projects are less likely to experience delays to the construction schedule and/or cost overruns related to substitution requests and requests for information.

Furthermore, the myth that all real estate development project budgets are crafted with the sole purpose of strictly adhering to a three-year ROI formula is false. Most project budgets reflect several goals including, but not limited to, the projected payback period. All of these goals can shift depending on the type of developer (e.g., for-profit, public sector, or non-profit), the tenant makeup (e.g., owner-occupied or speculative), the role the development is expected to play in its community (e.g., public-private partnership). and the scale of the development. Similarly, ArchEPI recommendations should reflect both the project's stated and implicit goals.

4.3.a Architectural Epidemiology within the Context of For-Profit, Public Sector, and Non-profit Developers

4.3.a.i For-Profit Developers

For-profit developers are the most likely group to rely heavily on the traditional three- to five-year ROI formula when they make decisions. They are primarily motivated by speeding up the development process, reducing risk that the development will not be approved for construction, and generating the maximum financial return for their investors.

As a result, ArchEPI recommendations should focus on generating two types of value:

1. Enhancing the project's marketability to prospective tenants, so that it leases up quickly
2. Using the health promotion aspects of the project to identify opportunities to expedite permitting, share construction costs with the authority having jurisdiction, and reduce real estate taxes[CC4.3]

4.3.a.ii Public Sector and Non-profit Developers

Public sector and non-profit developers often pursue parallel goals. Like for-profit developers, they must set a realistic ROI. But depending on the entity, they may be able to justify a longer payback period—such as 10 or more years. Their second goal for the project is often connected to their organization's mission.

ArchEPI recommendations may serve a variety of functions for this type of client:

CORE COMPETENCY 4.3

Epidemiology
Financial and Operational Planning

Real Estate Development
Capital Structure Modeling

1. All recommendations should reference relevant environmental public health indicators (EPHIs), so that the project can clearly show how it is improving environmental health conditions that are high priority for the public agency's or non-profit's stakeholders.
2. Public sector projects may be funded through specific appropriations that are designed to mitigate community risks, such as climate change, flooding, extreme heat, or air quality. Tracking EPHIs through the ArchEPI process will help a project demonstrate to policymakers and the public that it is meeting its obligations to the funding source.
3. Tracking EPHIs can serve a similar purpose for non-profits who may wish to position the project as a demonstration of innovative ways to address environmental health concerns through design. This process may also benefit for-profit entities who report environmental, social, and governance metrics.[SR4.5]

4.3.a.iii Architectural Epidemiology in Action

Boxes 4.2 to 4.7 compare financial and health goals for high-performance buildings developed by for-profit, public, and non-profit developers in the US, Australia, Canada, and the Netherlands. Both of the projects developed by for-profit developers (boxes 4.2 and 4.5) focused exclusively on the health and wellbeing of occupants. Meanwhile, the office building in Santa Monica, California, USA, the conference center in Vancouver (Canada), and the university buildings in Boston, Massachusetts, USA, and Australia (boxes 4.3, 4.4, 4.6, and 4.7) balanced indoor air quality and mental health and wellbeing for occupants with measures to improve community environmental health—such as active transportation infrastructure, access to healthy food, and brownfield mitigation.[CC4.4]

The metrics that are generated through an architectural epidemiology assessment can help for-profit developments share cost and risk with the public sector, so that they have more incentive to pivot towards emphasizing community benefit. These pivots allow for a single project to bring tangible benefits to the larger community and foster a development landscape that encourages community benefit design practices.

STAKEHOLDER ROLES 4.5

Opportunity for developers, local government, and community groups to align project goals with community climate, health, and equity goals

CORE COMPETENCY 4.4

Epidemiology
Community Dimension of Practice

Sustainability
Green and Healthy Building Certification Process; Integrative Strategies

BOX 4.2.

Architectural Epidemiology in Action
425 Park Avenue, New York City, New York, USA

For-Profit Developer: US Project

Overview
This 691,000 ft² (64,000 m²), 41-story, Class A office building, which was completed in 2021, is located in midtown Manhattan with retail on the ground floor, 12th floor, and 26th floor.[10,11] It achieved LEED Gold and WELL Gold building certification.

Financial Goals
The building has a 4- to 6-year payback period based on construction cost and a 10- to 14-year payback period if the total project development cost is included.

Health Goals and Indicators
- *Healthy indoor environment:* The building was constructed with low volatile organic compound (VOC) materials, increased outdoor air supply, high-efficiency filtration, and continuous commissioning.
- *Mental health:* The building has planted terraces on 12th and 26th floors, daylighting, a meditation center, and a wellness center.

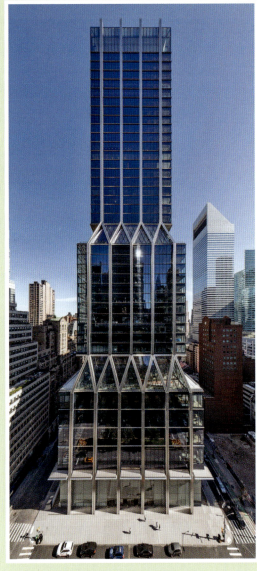

Image Credit: Nigel Young/Foster + Partners

Stakeholder Roles: 425 Park Avenue

Development team	**Local government**	**Community groups**
Positioned indoor air quality and wellness amenities as a market differentiator for a Class A commercial office building in a dense, highly urban setting	No information	Design focused on building users rather than providing community benefits to the surrounding neighborhood

232   ARCHITECHTURAL EPIDEMIOLOGY

Health Situation Analysis Snapshot

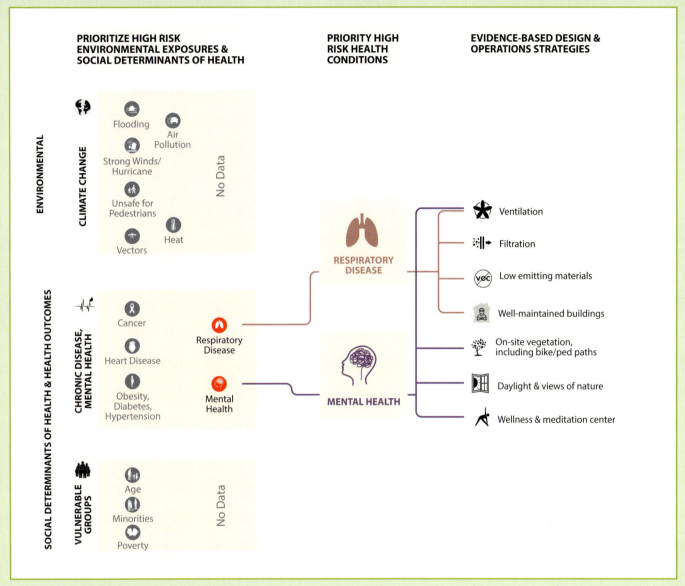

HSA 4.2. 425 Park Avenue

Note: This snapshot reflects the information in the case study. Additional research and data collection might uncover additional environmental risk factors, population health risk factors, priority health concerns, and/or evidence-based design strategies. For more examples, see figure T.4 in the toolbox to explore a crosswalk of climate change and community health co-benefits associated with common design and operations strategies.

BOX 4.3.

Architectural Epidemiology in Action
Santa Monica City Hall East, Santa Monica, California, USA

Public-Sector Developer: US Project

Overview
This new 50,000 ft² (4,650 m²) building, which was completed in 2020, brought a number of offices that had been dispersed across the city into a single administrative building next to city hall.[12–14] The site is exposed to several climate-related hazards. Traffic-related air pollution is a concern, because the site is across the street from the West Coast terminus of the Interstate 10 freeway. The neighborhood is in the 80th to 90th percentile for particulate and ozone burden in the State of California.[18] In particular, there is a high concentration of diesel particulate pollution, which is estimated at 20.39 kg/day.[19] The car culture in Los Angeles, which surrounds Santa Monica on three sides, has resulted in almost 60% of the land in Los Angeles County being covered with impervious surfaces.[20] Since the site is downhill from LA and only a block from the coast, it is vulnerable to stormwater flooding. On the other end of the precipitation spectrum, Santa Monica is vulnerable to drought, because the city does not have access to a dedicated water supply.[18] Social vulnerability in the neighborhood is concentrated in the high population of adults aged 65 and older (19.4%).[21]

The building demonstrated the city's sustainability, human health, and equity aspirations by seeking Living Building Certification—the first municipal building to achieve that goal. As such, it has net zero water and energy systems.

Financial Goals
The total cost of construction was $75 million and a 16-year payback period for a building designed with a 100-year lifespan. The project contributes to Santa Monica's goal of attaining water independence by 2023.

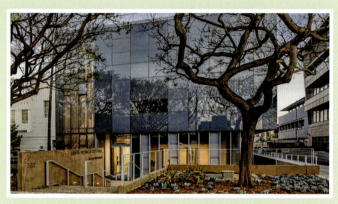

Image Credit: Randy Howard

Health Goals and Indicators
- *Passive survivability:* The 15,000 ft² (1,400 m²) solar array and net zero design allows the building to function during a power outage.
- *Water scarcity/flooding:* Rainwater is stored in a well and filtered for use on site. No water leaves the site during heavy rainfall events or as sewage.
- *Mental health:* The building attempts to extend the interior outside through daylighting, operable windows, and programming that signals that the courtyard outside is intended as an outdoor room that is an extension of open office spaces inside the building.
- *Respiratory health:* Operable windows provide natural ventilation to occupants.
- *Obesity prevention:* The courtyard outside the front door is planted with edible plants, which are designated for consumption by staff and local homeless shelters. Each floor includes a kitchen that doubles as a workspace.
- *Community test case:* This is the first building in California granted a permit to convert rainwater to potable water.

Stakeholder Roles: Santa Monica City Hall East

Development team	Local government	Community groups
City of Santa Monica developed the building with community benefit goals such as advancing social equity and converting the facility into an emergency shelter if needed	City of Santa Monica used the project to create precedents for advanced green and healthy building strategies such as compostable toilets, on-site water treatment, and net zero energy use	The design and operations of the building reflect the City's active outreach to support resident homeless populations and local civic and artist groups

Health Situation Analysis Snapshot

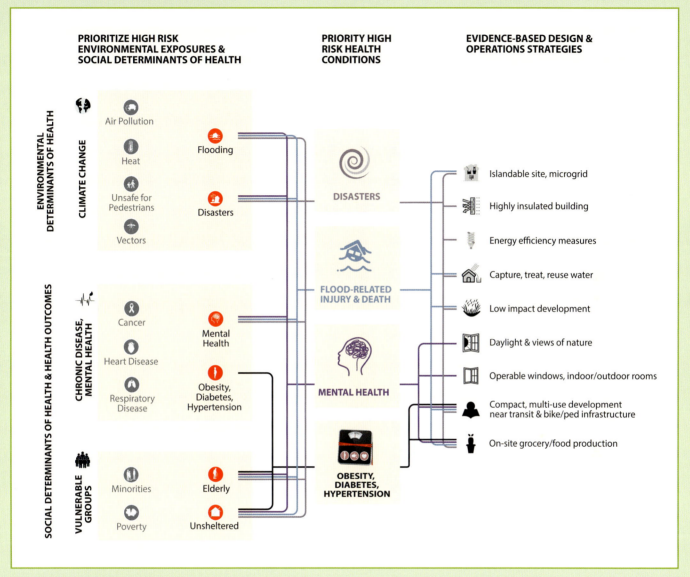

HSA 4.3. Santa Monica City Hall East

Note: This snapshot reflects the information in the case study. Additional research and data collection might uncover additional environmental risk factors, population health risk factors, priority health concerns, and/or evidence-based design strategies. For more examples, see figure T.4 in the toolbox to explore a crosswalk of climate change and community health co-benefits associated with common design and operations strategies.

DIFFERENT CONTRACT AND FINANCING STRUCTURES   **235**

BOX 4.4.

Architectural Epidemiology in Action
Harvard Science and Engineering Complex, Boston, Massachusetts, USA

Non-Profit Developer: US Project

Overview

This 445,350 ft² (41,400 m²), 8-story academic building, which was completed in 2020, houses classrooms, workshops, laboratories, 20,000 ft² (1,900 m²) of publicly accessible community and retail areas, and 400 covered bicycle parking spaces.[15–17] The project is part of a larger brownfield remediation project on the Harvard Allston campus. The design encourages pedestrians to pass through the building and campus to avoid roadways. The streets on all four sides of the property encourage safe walking, cycling, and transit use. The 70,000 ft² (6,500 m²) of publicly accessible green space on the south side of the building is designed to reduce flooding risk and the urban heat island effect. The project achieved LEED Platinum and Living Building Challenge Petal certification.

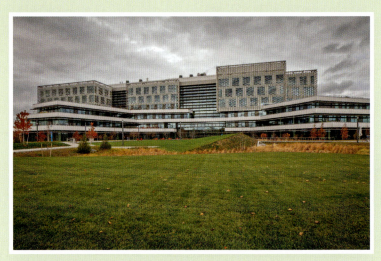

Image Credit: Rose Lincoln / Harvard University

Financial Goals

The total cost of construction was $1 billion. The project contributes to Harvard's obligations to the Allston neighborhood of Boston, its sustainability plan, and its climate action plan.

Health Goals and Indicators

- *Obesity prevention:* The design supports an expected high percentage of active transportation for commuting (79% walk, bike, or transit). Streets bordering the site are designed according to "complete streets" principles to prioritize walking, cycling, and transit over single-occupancy vehicles. An off-road, two-way cycling track is included in the development.
- *Mental health:* The building has natural ventilation and a double façade that both shades the building envelope and enhances daylighting.
- Reduced exposure to environmental toxins: Exposure to soil pollution was reduced through site remediation.
- *Flood safety:* Landscaping, a vegetated roof on the garage, and pervious pavement on sidewalks and pathways retain up to a 100-year rain event, which is stored and reused in flush fixtures, for irrigation, and in the cooling tower.
- *Futureproofing for extreme weather events:* The complex is connected to a new, high-efficiency central plant that has been designed as a micro-grid for the Allston campus, combining traditional electricity sources with rooftop solar on campus buildings.[22]

Stakeholder Roles: Harvard Science and Engineering Complex

Development team	Local government	 Community groups
Project developed by an owner-occupier, a private university who is implementing a long-term redevelopment plan that expands its core campus	Project located in a city (Boston, MA) with strict regulations around climate mitigation, resilience, and health equity	Resident groups in Allston have pushed Harvard to include design features in the new campus that simultaneously improve quality of life for existing residents and slow the process of gentrification

Health Situation Analysis Snapshot

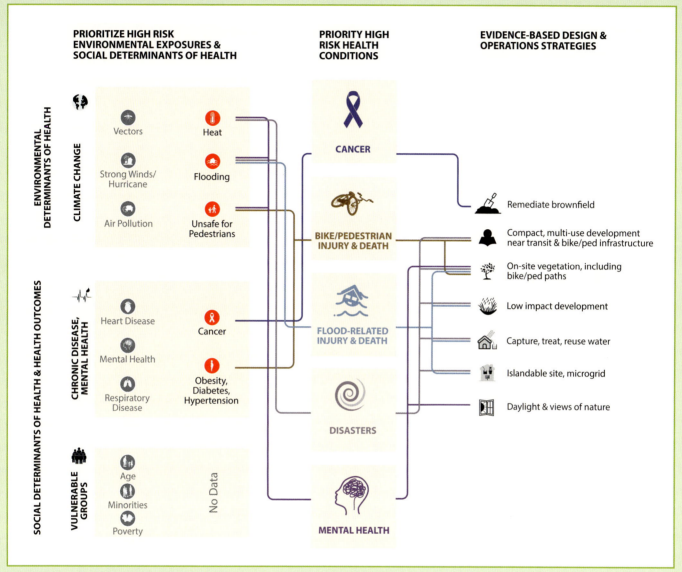

HSA 4.4. Harvard Science and Engineering Complex

Note: This snapshot reflects the information in the case study. Additional research and data collection might uncover additional environmental risk factors, population health risk factors, priority health concerns, and/or evidence-based design strategies. For more examples, see figure T.4 in the toolbox to explore a crosswalk of climate change and community health co-benefits associated with common design and operations strategies.

BOX 4.5.

Architectural Epidemiology in Action
Heerema Marine Contractors B.V. Headquarters, Leiden, Netherlands

For-Profit Developer: International Project

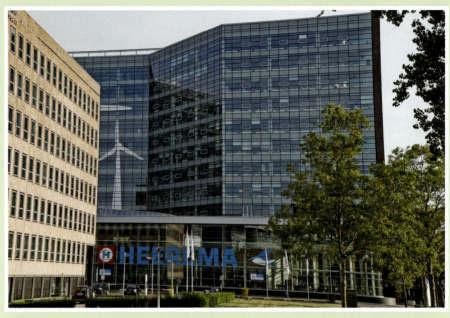

Image Credit: Luyi Yin

Overview
This 251,200 ft² (23,336 m²), 12-story urban infill office building, which was completed in 2015, serves 1,100 employees.[23–25] A three-story enclosed "plaza" contains a restaurant, fitness center, and conference center and is topped by a vegetated roof. A 575-space parking garage is planted with a vegetated façade. The development is certified BREEAM-NL "Excellent."

Financial Goals
The total project cost was: €60 million.[29] A KPMG True Value analysis yielded a net present value of €42 million over a 20-year leasing period due to reduced absenteeism and increased employee retention. The development is among the top 4% of office buildings worldwide for workplace productivity (Leesman index).

Health Goals and Indicators
- *Reduced exposure to environmental toxins:* The building is constructed of low VOC and Cradle to Cradle materials and features enhanced ventilation.
- *Mental health:* Daylighting is available throughout the buidling.
- *Occupant satisfaction:* A Leesman pre- and post-move survey found that satisfaction in total indoor environmental quality increased from 39% to 50%, satisfaction in indoor air quality increased from 36% to 54%, and satisfaction in daylighting and lighting increased from 59% to 84%.

Stakeholder Roles: Heerema Marine Contractors B.V. (HMC) Headquarters

Development team	Local government	Community groups
Developer intended for their company's staff to work in the building and emphasized strategies that would promote the mental and physical health of their employees	City encouraged the developer to improve the street-level experience along the road at an intersection that was previously inhospitable to pedestrians	No information

238 ARCHITECHTURAL EPIDEMIOLOGY

Health Situation Analysis Snapshot

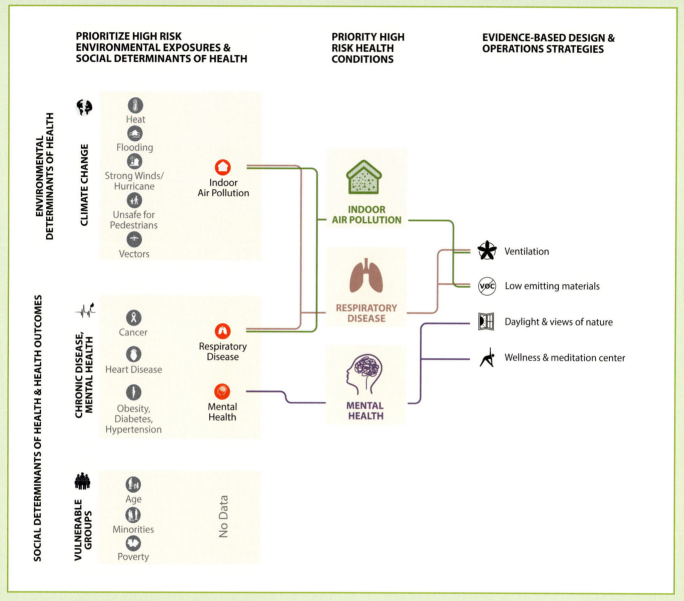

HSA 4.5. Heerema Marine Contractors B.V. Headquarters

Note: This snapshot reflects the information in the case study. Additional research and data collection might uncover additional environmental risk factors, population health risk factors, priority health concerns, and/or evidence-based design strategies. For more examples, see figure T.4 in the toolbox to explore a crosswalk of climate change and community health co-benefits associated with common design and operations strategies.

BOX 4.6.

Architectural Epidemiology in Action
Vancouver Convention Centre West, Vancouver, British Columbia, Canada

Public-Sector Developer: International Project

Overview
This 1.2 million ft² (111,500 m²) LEED Platinum convention center, which was completed in 2009, juts out into Coal Harbour.[26] The waterfront promenade is open to the public and features restaurants, retail, and public art.

Financial Goals
The construction cost was CAN $883 million.[30] The convention center generated CAN $2.4 billion public sector income in the first 10 years of operation.[30]

Health Goals and Indicators
- *Obesity prevention:* The project anchors the harbor greenbelt/waterfront hike and bike trail that links to 1,000 acre (405 hectare) Stanley Park. The complex draws the public from the central business district to the harbor walk by creating public access to the waterfront around the entire site—including 130,000 ft² (12,000 m²) of walkways/bikeways, 120,000 ft² (11,200 m²) of public plazas, and 90,000 ft² (8,400 m²) of retail space. In 2016, the convention center was accredited as a Healthy Venue by the World Obesity Federation in recognition of its promotion of active conferences and healthy food options.[31]

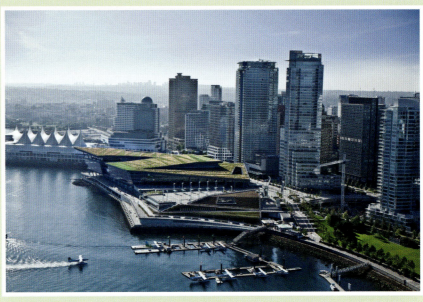

Image Credit: Nic Lehoux courtesy of LMN Architects

- *Reduced exposure to soil and water pollution:* An existing brownfield site was remediated, a 6-acre (2.4-hectare) vegetated roof to capture and filter rainwater was installed, and an artificial reef was created underneath the building to support native marine species and improve water quality.

Stakeholder Roles: Vancouver Convention Centre West

Development team	Local government	Community groups
Developer was a public entity—the City of Vancouver—who prioritized using the project to activate the waterfront and to provide access to opportunities for physical activity to existing residents	City used the project to anchor a greenbelt along the waterfront and reduce pollution in the harbor	The development highlighted the environmental, economic, social, and health promoting aspects of the project that were designed to benefit existing Vancouver businesses and residents—not only conference visitors

Health Situation Analysis Snapshot

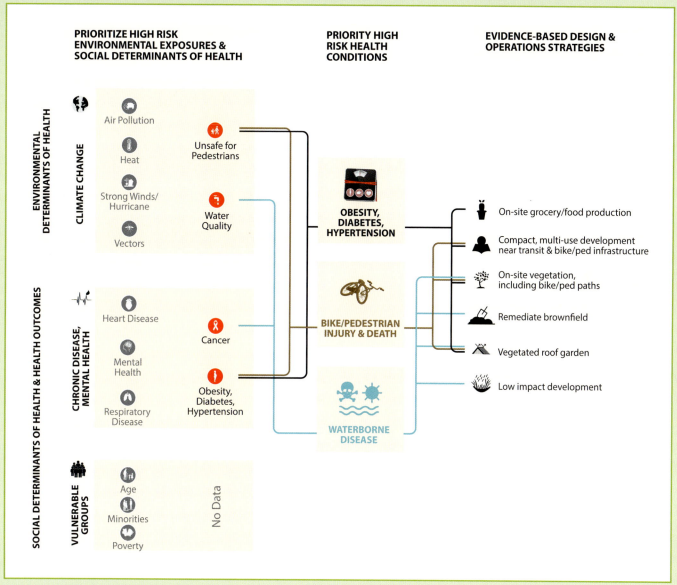

HSA 4.6. Vancouver Convention Centre West

Note: This snapshot reflects the information in the case study. Additional research and data collection might uncover additional environmental risk factors, population health risk factors, priority health concerns, and/or evidence-based design strategies. For more examples, see figure T.4 in the toolbox to explore a crosswalk of climate change and community health co-benefits associated with common design and operations strategies.

BOX 4.7.

Architectural Epidemiology in Action
School of Sustainable Development, Bond University, Robina, Queensland, Australia

Non-Profit Developer: International Project

Overview
This 14,300 ft² (1,331 m²), 3-story academic building, which was completed in 2008, is situated on a 49.86 hectare (123 acre) suburban campus on the Gold Coast of Australia.[27,28] It houses studio spaces, workshops, classrooms, office space, a living laboratory, and outdoor teaching and recreation spaces. The building orientation maximizes daylight and captures prevailing sea breezes as part of the mixed-mode ventilation system. Cross-ventilation design includes offices with operable interior and exterior windows and ceiling fans to maximize cross-ventilation and a double-loaded central corridor with vents and an air chimney to draw out hot air. Corridors and common areas are naturally ventilated. The building features solar hot water, a 18.375 kW photovoltaic solar array, and a 1 kW wind turbine. Rainwater capture, storage, and recycling are used for irrigation. The development achieved a 6-Star Green Star rating from the Green Building Council of Australia.

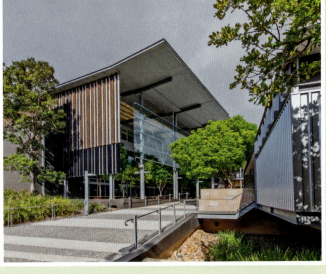

Image Credit: Bond University

Financial Goals
The construction cost was AUD $11 million with a 9-year payback on sustainability design features. The building provides additional value by acting as a living lab for student projects and faculty research.

Health Goals and Indicators
- *Obesity prevention:* Internal stairs are highly visible and conveniently located to encourage using them in lieu of the elevator. Pedestrian paths are marked leading to public transit and other nearby amenities. BUS questionnaires performed 4 and 10 years post-occupancy found a 15% increase in active transportation commuting among building users.
- *Reduced exposure to environmental toxins:* The building has mixed-mode ventilation (mechanical and natural) and contains low-VOC materials.
- *Mental health:* Daylighting and views of nature are available throughout the building.
- *Occupant satisfaction:* BUS questionnaires performed 4 and 10 years after occupancy returned moderately above average results for all indoor environmental quality questions. Overall satisfaction with the building and satisfaction with indoor air quality, noise levels, and thermal comfort in the winter remained steady across the two questionnaires. But satisfaction with lighting improved slightly, and thermal comfort during the summer fell slightly.

Stakeholder Roles: School of Sustainable Development, Bond University

Development team	Local government	 Community groups
Project developed by an owner-occupier, a private university, on its campus to be both a functioning facility and a living lab used by students and faculty members	No information	Project designed to reduce exposure to toxic chemicals, promote physical activity, and provide access to daylight and views for students and faculty who use the building on a regular basis

Health Situation Analysis Snapshot

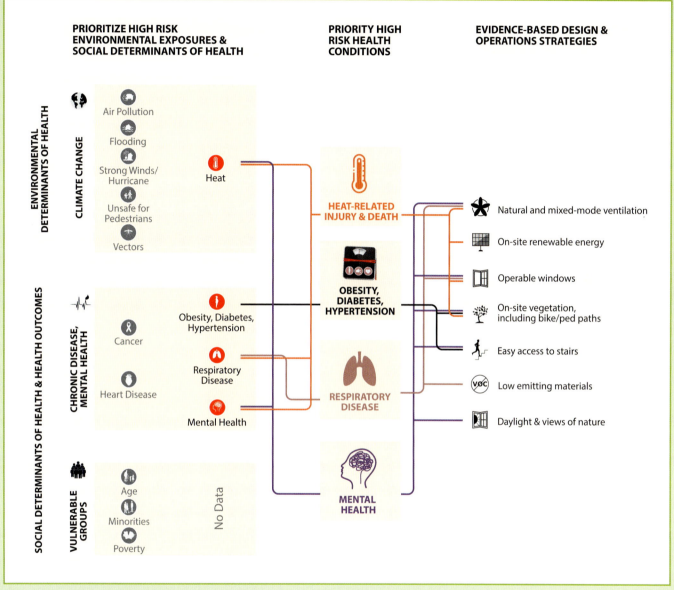

HSA 4.7. School of Sustainable Development, Bond University

Note: This snapshot reflects the information in the case study. Additional research and data collection might uncover additional environmental risk factors, population health risk factors, priority health concerns, and/or evidence-based design strategies.

4.3.b Architectural Epidemiology within the Context of Speculative Development versus Owner-Occupied Development

Many for-profit developers build projects for prospective tenants or future owners. So-called "speculative" developments may range from office buildings to single family homes to mixed-use mega projects that combine retail, office, and residential in a single complex. These projects represent a higher financial risk than real estate developments that are designed for a single owner-tenant. As a result, the decision-making process for speculative and owner-occupied projects often prioritize different objectives.

4.3.b.i Speculative Development

Speculative development projects are often the projects with the least flexibility in terms of budget or design innovation. Because the lessee or purchaser is hypothetical, the developer must rely on real estate trends to make decisions about which aspects of the design to prioritize.

Similar to the for-profit developer section above, ArchEPI recommendations will be most successful if they

1. demonstrate that the health-promoting aspects of the design will increase the project's marketability and/or
2. focus on tapping into unconventional funding streams (e.g., a speculative condominium tower located in a neighborhood that has been designated as an urban heat island by the city might be able to use public funds to pay for installing vegetative roofs).

4.3.b.ii Owner-Occupied Development

Owner-occupied development projects vary as widely in their approach to decision-making as the owners who are making those decisions. Some owners approach the design and construction process with goals that are similar to speculative developers. Others take a long view and, therefore, are willing to invest in design innovations that may take years to generate a return.

ArchEPI recommendations for these projects should be tailored to the needs and goals of the owner, which could range widely:

1. The ArchEPI project should be informed by the goals stated by the owner.
2. In some cases, the owner's goals may not align with the empirical results of the health situation analysis in terms of which health issues to prioritize. If that occurs, it can be helpful to share information linking the topics of interest to the owner with the health issues generated through the health situation analysis. For example, many times, the design recommendations coming out of the health situation analysis or health impact assesssment also advance other health and sustainability goals. A handful of design features might therefore simultaneously help the owner achieve their goals for the project and contribute to the larger goals of a local climate action plan or community health needs assessment.
3. Owner-occupied buildings often serve a marketing role for their occupants. ArchEPI recommendations can enhance the owner's visibility as a community leader by highlighting the ways in which the new facility benefits the larger community.[SR4.6]

STAKEHOLDER ROLES 4.6

Opportunity for the development team to demonstrate leadership in community-benefit design

4.3.b.iii Architectural Epidemiology in Action

Boxes 4.8 and 4.9 compare two wellness centers in the US—one of which was developed as a speculative development and the other, as a corporate employee center. The speculative development, Health and Wellness District at Frisco Station (under development), occupies 35 acres of a $1.8 billion, 242-acre mixed-used development in Frisco, Texas, USA, called Frisco Station (box 4.8). The development team are using the Health and Wellness District and 32 acres of the larger property that are set aside for parks and trails as a market differentiator in a hot real estate market. The same attributes may also have contributed to the City of Frisco's decision to support the project financially. As of 2023, the City had entered into a 25-year agreement with Frisco Station to rebate a proportion of the development's sales tax and property tax back to the developer. The City also allocated $1.5 million in capital improvements to support the construction of the Frisco Station park. Genentech's decision to expand the services provided by its Employee Center, on the other hand, were motivated by internal considerations (box 4.9). The project started out as a fitness center and cafeteria. In response to internal surveys, it ultimately expanded to include a primary health care center, a career center, a nursing mother's room, and a Zen garden. The financial considerations behind the decision to expand the range of services offered by the Employee Center were based on internal tracking of value on investment—specifically, the extent to which the added services improved employee recruitment and retention and lowered the company's health care costs. An internally performed post-occupancy survey tracked metrics such as staff satisfaction with the new building and level of use.

The two international projects showcased in boxes 4.10 and 4.11, the JLL Shanghai Office located in a speculative mixed-use development in China, and the stand-alone Floth Office building in Brisbane, Australia, demonstrate the different ways environmental service companies are using their headquarters to highlight their leadership position in the market. JLL is a global real estate services firm in commercial property and investment management. Their contribution to community benefit was the act of leasing space in a mixed-use development, HKRI Taikoo Hui Shanghai, that had taken steps to protect a culturally significant historic building; designed the landscaping to create a spiritual retreat in the middle of the city; and signed the first WELL-certified supermarket as a tenant (box 4.10). JLL also uses its office as a showcase to clients, demonstrating that they are experts both at selecting rental spaces and helping clients customize the space as a market differentiator. Floth, an environmental consulting company in Australia, used their building in a similar way. However, they built a stand-alone office so that they could showcase their expertise in designing net zero carbon building envelopes and systems that also protect indoor air quality and provide access to views of nature (box 4.11).

Architectural epidemiology could add value to both sets of examples by helping the development teams craft evidence-based storylines explaining how their projects are tailored to amplify changes to the built environment that are designed to address the specific environmental exposures and health vulnerabilities present among occupants and the surrounding community.

BOX 4.8.

Architectural Epidemiology in Action
Health and Wellness District at Frisco Station, Texas, USA

Speculative Developer: US Project

Overview
This 35-acre health and wellness district north of Dallas contains a mix of medical office, life science, wellness amenities, multi-family, and mixed-use spaces.[32–34] The first building in the district was completed in 2015, and development of the site is ongoing. The district is part of a 242-acre mixed-use development that includes 32 acres of parks and trails.

Financial Goals
The development cost was $1.8 billion for the full project (Frisco Station). The developer negotiated a 25-year 380-Grant Sales Tax and Property Tax Agreement with the City of Frisco. The City also contributed $1.5 million in capital improvements to support park construction.[33]

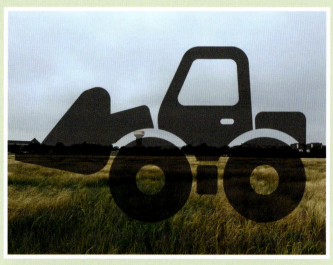

Image Credit: Adele Houghton

Health Goals and Indicators
- *General health:* The site is across the street from Baylor Scott + White Frisco Medical Center. Outpatient medical care and wellness amenities can also be accessed directly on site. High-speed wireless infrastructure is available across the entire development to promote apps that monitor health and wellness status.
- *Obesity prevention:* The site provides healthy food options, fitness amenities, and a 3-acre linear park. It is adjacent to 32 acres of parks and trails on the larger Frisco Station property and connected to the Frisco regional trail system. Developer Cambridge Partners' design criteria encourage the use of stairs and the installation of complete streets, which support safe travel for multiple modes of transportation.
- *Mental health:* Activated outdoor spaces promote outdoor living and community connections. Multi-family housing in sections of the larger development activates the space in the evenings and on weekends (https://www.friscostation.com/health-wellness/). Developer Cambridge Partners' design criteria encourage enhanced access to daylight and views of nature.
- *Reduced exposure to environmental toxins:* Developer Cambridge Partners' design criteria include low VOC materials and enhanced indoor air filtration.
- *Climate change:* Developer Cambridge Partners' design criteria include energy efficiency measures, which reduce the development's contribution to climate change; green infrastructure, which can reduce the risk of flooding; and green roofs, which can reduce heating and cooling loads and reduce the risk of flooding.

Stakeholder Roles: Health and Wellness District at Frisco Station

Development team	Local government	Community groups
Developer focused on green and health-promoting strategies that would help it attract leaseholders and development residents with aligned values	Local government granted tax breaks to the development and committed public capital improvement funds to help build a park that is central to the development's identity	Project caters to a highly educated and health-conscious clientele

246   ARCHITECHTURAL EPIDEMIOLOGY

Health Situation Analysis Snapshot

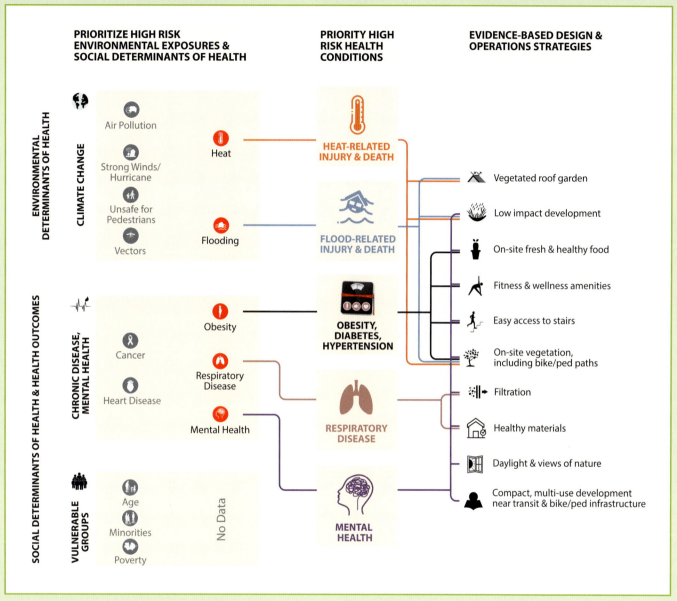

HSA 4.8. Health and Wellness District at Frisco Station

Note: This snapshot reflects the information in the case study. Additional research and data collection might uncover additional environmental risk factors, population health risk factors, priority health concerns, and/or evidence-based design strategies.

BOX 4.9.

Architectural Epidemiology in Action
Genentech, South San Francisco, California, USA

Owner-Occupied Development: US Project

Overview

The Employee Center (Building 34, The Hub)—a 68,000 ft² (6,300 m²) amenity building on the Genentech campus that was completed in 2016—is LEED version 4 Gold and WELL Building Gold certified.[35,36] The site includes a cafeteria, fitness center, wellness center, primary health care center, career center, nursing mother's room, and Zen garden.

Financial Goals

Internal tracking of value on investment showed improvement to employee attraction and retention, better staff health, and lower health care costs. An internal post-occupancy survey found high staff satisfaction as well as increased use of the fitness center, health center, ergonomics showroom, and career lab.

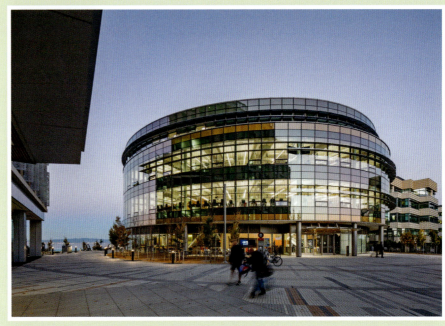

Image Credit: Tim Griffith. All rights reserved. Used with permission.

Health Goals and Indicators

- *General health:* Access to primary health care services is provided on site.
- *Obesity prevention:* The building has a central staircase and a fitness center. Healthy food options are available.
- *Accessibility:* The site was designed according to universal design strategies.
- *Reduced exposure to environmental toxins:* Building materials were screened using Perkins+Will precautionary list. The building has natural ventilation.
- *Mental health:* Daylighting and views of nature are available throughout the building.

Stakeholder Roles: Genentech Employee Center

Development team	Local government	 Community groups
Project developed by an owner-occupier whose goal is to promote staff productivity and retention on a self-contained campus	No information	Facility services a large campus and a range of genders, ages, and income levels that was reflected in the final list of programming, which was expanded beyond a fitness center and cafeteria after surveying Genentech staff

Health Situation Analysis Snapshot

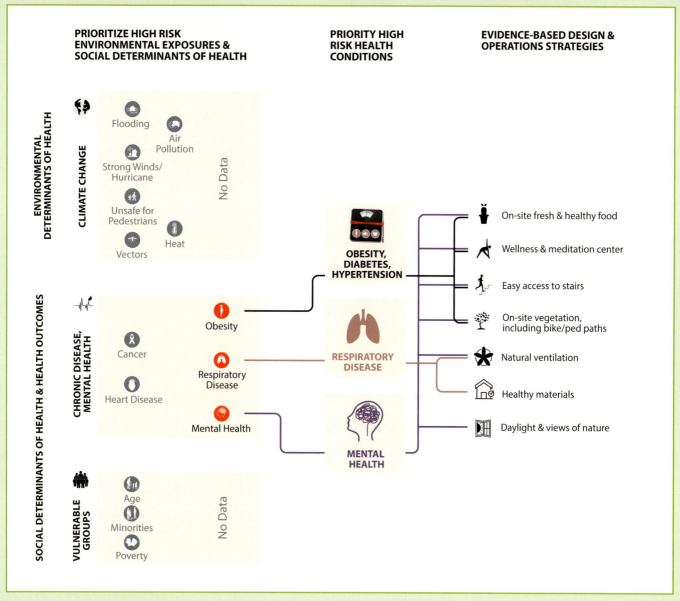

HSA 4.9. Genentech Employee Center

Note: This snapshot reflects the information in the case study. Additional research and data collection might uncover additional environmental risk factors, population health risk factors, priority health concerns, and/or evidence-based design strategies.

DIFFERENT CONTRACT AND FINANCING STRUCTURES

BOX 4.10.

Architectural Epidemiology in Action
JLL Shanghai Office, Shanghai, China

Speculative Developer: International Project

Overview
HKRI Taikoo Hui is a 3.45 million ft² (322,000m²) mixed-use development in the Jing'an District of Shanghai comprising two Class A office buildings, a mall, two luxury hotels, and a serviced apartment building.[39,40] The office building where JLL built out its 50,720 ft² (4,712 m²) Shanghai office headquarters[41] was certified LEED Platinum.[39,40] JLL's office has been certified WELL Platinum and LEED Platinum.

Financial Goals
The office buildings and mall were designed to attract tenants/customers (HKRI Taikoo Hui)[39] and were 95% occupied by opening day. And both hotels in the complex were included on the list of the world's leading new hotels by Conde Nast Traveler.

JLL selected and fit out office space in the HKRI Taikoo Hui to demonstrate their expertise in creating market differentiation in the real estate sector.[41–43] The company holds 30% of its events in its public office space, which both reduces venue rental costs and showcases the company to clients. The office fit out has reduced JLL's operational costs[41–43] by using 41% less electricity compared with their previous office space, in spite of increasing the square footage by 25.8%. The flexible layout also allows JLL to maintain 80% utilization rate and 1:1.3 proportion of office space to number of employees.

Health Goals and Indicators
- *Physical health (JLL):*[41–43] Sick leave was reduced by 20% compared with previous office space

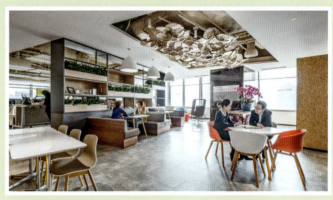

Image Credit: JLL

- *Reduced exposure to environmental toxins (JLL):*[41–43] Air filtration removes PM$_{2.5}$, and the building was constructed using low-VOC materials.
- *Obesity reduction (JLL):*[41–43] Height-adjustable desks are available on 30% of the workstations. Space that would have gone to closed offices was reallocated as collaboration spaces, the gym, showers, and lockers
- *Mental health (JLL):*[41–43] Office space has a mix of options for working alone or in groups, which fosters cross-departmental collaboration. Views of nature are available inside the office space, including an eco-wall along the staircase between two floors. Most staff (84%) reported that they are very satisfied with the new space.
- *Historical and cultural context (HKRI Taikoo Hui):*[44] The development moved an historic school from the 1920s to a corner of the site and converted it into a cultural center. Thirty percent of the site is covered with native vegetation and sculptures to create a spiritual retreat in the heart of the city.

Stakeholder Roles: JLL Shanghai Office

Development team	Local government	 Community groups
Project built by the lessee/occupier with the goal of demonstrating JLL's expertise in selecting prime locations in developments at the forefront of green and healthy design	Large, mixed-use development where the office is located partnered with the City of Shanghai to protect an historic structure as part of the development plan	Community served by this office space consists of JLL staff and clients; location and design reduce exposure to toxic chemicals and increase access to active transportation and sustainable, healthy food

Health Situation Analysis Snapshot

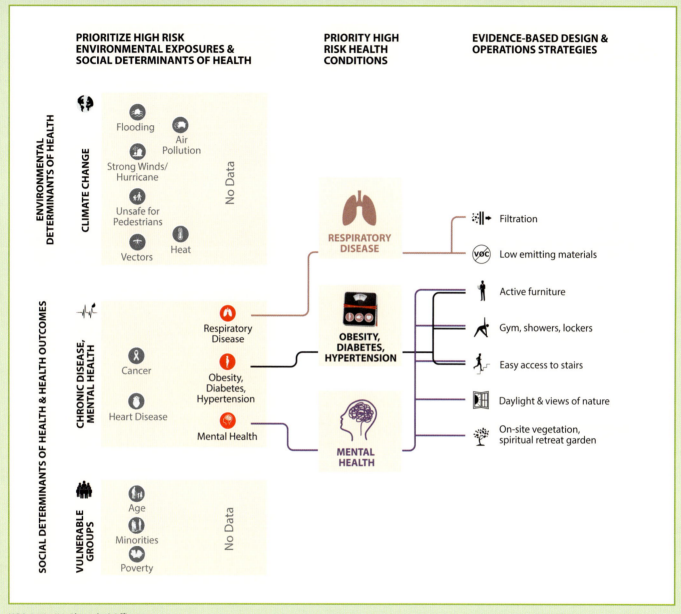

HSA 4.10. JLL Shanghai Office

Note: This snapshot reflects the information in the case study. Additional research and data collection might uncover additional environmental risk factors, population health risk factors, priority health concerns, and/or evidence-based design strategies.

DIFFERENT CONTRACT AND FINANCING STRUCTURES   **251**

BOX 4.11.

Architectural Epidemiology in Action

Floth Headquarters, Brisbane, Queensland, Australia

Owner-Occupied Development: International Project

Overview
This 10,700 ft² (1,000 m²) new construction, which was completed in 2015, is headquarters to an engineering firm dedicated to sustainable development.[37,38] The project received the first 6-star rating under Green Star Design and As Built v1.1, the first WELL v2 Platinum certification, and the first 6-star National Australian Built Environment Rating System (NABERS) Indoor Environment rating in Queensland.

Financial Goals
The building was developed as a market differentiator that demonstrates the company's innovative approach to green and healthy buildings, including its ability to minimize additional construction cost. Operational costs are reduced by insulation, efficient HVAC equipment, LED lighting controlled by occupancy and daylight sensors, and a 15-kW roof-mounted solar array, the combination of which have reduced the building's operational carbon emissions by 66%.

Health Goals and Indicators
- *Water scarcity/drought:* Rainwater capture on the roof is used for irrigation and to flush toilets.
- *Respiratory health:* The building has a 97% score from NABERS for air quality due to low-emitting materials and a 50% increase in outside air supply over code requirements. CO_2 and PM_{10} sensors monitor indoor air quality.
- *Mental health:* Drought-tolerant vines grow up green trellis walls in the light well. Thermal comfort is enhanced using insulation, double-glazed low-e glazing, shading devices, and zoned air con-

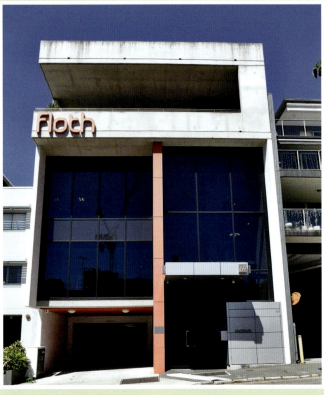

Image Credit: John Salomon

ditioning. Staff satisfaction with overall performance, health, and productivity of the building is 94.5%.
- *Historical and cultural context:* The historic Queenslander home previously on the site was moved 60 miles (100 km) to the town of Esk to replace a home that had been lost to fire.

Stakeholder Roles: Floth Headquarters

Development team	**Local government**	**Community groups**
To showcase the owner-occupier's expertise in sustainable engineering, the project was designed to focus on achieving high ratings in third-party green and healthy building rating systems	City allowed the owner-developer to move an historic structure to a new location and permitted a project that attempted to achieve close to net zero energy and water use	Owner-developer moved an historic structure 60 miles away to replace a home that had been destroyed by fire, in recognition of the need to preserve the region's architectural heritage

Health Situation Analysis Snapshot

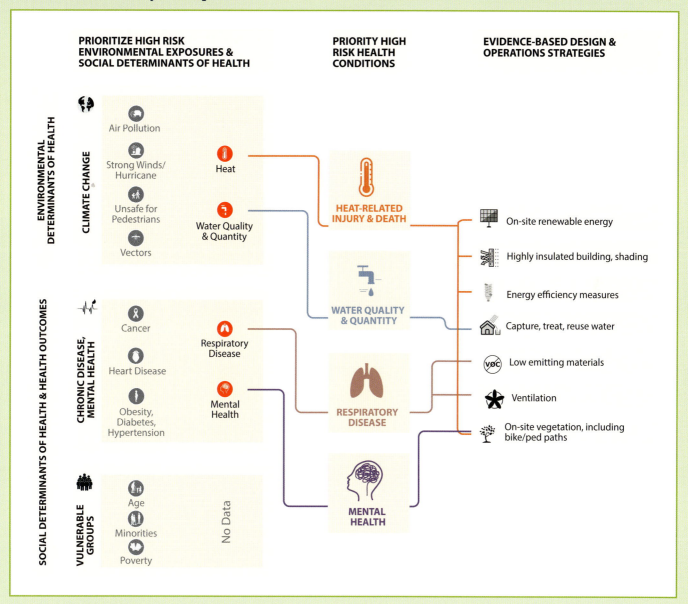

HSA 4.11. Floth Headquarters

Note: This snapshot reflects the information in the case study. Additional research and data collection might uncover additional environmental risk factors, population health risk factors, priority health concerns, and/or evidence-based design strategies.

DIFFERENT CONTRACT AND FINANCING STRUCTURES   253

STAKEHOLDER ROLES 4.7

Opportunity for developers, local government, and community groups to align project goals with community climate, health, and equity goals

CORE COMPETENCY 4.5

Real Estate Development
Capital Structure Modeling

Philanthropy
Collaboration, Partnership

4.3.c Public-Private Partnership

Public-private partnerships (PPPs) refer to collaborations between public entities and the private and non-profit sectors to develop a plot of land, a neighborhood, a community, or an infrastructure network. PPPs are usually formalized through non-binding memoranda of understandings or memoranda of agreement. They may also be formalized through a contract.[45,SR4.7]

PPPs are an ideal organizational structure for ArchEPI projects. Since a public entity is funding a portion of the project, the private developer (and, by extension, the design team) is strongly incentivized to demonstrate how the project is advancing the community's environmental health goals.[CC4.5] This is particularly true in communities that have committed to meeting measurable objectives laid out in their community health needs assessment and implementation plan, climate action plan, and other environmental health policies.

Building a coalition that advances the goals of both the public and private sectors can increase the PPP's long-term financial sustainability. For example, a study of 25 communities in Colorado, USA that implemented Healthy Eating and Active Living (HEAL) strategies over a period of 9 years found that 70% of the strategies that were sustained after grant funding phased out involved a mix of three or more partners representing community members, service providers, and government entities. The HEAL program is cross-disciplinary and combines programmatic, environmental, and policy-related strategies. One-third of the interventions made changes to the built environment, such as installing playground equipment, improving parks, and constructing bike paths. One-half of the environmental interventions were sustained in school settings (compared with 45% of programs and 100% of policies). And 37% of the environmental interventions in the community were sustained (compared with 21% of programs).[46]

ArchEPI recommendations for PPPs will be most successful if they

1. help shape the stated goals of the partnership to reflect the results of the health situation analysis and
2. generate baseline, design/construction phase, and operations phase data demonstrating how the project is contributing to the community's environmental health goal(s).

4.3.c.i Architectural Epidemiology in Action

Boxes 4.12 and 4.13 share two examples of hospital projects that were developed using PPPs. Public sector involvement in the Dell Children's hospital and New Karolinska Solna University Hospital projects likely influenced the emphasis that both projects placed on integrating their campus into the surrounding neighborhood. The hospitals benefited, because community members enter their grounds on a daily basis to use their parks and hike and bike trails. In the case of the New Karolinska Solna University Hospital, a commuter subway stop is located directly under the building (box 4.13). In addition to reducing barriers to community access to medical services, both projects' campus design supports the hospitals' and the communities' goals for reducing rates of obesity and poor mental health.

Finally, the PPP created an opportunity for both projects to use unconventional financing structures to achieve the combined goal of a traditional financial return and community benefit. Dell Children's anchors the Mueller Redevelopment Campus, which codified a 25% affordable housing goal in its development master planning agreement (box 4.12). Almost 25 years after opening, a foundation created by the developer continues to manage sales of affordable housing properties in the redevelopment so they transfer from one eligible family to the next.

The Healthy Neighborhoods Equity Fund (HNEF; see chapter 1) offers an example of a similar approach spearheaded by private equity. The HNEF makes concessionary debt financing available to real estate development projects that incorporate community benefits into their design that the fund has identified as particularly needed in the target neighborhood.

4.4 Scale of Development

Scale is a major factor in the health situation analysis that underpins the ArchEPI process. Because ArchEPI methods combine population data with environmental data to estimate the site-specific risk of vulnerability to certain environmental health hazards, the results of health situation analyses are generally more accurate for larger project sites. ArchEPI teams can overcome this constraint by working with anchor institutions in the private realm—such as universities (box 4.14) and health systems (boxes 4.12 and 4.13 above)—as well as public institutions (boxes 4.3 and 4.6 above) to develop neighborhood- or community-scale vulnerability indices that allow comparisons down to the census block group or census block level. If these vulnerability maps are integrated into larger planning products—such as community health needs assessments, climate action plans, and emergency preparedness plans—even the smallest projects will know which design and operations strategies they should prioritize to help the community meet its environmental health goals.[SR4.8]

STAKEHOLDER ROLES 4.8

Opportunity for local regulators to tailor requirements and incentive programs to address neighborhood needs

BOX 4.12.

Architectural Epidemiology in Action
Dell Children's Hospital, Austin, Texas, USA

Public-Private Partnership: US Project

Overview
This 600,000 ft² (55,700 m²) acute care pediatric hospital, which was completed in 2007, anchors the 700-acre (283-hectare) Mueller redevelopment project, a PPP between the City of Austin and Catellus Austin, LLC.[47–51] The full development remediates the old municipal airport site into a planned community with 4 million ft² (371,600 m²) of office and retail, 6,200 homes, and 140 acres of green space in central Austin, Texas, USA. The site is located in a neighborhood with moderately high heat exposure and population vulnerability to heat-related injury and death.[54] Its location across the street from a major freeway also exposes occupants to traffic-related air pollution (TRAP). The northwest corner of the Mueller Redevelopment—which is the main route for crossing the freeway from Central Austin to access Mueller—has been designated by the City of Austin as a hotspot for severe injury and fatal pedestrian crashes.[55]

The PPP mandated 25% affordable housing, mixed-scale retail, safe pedestrian and cycling infrastructure, and publicly accessible green space. As a result, the development is home to a moderately high percentage of families living in poverty[56]—a population which traditionally has had lower access to healthcare and other opportunities that can support health and wellbeing. The development is also home to a moderately high percentage (8.8%) of children under 5 years of age.[21] Young children are more vulnerable to poor health outcomes after exposure to environmental hazards like extreme heat, air pollution, and pedestrian or cycling accidents. Refer to the toolbox for additional details.

The PPP helped finance the combined heat and power microgrid that powers the site and is responsible for a large percentage of the hospital's energy efficiency. All buildings in the redevelopment are required to achieve green building certification. Following the aspirational spirit of the development, Dell Children's Hospital was the first hospital in the world to achieve LEED Platinum certification.

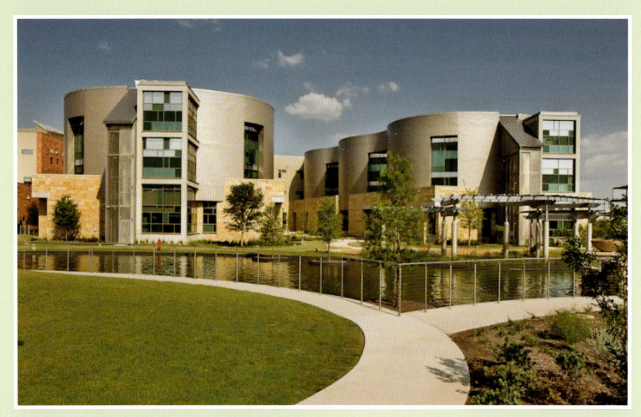

Image Credit: John Durant. All rights reserved. Used with permission.

Financial Goals

The hospital's construction budget was $200 million, and the Mueller Redevelopment infrastructure financing was $265 million. The hospital anchored both the development as a whole and the financial investment from the local energy utility, Austin Energy, to construct an efficient combined heat and power plant, which provides electricity to much of the site as well as district heating and cooling for the hospital and several nearby office buildings. The hospital uses 35% less energy than baseline; water consumption fell 17% during the first 3 years of operation (primarily due to reduced irrigation). A post-occupancy evaluation comparing the new hospital to the facility it replaced found a 14% decrease in average length of patient stay and a 2.4% nurse turnover rate compared with 10%–15% nationally. The promise of a green, mixed-income, mixed-use, and healthy development enhanced the desirability of purchasing a home in the neighborhood. The major home builder active in the development reported that Mueller had the highest absorption rate and the highest price per square foot for market-rate housing of all of their concurrent projects.

Health Goals and Indicators

- *General health:* The development increases access to green, affordable housing and safe spaces for outdoor recreation in the center of Austin, which can lower the risk of asthma, obesity, and poor general health status, particularly among low-income individuals.
- *Obesity prevention:* The hospital is designed to encourage patients to walk inside the facility and for visitors and staff to take advantage of the parks, walking trails, and protected bike lanes just outside. Studies have found that Mueller residents have increased their average weekly walking and/or cycling activity by 40–50 minutes. And almost one-third of residents' total physical activity is attributable to the social and physical environment at Mueller.[57,58]
- *Reduced exposure to environmental toxins:* The hospital is located on a brownfield (airport) that was remediated to residential level. The green building requirements in the redevelopment encourage low-VOC composite wood and finishing materials and enhanced ventilation in all buildings on the campus. The hospital also avoided halogenated organic compounds in materials selection.
- *Mental health:* The hospital is located next to the Mueller Redevelopment linear parks. Patients, families, and staff make use of the extensive interior courtyards within the hospital, and a 3.5-acre healing garden just outside. The building is designed with abundant natural light and easy access to the courtyards.
- *Heat island reduction:* The hospital's seven interior courtyards, two roof gardens, and 3.5-acre healing garden mitigate the urban heat island effect. The extensive linear park system and street tree planting program in the larger Mueller Redevelopment contribute to that goal.

Stakeholder Roles: Dell Children's Hospital

Development team	Local government	Community groups
New hospital acted as the anchor development, which made it possible for the City to attract retailers, residential and multi-family builders, and speculative mixed-use developers to fill out the remainder of the campus	City of Austin participation in the partnership supported the master plan's emphasis on integrating the Mueller redevelopment campus into the surrounding neighborhoods	Since surrounding neighborhoods were historically minority and low to middle income, the project was developed with a long-term financing structure that is designed to maintain the mix of incomes among residents as one way to try to counteract the tendency for infrastructure improvements and park construction to displace existing residents

DIFFERENT CONTRACT AND FINANCING STRUCTURES

BOX 4.12. (cont.)

Health Situation Analysis Snapshot

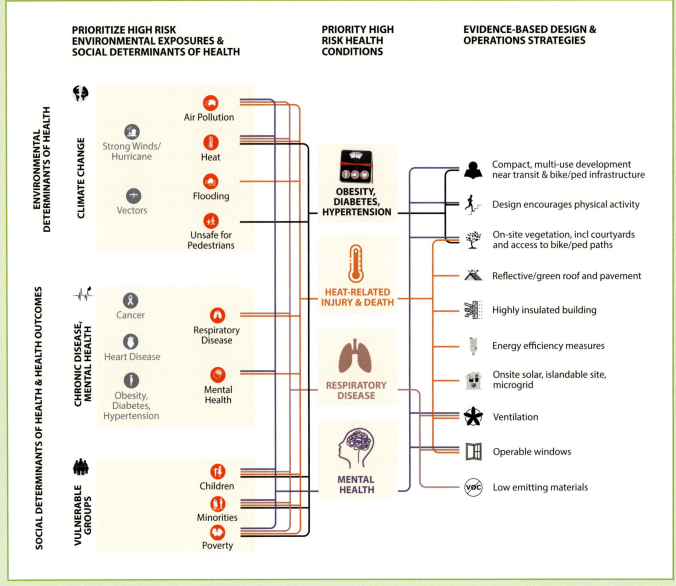

HSA 4.12. Dell Children's Hospital

Note: This snapshot reflects the information in the case study. Additional research and data collection might uncover additional environmental risk factors, population health risk factors, priority health concerns, and/or evidence-based design strategies.

BOX 4.13.

Architectural Epidemiology in Action
New Karolinska Solna University Hospital, Solna, Sweden

**Public-Private Partnership:
International Project**

Overview

This 2 million ft² (185,806 m²) inpatient hospital, outpatient services, hotel, research lab, and parking garage is a PPP between the City of Stockholm and Swedish Hospital Partners (a joint venture of Skanska Infrastructure Development and UK pension fund Innisfree).[48(pp147–49),52,53] The project is broken into five connected buildings interspersed with green spaces to allow the existing street grid to permeate the site. A new urban commuter subway station increases access to active transportation options. The project used a BIM platform that bridges design, construction, and operations. The web platform lists the installation date and owner's manuals for equipment in the building to support ongoing preventive maintenance. The project achieved Miljöbyggnad Gold and LEED Gold certification.

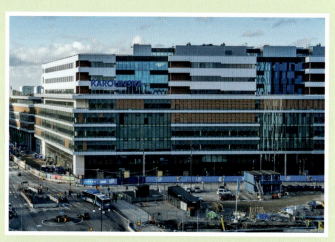

Image Credit: Skanska

Financial Goals

The total project budget was $3 billion, and the construction budget was $1 billion. Stockholm City Council issued a green bond to partially finance the project. The development supports the achievement of the Stockholm City Council's stringent environmental and climate change goals for the region. The hospital complex anchors community development in the surrounding neighborhood and provides a link between Solna and Stockholm. Operational efficiency is emphasized, in part because Skanska was on the development team, acted as General Contractor, and will operate the building until at least 2040.

Health Goals and Indicators
- *General health:* The development increases community access to outpatient and inpatient health care services.
- *Obesity prevention:* Active transportation is encouraged by integrating into the urban street grid, making green space publicly accessible, and locating a bus stop and a commuter subway stop at the entrance to the site.
- *Reduced exposure to environmental toxins:* Building materials were screened using Miljöbyggnad certification system. The HVAC system uses a ground-source heat pump and "free" cooling from the outside air to reduce energy use while enhancing indoor air quality.
- *Mental health:* The double-skin envelope and automatic blinds reduce energy demand and enhance daylighting.

Stakeholder Roles: New Karolinska Solna University

Development team	Local government	Community groups
Hospital anchored a new commuter subway stop, which was constructed underneath the facility	Stockholm City Council issued a green bond to partially finance the project, because it supports achievement of local environmental and climate change goals	Development designed to continue the block and street layout around the hospital campus to encourage community members to pass through the campus and use the commuter rail station

BOX 4.13. (cont.)

Health Situation Analysis Snapshot

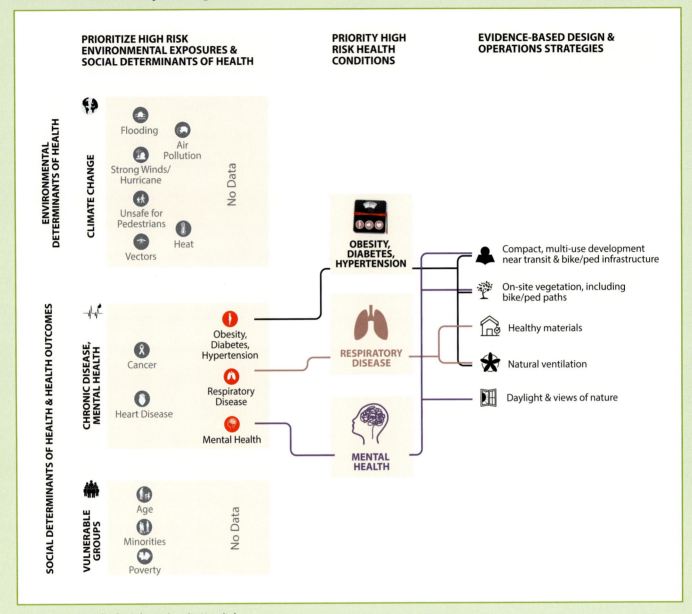

HSA 4.13. New Karolinska Solna University Hospital

Note: This snapshot reflects the information in the case study. Additional research and data collection might uncover additional environmental risk factors, population health risk factors, priority health concerns, and/or evidence-based design strategies.

BOX 4.14.

Architectural Epidemiology in Action
Texas Woman's University Master Plan, Denton, Texas, USA

Texas Woman's University (TWU) was founded in 1901 with the goal of training women in both liberal arts and technical careers that would help them attain financial independence for themselves and their families. Today, it is the largest university in the US with a focus on educating women. And its student body is highly diverse in terms of race, ethnicity, cultural background, income level, age, and parental status.

A comparison of the resident student population in 2017 with the City of Denton and the State of Texas found that 32% of resident TWU students self-identified as Hispanic or Latinx, 46% self-identified as non-Hispanic White, 14% self-identified as non-Hispanic Black, and 6% self-identified as Asian (compared with 19.6% Hispanic/Latinx, 73.9% non-Hispanic White, 10% non-Hispanic Black, and 9.6% Asian in Denton; and, 39.7% Hispanic/Latinx, 73.4% non-Hispanic White, 12.3% non-Hispanic Black, and 5% Asian in Texas). The percentage of people living in poverty was 147% higher on TWU campus compared with Denton County (22% among resident students on TWU campus, 8.9% in Denton County, 17.7% in Texas, and 15.6% in US).[59]

It is within this context that TWU commissioned Author Adele Houghton to perform a health situation analysis (HSA) of their living master plan. The goal of the HSA was to inform both the master plan and ongoing health and wellbeing initiatives, both of which integrated engagement with student groups and professors interested in integrating environmental health into their course curriculum.

After reviewing federal, state, and local data sets and reports on chronic disease, mental health, climate change, and population demographics, the HSA recommended focusing master planning efforts on activities that would address three priority health topics: obesity/diabetes/hypertension, mental health, and air quality.

Figure 4.2 displays the full set of EPHIs that were considered by the HSA and links high priority indicators with the priorities that were identified for the campus. The diagram also identifies the evidence-based strategies in the previous version of the master plan demonstrating TWU has already begun to integrate both design and programmatic elements into the campus that can help reduce the risk factors. Finally, the HSA calls out key performance indicators in the TWU Health & Wellbeing Initiative, 2020 Denton Mobility Plan, Denton Simply Sustainable Framework, and Denton County Community Health Improvement Plan that could benefit from actions proposed by the TWU master plan.

By quantifying and visually representing the environmental exposures and population health needs on and around the TWU campus, the HSA furthered collaboration and active sharing between the campus facilities department at the university and the more student-facing and program development department leading the university's health and wellbeing initiative.

While the final output—an infographic and backup documentation—will provide a meaningful contribution to the next version of the campus master plan, the process of getting there may be the most profound and long-lasting outcome of this project. The HSA has helped departments who were working in parallel towards common goals connect the dots between their own goals and activities and the goals and activities of other departments, as well as university-wide community advocacy.

The leadership message of this project is that understanding the environmental, social, and health context of their campus and community can amplify the reach of university investments. Rather than duplicating efforts in multiple departments, an HSA can help anchor institutions identify opportunities to connect investment horizontally and ultimately increase the co-benefits they deliver to the community they serve.

BOX 4.14. (cont.)

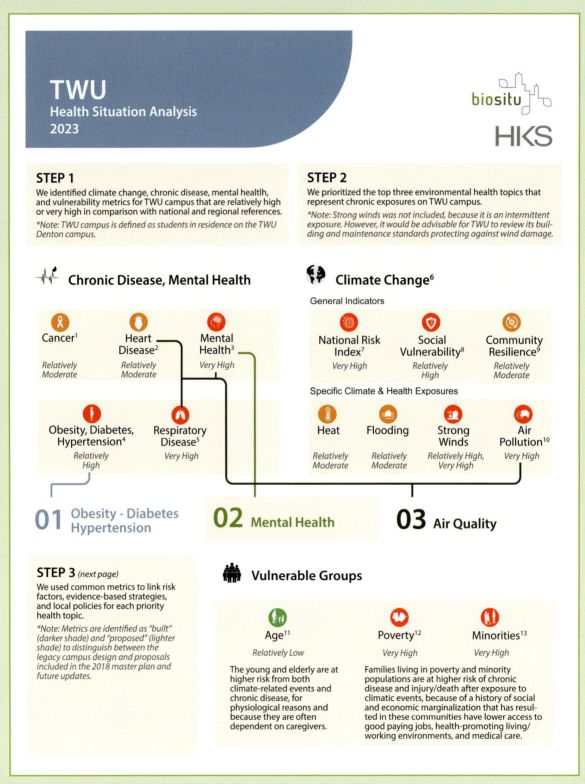

Figure 4.2. Texas Woman's University, Denton, Texas, USA, Master Plan: Health Situation Analysis

Acknowledgments: Thanks to Texas Woman's University for its assistance with this project

01 Obesity - Diabetes - Hypertension

Risk Factors

TWU campus 37.1%
Denton 34.7%
Texas 34.8%
HP2030 Goal 36.0%

Adult Obesity Rates
Obesity is a risk factor for hypertension & diabetes.

TWU campus 28.8%
Denton 22.5%
Texas 25.6%
HP2030 Goal 21.2%

Physical Inactivity
Physical activity can reduce the risk of obesity, diabetes, and hypertension.

Denton 12.0%
Texas 13.3%
HP2030 Goal 6.0%

Food Insecurity
Food insecurity, uncertain access to enough food to meet nutritional needs, is a risk factor for obesity.[1]

Evidence-Based Design Strategies

Built | Proposed

Multi-modal Transportation
- 1 bus line linking TWU campus to surrounding areas. Campus is also serviced by GoZone
- 1,000 average daily trips on bus lines passing through/adjacent to TWU campus
- Promote pedestrian/bike safety on/around TWU campus, particularly on N Bell

Public Hike/Bike Trails
- Number of linear miles public hike/bike trails on TWU campus
- Number of linear miles of publicly accessible sidewalks on/adjacent to TWU campus

Access to Fresh/Healthy Food
- Proposed: Protected bike path linking TWU campus with Shiloh Field community garden
- Number of meals served by TWU mobile food pantry each week
- Number of meals served by TWU on-campus food pantry each week

02 Mental Health

Risk Factors

TWU campus 20.3%
Denton 11.8%
Texas 11.7%

Percentage of adults with mental health that was not good for ≥14 days

Denton County Community Health Improvement Plan[5]
Behavioral Health Objectives 1.1 & 1.3

Evidence-Based Design Strategies

Built | Proposed

Multi-modal Transportation
- Number of linear miles of publicly accessible sidewalks on/adjacent to TWU campus

Public Hike/Bike Trails
- Number of linear miles public hike/bike trails on TWU campus

Biophilia
- 1/2 acre of existing publicly accessible gardens on TWU campus

03 Air Quality

Risk Factors

Denton 9.4μg/m3
Texas 7.3μg/m3
U.S. 7.8μg/m3

Particulate Matter (PM2.5)

TWU campus 11.9%
Denton 8.4%
Texas 7.1%
U.S. 8.0%

Adult Asthma Rates (Current)

TWU campus 92-100
Denton 89

Tree Equity Score
A score of 100 indicates that all socioeconomic groups have equal access to tree canopy.

Evidence-Based Design Strategies

Built | Proposed

Support Multi-modal Transportation
- Bus line linking TWU campus to surrounding areas. Campus is also serviced by GoZone
- 1,000 ave daily trips on bus lines passing through/adjacent to TWU campus
- Number of linear miles of publicly accessible sidewalks on/adjacent to campus

Protect Campus Bike/Ped from Emissions
- Reduce exposure to traffic-related air pollution on N Bell
- Number of linear miles public hike/bike trails on TWU campus
- Proposed: Protected bike path linking TWU campus with community garden

Separate Buildings & Trails from Emissions
- Number of linear feet vegetative barrier on west & north edges of TWU campus
- No idling policy on campus
- No smoking policy on campus

Air Filtration
- Percent TWU buildings participating in an annual IAQ occupant survey and annual IAQ measurement of CO_2 & TVOC

DIFFERENT CONTRACT AND FINANCING STRUCTURES

4.5 Summary

This chapter has placed architectural epidemiology within the context of different contract structures and different financing structures. In each case, an architectural epidemiology analysis of the environmental exposures and human health needs on and around a building site can generate value for private investors, the local government, and community members. Fundamentally, architectural epidemiology is focused on finding those win–win opportunities so that every building project is strategically designed to improve the quality of life of its occupants and the surrounding neighborhood, reduce their risk of injury and death during climatic events, and accelerate community progress toward addressing their most intractable concerns around population health and social equity.

In the next chapter, we conclude the book with a vision for bringing architectural epidemiology to scale—and the promise such a future world would hold for the human race and for the future health of our planet.

4.5.a Core Competencies by Discipline

Architectural Epidemiology within the Context of Different Contract and Financing Structures: Core Competencies

Field	Core Competencies
Epidemiology	• Community dimension of practice • Financial and operational planning and management
Real estate development	• Capital market analysis • Capital structure modeling
Facility design, construction, operations	• Project management
Sustainability	• Green and healthy building certification process • Integrative strategies
Philanthropy	• Collaboration/partnership

DISCUSSION QUESTIONS

1. Describe the ways ArchEPI can assist for-profit developers in moving their projects forward.
2. Identify two ways the Design-Bid-Build process could create obstacles for an architectural epidemiology project and how to overcome them.
3. What is the main advantage of Integrated Project Teams compared with other PDMs?
4. Describe the role of ArchEPI metrics/data in helping two different project delivery models in delivering a building project on time and on budget.

CHAPTER 5

Looking Ahead to the Future of Architectural Epidemiology

KEY MESSAGES

1. With great power comes great responsibility—the real estate sector has the power to create healthy places that act in concert with other properties to improve health outcomes for whole communities while also creating value for the developer's bottom line.

2. Connecting site-specific improvements to larger scale planning and community goals leverages investments to scale jump and create value for areas outside of their property boundaries.

3. Architectural epidemiology sits within a growing body of literature and scientific endeavor that is increasing our understanding of the role that design, development, and facilities operations play in the environmental health of our communities.

4. While researchers are continually working to build the evidence base around the relationship between individual design strategies and health outcomes, a research agenda for architectural epidemiology should be fleshed out and funded to fill in the many gaps in knowledge.

5. Climate change is both a contributor to negative health outcomes and a result of non-sustainable/non-adaptive real estate development. Real estate has a great opportunity to improve the health of our planet and of our people while also improving the bottom line.

5.1 Introduction

We introduced this book with a vision of today. Even as more and more green and healthy buildings come online, in aggregate, they cancel each other out on the topics they care about—greenhouse gas emissions, air pollution, heat, flooding, obesity, asthma, mental health, etc. Individual building projects cannot tackle these societal problems on their own. But, working in concert, they can galvanize rapid and profound change. Returning to the analogy of the flock of birds from chapter 1, if one bird in a flock slightly shifts direction but its neighbors do not, nothing happens to the flock. It is when a small group of birds shift their direction in concert that rapid change courses through the community. We can visualize the same potential in the building sector by returning to the street where this book began.

Imagine a street with three buildings under construction, one next to the other. The local government requires all buildings over a certain size to achieve LEED® Gold certification. The community has also committed to meeting the terms of the Paris Climate Agreement for mitigation and adaptation and the US Healthy People 2030 goals for chronic disease. An internal task force has identified the private real estate sector as an essential partner in meeting those goals. In response, the sustainability, climate change, and public health departments worked together to identify the climate and chronic disease concerns that each neighborhood should prioritize, given its environmental, social, and economic context. They also reviewed their funding streams to consider how improvements to the built environment could be identified as eligible for financing. And they asked their sister agencies in zoning, permitting, and public works to do the same. In this way, when each of the three building projects began conversations with the permitting department, the local government was prepared to talk about opportunities for entitlement concessions for projects that demonstrated how they would improve quality of life in the neighborhood and contribute to the community's goals around climate change and chronic disease.

The three building projects use architectural epidemiology to develop project-specific goals for addressing climate change and chronic disease. From the neighborhood community health needs assessments provided by the city health department and local hospitals, they see that neighborhood residents are not meeting the Healthy People 2030 goals for heart disease, respiratory disease, or diabetes. The neighborhood is also an urban heat island, at high risk of flooding, and suffers from poor air quality. All three of these risks are associated with the high percentage of impervious surface—in the form of streets with a high-volume of traffic and large parking lots.

The first property, an office building, retains its commitment to $0 electricity bills for tenants. Given what the owner now knows about the needs of the community, the team expands that commitment beyond the building itself. They increase vegetation on site to help lower ambient air temperature in the neighborhood—thereby reducing everyone's summer electricity bill. The vegetation along the road also helps screen a portion of the traffic-related particulate matter generated by passing cars. And they reorient the building and redesign the parking area to promote active transportation rather than single-occupancy cars with combustion engines.

The second property also tailors their landscape design to screen pedestrians and cyclists from traffic-related air pollution. And they reach out to the neighbors on either side to talk about opportunities to pool their three landscaped areas to create a semi-public park/detention pond. They also ask the owner of the first property if they could create an agreement that would allow occupants in the second and third building to congregate in the first building's lobby and atrium if the power ever goes out in the other two buildings during a heat or flooding emergency.

The owner of the wellness center on the third property is thrilled to expand the hike and bike trail that had been planned for just one site to encompass three. They reorient the building to encourage casual passersby to enjoy the new pocket park behind the three buildings. And, in order to align aesthetically with the other two buildings, the third building increases its insulation and other energy efficiency measures, which it had previously downplayed.

The local zoning and public works departments chip in by turning the street in front of the three buildings into a complete street, which reduces the car traffic and increases access to transit and active transportation options. The three projects submit metrics to the permitting department to demonstrate neighborhood environmental and health benefits. The permitting department works with the zoning and code enforcement departments to grant entitlement concessions. And all three developments are also able to tap into funding that was pooled from the sustainability, climate change, and public health departments to advance progress on those topics.

Community groups, who had originally opposed new development on the neighborhood's main thoroughfare, weigh in on the projects' designs, enhancing their inclusivity of and cultural relevance to the existing population.

Ten years after issuing the permits for the three buildings, the local government reviews its progress towards meeting its climate and chronic disease commitments. All three buildings have been operational for five years at that point. And local metrics show that the neighborhood they serve has weathered heat and flooding events better than other parts of town. A quality-of-life survey conducted by the local university shows a marked increase in self-reported physical and mental health in the neighborhood compared with other neighborhoods. And community groups report that long-standing residents have been able to enjoy the benefits of the new investment without being priced out and forced to relocate to a lower income area. On the contrary, neighborhood-grown businesses have proliferated, because this new approach to development gave community members a seat at the table with developers and local government that previously had not included them.

5.2 What Will It Take to Turn a Ripple into a Wave?

Shifts both inside and outside the real estate industry are beginning to make the vision described in the previous section feel more like a realistic possibility than a fairy tale.

Within the industry, there is growing frustration among practitioners that so little has changed in the built environment after 20 years of mainstreaming green building. The industry has evolved over time from a laser focus on energy and water efficiency to taking on the mantle of combatting climate change to embracing more holistic approaches like biophilia to recognizing the fundamental role that design plays in setting the context for healthy (or unhealthy) living. What the green and healthy building industries have not done is recognize that the lack of coordination from one building project to the next stands in the way of their combined mitigation of larger scale environmental and health challenges like flooding, air pollution, obesity, and mental health. The good news is that a growing number of practitioners are looking for a method to respond to their projects' context—environmental, social, and economic. They are looking for a way to scale their impact so that an investment made at the project level investment coordinates with its neighbors to have an outsized impact on larger systems like flood risk, air pollution, animal habitat, and economic development.

Chapter 2 of this book outlines a pathway for projects to bridge the property boundary, encouraging individual project teams to reflect on and activate planning concepts to achieve neighborhood, city, and regional planning goals. Chapter 1 arms you with a value proposition you can present to the local government demonstrating that your project will both improve quality of life in the surrounding neighborhood and help the community make progress towards its environmental and social priorities. Local governments who see the value of architectural epidemiology as a mechanism for accelerating progress on climate, health, and equity goals should use it as a mechanism to convert one-size-fits-all green building regulations into opportunities to integrate neighborhood needs and priorities into community-wide efforts.

External forces are also nudging the real estate sector in this direction. Starting in 2023, signatories to the Paris Climate Agreement are required to issue increasingly ambitious action plans every five years explaining how they will achieve three goals by 2050: a carbon neutral economy, climate adaptation, and climate equity. Most countries focused on government holdings and highly regulated industries like the power sector in the first round of commitments from 2015–2023.[1] Private real estate is under increasing pressure to contribute to subsequent action plans, because buildings emit 39% of global greenhouse gas emissions,[2] they shelter occupants during disasters, and they create the physical conditions that can lead to or help break down structural inequities.[3]

While the Paris Agreement itself pertains only to national governments, groups like America Is All In[4] have amplified the Agreement's reach by organizing local governments and private companies to pledge to meet the same goals. As of 2023, over 340 cities and counties, 2,800 private companies, 800 faith groups, 400 higher education institutions, 50 health care organizations, 160 investors, 10 states, and 12 Tribal Nations in the US have joined the effort. Local governments track their progress through climate action plan reports. Companies have integrated their climate commitments into annual environment, social, and governance reports. Consulting company Deloitte found that the widespread adoption of the Paris Agreement and the U.N. Sustainable Development Goals (SDGs) among private companies has led to increasing demands from capital investors; employees, customers, and tenants; and local governments that the real estate sector accelerate decarbonization.[5] Adoption of the UN SDGs is a particularly significant development, because they address both climate change (SDG 13) and chronic disease/mental health (SDG 3.4).

5.3 Envisioning a Research Agenda for Architectural Epidemiology

While this book proposes a new, transdisciplinary field, it stands on the shoulders of thought leaders in the fields of public health, environmental justice, community planning, architecture, engineering, and green and healthy building who have spent decades patiently building an evidence base linking design interventions with health outcomes and measuring disparities associated with the social determinants of health.

Arguably the most influential text at the intersection of public health and the built environment is *Making Healthy Places*.[6] Edited by pioneers in the fields of public health and planning, *Making Healthy Places*—now in its second edition—has expanded the definition of a healthy building beyond indoor air quality to include traffic-related injuries, exposure to outdoor air pollution, water quality, mental health, and social capital. It also introduced the building sector to their role in addressing the social determinants of health— the social, economic, and environmental factors that influence an individual's health outcomes and wellbeing.

Health and Sustainability: An Introduction,[7] *Health, Sustainability and the Built Environment*,[8] and *Health and Well-Being for Interior Architecture*[9] all use an environmental health approach to identify the links between building design, material selection, and occupant behavior and health outcomes. *Sustainable Healthcare Architecture*[10] applies a similar approach to the health care sector, which has been a leader in the healthy building movement because it aligns with their mission to advance community health.

This book builds on the work of those scholars by introducing an epidemiological methodology that translates public health research into actionable, location-specific strategies that can be implemented on building design and operations projects.

The confluence of two major developments over the past decade has made it possible for this book to take the additional step of proposing a methodology for activating public health concepts through individual building projects. First, there has been an explosion of scientific studies quantifying the co-benefits and co-harms of building and land use strategies to human health and the natural environment. The growing body of evidence makes it possible for the first time to recommend building strategies as an antidote to specific health concerns.

Second, it is becoming easier and easier to map environmental, health, and social considerations down to the neighborhood level. Until very recently, data was either not available or very hard to access. Today, 479 communities in the US have established open data portals.[11] And, as portals like CDC PLACES[12] and the National Environmental Public Health Tracking System[13] offer ever more granular datasets, the problem for project teams and local government has shifted from trying to locate data to understanding how to deploy the most appropriate data to answer a research or design question in a specific location.

Now that both evidence is available to link building design and operations to specific health outcomes and metrics are available to identify which health concerns are most relevant to their site and population, architectural epidemiology has become a viable pathway for increasing the effectiveness with which building projects contribute to the environmental, health, and economic wellbeing of their communities.

While the minimum research and technology requirements have been met to allow architectural epidemiology to enter general practice, we have a long way to go before it is considered standard practice.

- *Foundational research:* A great deal of progress has been made over the past decade linking general design themes with environmental exposures like heat waves and behaviors that contribute to chronic disease. The next step in building a strong evidence base for architectural epidemiology will be to leverage the growing sophistication of computer modeling to quantify the relative benefits of certain strategies as the building geometry, its siting, and the sources of environmental exposure shift from one project to the next. Tong and others offer a glimpse into this nascent field with their model testing window size and placement and room configurations in a naturally ventilated building exposed to traffic-related air pollution.[14]
- *Translational research:* Architectural epidemiology translates between public health and real estate in two ways. It uses public health methods and data sets to help real estate teams learn about the environmental and human health needs specific to a property. It also helps teams develop a conceptual framework linking design and operations strategies to desired health outcomes. To mainstream those two translational moves, more research is needed to investigate the ways in which the history, theory, and practice of architecture have intersected with, influenced, and been influenced by public health. In chapter 1, we presented an abbreviated version of this history. We demonstrated that the field of public health finds its origins in the sanitary movement of the 19th century that was, in turn, a reaction to unhealthy land use and design decisions. Additional research is necessary to trace that shared history up until today, where climate change and chronic disease are widely acknowledged as a crisis for both fields. But the ways in which public health and real estate practice have brought about those crises (both separately and in dialog with each other) have not been fully investigated.
- *Longitudinal research:* The evidence is clear that the current, non-site-specific application of green and healthy building standards has not moved the needle on either climate change or chronic disease, in spite of the influence of the building sector on both of these topics. What is less

clear is how tactical interventions in the built environment lead to long-term change. As projects begin to implement architectural epidemiology and as local governments begin to promote it as a strategy for achieving their climate- and chronic-disease-related goals, opportunities will arise to track the long-term impact of these projects. This research is a critical step in the development of architectural epidemiology as a field. It will help practitioners make evidence-based decisions about how to tailor their application of the method to the unique circumstances of a site, its neighborhood, and the population it serves.
- *Practice- and policy-focused research:* While architectural epidemiology is designed to fit into the current project delivery process, it will open new conversations both within the real estate project team and between the developer, the local government, and community groups. Research tracking these conversations will help practitioners learn from their peers about the most efficient and effective ways to use architectural epidemiology to improve the project delivery process, the community engagement process, and the permitting process for development projects.

It is an exciting time for research in both public health and the allied fields that together comprise the real estate industry (development, architecture, engineering, community planning, etc.). As more and more students pursue dual or sequential degrees in both sectors, we are collectively building the capacity and the knowledge base that will be required to transform our communities into healthy, sustainable places to live, work, and play.

5.4 Closing Thoughts

In some ways, we have come a long way since the founding of public health practice in the 1850s. Most of the world is governed by building codes that set minimum health, safety, and welfare requirements that are designed to prevent structural failures and the airborne and waterborne diseases that led to preventable suffering and death in earlier times. In some ways, the success of environmental public health systems in preventing infectious disease outbreaks has created a dangerous feeling of complacency that human society has somehow innovated its way out of vulnerability to threats to environmental public health. But, as one of Adele's colleagues from the CDC told her once, all it takes is a hurricane to transport us back to 1830.

The dual challenges of climate change and chronic disease have created an urgent need for public health and real estate development to work in concert. Many climatic events raise the specter of upticks in infectious diseases that, until recently, were talked about as historical events. Protective building design can minimize the risk of health effects from climatic events by protecting occupants and, in the case of vector-borne disease, eliminating habitat for mosquitoes, ticks, and other vectors of disease. Until the repeated disruptions to utilities after hurricanes and the COVID pandemic reminded residents of industrialized nations that infectious disease is not, in fact, a thing of the past, chronic disease was their primary concern. Blame for the sedentary lifestyle and poor eating habits that led to the chronic disease crisis has been squarely placed on land use and zoning decisions that accelerated in the 1960s and did not slow down until the green building movement began to question the wisdom of placing cars before pedestrians during the first decade of the 21st century. Now that local public health departments are seeking out partnerships with their counterparts in local government (zoning, permitting, etc.), private real estate developers, and community-based environmental justice organizations, the real estate industry has reached a turning point.

It is time for public health and real estate to work together to meet the environmental and health challenges of the 21st century. Architectural epidemiology can help make that collaboration possible. But it will be up to each project team, each permitting office, and each community partner to recognize the value that could be generated by working together to address climate, health, and equity in their community. No one can do this work alone. It will take a global village to make it happen.

DISCUSSION QUESTIONS

1. How did the three buildings from chapter 1 change when an architectural epidemiology framing was applied to the design and development process?
2. How does architectural epidemiology build on existing research about the links between the built environment and health?
3. What problems have project teams faced in the past when they tried to use environmental health data to inform the design and facilities planning process? How is the problem of data shifting?
4. What is the ultimate opportunity for the real estate sector with regard to human health? How can architectural epidemiology support the industry in achieving that goal?

Glossary

architectural epidemiology: A transdisciplinary subfield that uses building design and operations as a social mechanism for addressing environmental hazards.

built environment: For the purposes of this text, built environment is defined as structures, sites, landscapes, streetscapes, zoning, transportation options, food access and other physical attributes designed, constructed and maintained by humans for human activity including living, working, and recreation day to day.

community-based participatory research: Scientific enquiries in which scientific and community researchers collaborate on all aspects of the study, including defining the research question, establishing methods, data collection, data analysis, forming conclusions, and implementing actions based on the study results. (See appendix A for more details.)

environment: In public health, environment can have at least two meanings. In this case, it means the localized physical environment such as you would find within the building, area, or region of a particular location. Environmental supports include anything in the localized physical environment that guides or supports behaviors, or creates conditions that lead to healthier outcomes. Environment can also mean the larger ecosystem primarily of the natural features of the world. Environmental health is concerned with both the natural and man-made physical surroundings that have an effect on health.

environmental determinants of health: The elements in the built and natural environment that influence population health outcomes. (See section 2.3.b.ii for more details.)

environmental epidemiology: The study and application of interventions to control "the health effects on populations of physical, chemical, and biological processes and agents external to the human body." Porta M, ed. *A Dictionary of Epidemiology*. Sixth Edition. Oxford University Press; 2014.

environmental public health hazard: An environmental situation or agent that is capable of causing harm to a population's health.

environmental public health indicators: Data that provide "information about a population's health status with respect to environmental factors." US CDC, National Environmental Public Health Tracking, 2022. https://ephtracking.cdc.gov/indicatorPages.

epidemiology: "[T]he study of the occurrence and distribution of health-related events, states, and processes in specified populations, including the study of the determinants influencing such processes, and the application of this knowledge to control relevant health problems." Porta M, ed. *A Dictionary of Epidemiology*. Sixth Edition. Oxford University Press; 2014.

gentrification: A process by which low-income families are forced to relocate due to rapidly rising property values.

grey literature: Publications that did not go through the peer-review process prior to publication. They can be useful for integrating anecdotes and case studies into a body of knowledge. But they are generally not considered generalizable beyond the specific situation they describe. (online)

health impact assessment (HIA): "[A]n analysis, evaluation, and assessment of the consequences and implications for public health of specific social or environmental interventions or processes. . . . A combination of procedures, methods, and tools by which a policy, program, or project may be judged as to its potential effects on the health of a population. Considered an opportunity to integrate health into all policies, HIA aims to influence the decision-making process, addressing all determinants of health, tackling inequities, and promoting participation and empowerment in health." Porta, M. *A Dictionary of Epidemiology*. Sixth Edition. Oxford University Press; 2014.

health mission statement: A short declaration stating a real estate project's objectives for promoting health and wellbeing.

health situation analysis (HSA): "Study of a situation that may require improvement. This begins with a definition of the problem and an assessment or measurement of its extent, severity, causes, and impacts upon the community; it is followed by appraisal of interactions between the system and its environment and evaluations of performance." Porta, M. *A Dictionary of Epidemiology*. Sixth Edition. Oxford University Press; 2014.

participatory action research: Scientific enquiry that "seeks to understand and improve the world by changing it." It is characterized by involving study participants in collecting and analyzing data, as well as implementing actions to improve their own and their community's health. Baum F, MacDougall C, Smith D. Participatory action research. *Journal of Epidemiology and Community Health*. 2006;80(10):854–857.

peer-reviewed literature: Articles, reports, and books that have gone through a layer of review by experts in the field prior to publication. These publications are generally accepted in the scientific community as more credible than publications that have not gone through that extra step. (online)

population: In Public Health, population refers to a group of people in a particular area, ethnic group, or other defining characteristic. It could also mean an entire population for a region, city, etc.

program: A list of the space functions, square footage, budget, and schedule required to meet the project's vision.

project delivery: The process of performing design and construction services on a capital development project.

project delivery model: The way project team members are organized contractually to deliver a building project.

real estate: The term real estate is defined in this book to be inclusive of the entire sector that creates, finances, develops, designs, builds and maintains buildings, sites, landscapes, streetscapes, infrastructure, and other elements of the built environment. It includes developers, architects, engineers, public health professionals, environmental consultants, contractors, program managers, property managers, maintenance engineers, code officials, and zoning boards, as well as officials and others who govern and influence the built environment.

social determinants of health: The underlying demographic, political, social, and economic factors that influence population health outcomes.

social epidemiology: "Studies the role of social structures, processes, and factors in the production of health and disease in populations. It uses epidemiological knowledge, reasoning, and methods to study why and how the frequency and distribution of a health state is influenced by factors such as ethnicity, socioeconomic status and position, social class, or environmental and housing conditions." Porta M, ed. *A Dictionary of Epidemiology*. Sixth Edition. Oxford University Press; 2014.

Index

Figures, tables, and boxes are indicated by "f," "t," and "b" following page numbers.

acute lower respiratory infections, 89, 92, 93, 93*t*, 95–97
ADHD. *See* attention-deficit hyperactivity disorder
aeroallergens, 144, 145, 147
Aerotropolis Atlanta, 200–201*b*, 200*f*
affordable housing, 31, 32, 179*b*, 206, 254, 256–57*b*
airborne allergens, 144, 145, 147
airborne diseases, 16, 81, 270
air filtration, 9*b*, 25, 176*b*, 215*b*, 246*b*, 250*b*
air pollution: built environment and, 146; cancer and, 94, 110; cardiovascular diseases and, 86, 178; construction sector and, 215*b*; design strategies for mitigation of, 146–47; diabetes and, 102; extreme heat and, 50*b*; health effects of, 144–45, 145*t*; hypertension and, 102; mental health and, 119–22, 147; obesity and, 102; reduction strategies, 141, 144; respiratory diseases and, 94; siting process and, 29; sources and exposure pathways, 9*b*, 15*f*; vulnerability to, 147–48. *See also* traffic-related air pollution
air quality: cancer and, 94, 110; cardiovascular diseases and, 86, 178; climate change and, 124, 141, 142–43, 144–48; diabetes and, 102; environmental determinants of health for, 61*t*; example queries on, 67, 67*t*; health outcomes and, 61*t*; hypertension and, 102; infographic on, 142–43; Jack London Gateway project and, 198*b*; North Houston Highway Improvement Project and, 48*f*; obesity and, 102; respiratory diseases and, 94, 178; thresholds for, 141, 144*t*. *See also* indoor air quality
allergens, 144, 145, 147
Alzheimer's disease, 115, 119, 120
America Is All In, 268
American Institute of Architects, 2, 33
Ames Research Center, 203*b*, 203*f*
anxiety: cancer diagnosis and, 107; cardiovascular diseases and, 88; disasters/storms and, 102, 153, 156; hypertension and, 101; prevalence of, 114; symptoms of, 115
architectural epidemiology (ArchEPI): collaboration in, 5–7, 19, 270–71; conceptual framework, 20, 21*f*; in construction administration phase, 74, 209; in construction documents phase, 74, 209; core competencies relevant to, 40; defined, 20, 273; in design development phase, 74, 202, 206; epidemiological aspects, 19–20, 20*t*; flexibility of, 7–8; integration into project delivery process, 74, 174; need for, 1–2; objections to, 38–39; in occupancy phase, 216, 219; in programming/visioning phase, 74, 191, 194–95; project delivery models and, 221–26, 223–24*t*; real estate investment models and, 230–60, 232–43*b*, 246–53*b*, 256–60*b*; research agenda for, 268–70; role of space and time in, 21–22, 22*f*; scalability of, 6–7; in schematic design phase, 74, 195; value proposition for, 4, 34–38, 37*t*, 221, 267

architectural epidemiology assessments, 41–78; Bruce Elementary School, 61–62*b*, 61*t*; conceptual framework for, 46–49, 47–48*f*, 65; core competencies for, 46, 54, 66, 68, 70, 77; correlation vs. causation in, 42–43; data sources and data analysis, 53–54, 60, 63–65; defining problems, 43–46, 50*b*; developing strategies to prevent or mitigate problems, 66–68; EPHIs and, 49, 51–52, 60, 65–66, 73; establishing trust and credibility with stakeholders, 72–73; geographic scales for, 52, 53*f*; Guyer Problem-Solving Framework for, 41–43, 66–67, 69, 77; health effects of climate change in Kentucky, 56*b*, 57–59*t*; health situation analyses and, 43–45, 73; implementing and evaluating interventions, 70–77, 71–72*t*, 75–76*b*, 75*b*; measuring magnitude of problems, 48–49, 51–54; public health definitions and, 45; recommending policies and strategies, 69–70; understanding determinants of health, 54–56, 60, 63–66
asthma: air pollution and, 25, 94, 144, 147, 178; Breathe-Easy homes and, 185*b*; built environment and, 94; disasters/storms and, 149; extreme heat and, 93, 124; flooding and, 130; health impact bonds and, 29–30; monitoring activities, 215*b*; prevalence of, 89, 95, 179*b*; symptoms of, 92, 93, 93*t*; vulnerability to, 95–97
attention-deficit hyperactivity disorder (ADHD), 104, 115, 118, 118*t*, 121

Bartlett Station redevelopment (Boston), 31
behavioral disorders, 104, 115, 118, 118*t*, 121
biases, 68
bidding process, 222
BIM. *See* building information modeling
blood cancer, 107, 110, 110*t*, 111
Bond University School of Sustainable Development, 242–43*b*
Bon Pastor redevelopment (Barcelona), 188–90*b*, 188*f*, 190*f*
breast cancer, 106, 107, 110, 110*t*, 113, 114
Breathe-Easy homes, 185*b*, 185*f*
brownfields, 31, 178, 200*b*, 231, 236*b*, 240*b*, 257*b*
Bruce Elementary School (Houston), 25, 26*f*, 61–62*b*, 61*t*
Buckingham County Primary and Elementary Schools (Dillwyn, Virginia), 227–29*b*, 229*f*
building codes, 24, 35, 72, 139, 141, 178, 202, 205, 270
building information modeling (BIM), 202–5, 203–4*b*, 203–4*f*, 226
built environment: air pollution and, 146; cancer and, 111; cardiovascular diseases and, 82, 82*t*, 86; defined, 1, 273; diabetes and, 82, 82*t*, 102; disasters/storms and, 155; epidemiology's roots in, 23–24; extreme heat and, 125–28; flooding and, 134, 136–37; health and, 5–6, 24–29, 25*f*, 39; health outcomes and, 49–52, 50*b*; hypertension and, 82, 82*t*, 102; mental health and, 120; modifications to, 176*b*, 254, 266; obesity and, 82, 82*t*, 102; resilience of, 32; respiratory diseases and, 82, 82*t*, 94; societal interests in, 35; vector-borne diseases and, 164

275

built environment determinants of health, 20–21, 28, 49, 50b, 61t
Bulgari Manufacturing Plant (Valenza, Italy), 204b, 204f
Bullitt Center (Seattle), 195, 205

cancer: air quality and, 94, 110; blood, 107, 110, 110t, 111; breast, 106, 107, 110, 110t, 113, 114; built environment and, 111; climate change and, 110–11; colorectal, 106–7, 110t, 112; community planning and, 111; disasters/storms and, 110, 156; flooding and, 110; infographic on, 108–9; mental health and, 107, 112–13; mortality rate, 106; mouth and throat, 107, 110t; symptoms of, 107, 110t; vector-borne diseases and, 110–11; vulnerability to, 97, 111–14. *See also* lung cancer
carbon offset projects, 9b, 10–11t, 12–13f, 191
cardiovascular diseases: accessing data on, 50b; air quality and, 86, 178; baseline indicators for, 55–56; built environment and, 82, 82t, 86; climate change and, 83–86; community planning and, 86–87; disasters/storms and, 83–86, 149, 156; economic costs of, 83; example queries on, 67, 67t; extreme heat and, 83, 87, 124; infographic on, 84–85; mortality rate, 82–83; symptoms of, 83, 83t; TRAP exposure and, 176b; vulnerability to, 82, 87–89. *See also* heart attacks; stroke
causation vs. correlation, 42–43
Centers for Disease Control and Prevention (CDC): on cancer deaths, 106; on cardiovascular and stroke deaths, 83; on COPD deaths, 92; *Field Epidemiology Manual*, 70–73, 71–72t; Healthy People program, 45; National Environmental Public Health Tracking System, 50b, 64b, 64f, 269; PLACES data portal, 50b, 56, 269; population health data, 32; on West Nile virus, 160. *See also* Fitwel certification
certificates of occupancy, 215, 219
certifications. *See specific certifications*
Chadwick, Edwin, 24
Chai Wan campus of the Technological and Higher Education Institute (Hong Kong), 212–13f, 212–14b
children: air pollution and, 147; cancer and, 111–12; developmental delays in, 118t, 119; disasters/storms and, 155–56; extreme heat and, 128; flooding and, 140; obesity among, 103–5; respiratory diseases and, 95; vector-borne diseases and, 165. *See also* behavioral disorders
cholesterol, 87–89
chronic diseases: air pollution and, 147; built environment and, 81, 82, 82t; community goals related to, 7; COVID-19 pandemic and, 24; disasters/storms and, 149, 156; economic costs of, 81; environmental exposures and, 81, 82; extreme heat and, 128; flooding and, 140; health outcomes and, 30; mental health and, 121–22, 147; preventable deaths from, 23; Sustainable Development Goals on, 56, 268; as wicked problem, 3. *See also specific diseases*
chronic obstructive pulmonary disease (COPD), 89, 92–97, 93t, 144–45, 147
Clean Air Act Amendments of 1990, 144
climate change: air quality and, 124, 141, 142–39, 144–48; cancer and, 110–11; cardiovascular diseases and, 83–86; co-impact pathways linking building design with, 80f; community goals related to, 7; diabetes and, 101–2;

disasters/storms and, 124, 148–49, 150–57; extreme heat and, 123, 124–29; flooding and, 123, 129, 130–41; GHGs and, 9b, 23, 123, 125, 146, 154, 268; health effects in Kentucky, 56b, 57–59t; hypertension and, 101–2; Intergovernmental Panel on Climate Change, 125, 133, 146; mental health and, 119–20; obesity and, 101–2; Paris Climate Agreement and, 6, 23, 265, 267–68; resilience to, 191; respiratory diseases and, 93–94; Sustainable Development Goals on, 268; US National Climate Assessment, 125, 134; vector-borne diseases and, 124, 157, 158–67; vulnerability to, 56b, 57–59t, 60; as wicked problem, 3, 123, 124
climate equity, 267
CM-at-Risk project delivery model, 224t, 225–26
co-benefit design process, 167
cognitive ability, 114–15, 118t, 119–21
colorectal cancer, 106–7, 110t, 112
combined sewer overflows (CSOs), 129, 175, 177b, 205, 217b
communicable diseases. *See* infectious diseases; *specific diseases*
community-based participatory research, 44, 55, 219b, 273
community groups: Aerotropolis Atlanta and, 200b; Bond University School of Sustainable Development and, 242b; Bon Pastor redevelopment and, 190b; Buckingham County Primary and Elementary Schools and, 227b; Chai Wan campus and, 212b; Dell Children's Hospital and, 257b; education campaigns for, 215b; engagement with, 66, 79, 195, 206, 270; Family Health Center on Virginia and, 196b; Floth Headquarters and, 252b; 425 Park Avenue and, 232b; Genentech Employee Center and, 248b; Gillett Square and, 184b; Harvard University Science and Engineering Complex and, 236b; Health and Wellness District at Frisco Station and, 246b; High Point redevelopment and, 187b; Jack London Gateway project and, 198b; JLL Shanghai Office and, 250b; New Karolinska Solna University Hospital and, 259b; resilience of, 23, 175, 217b; Santa Monica City Hall East and, 234b; South Bronx Neighborhood and, 181b; Uberlândia housing development and, 219b; value streams for, 28, 35–38, 37t; Vancouver Convention Centre West, 240b; Via Verde housing complex and, 210b
community health: assessment of, 30, 55, 266; data sources for, 44; prioritization of, 4, 35; promotion of, 176b, 268; responsibility for, 33
Community Health Initiative (Kaiser Permanente), 176b
community planning: cancer and, 111; cardiovascular diseases and, 86–87; diabetes and, 103; disasters/storms and, 155; extreme heat and, 128; for green and healthy buildings, 21; health impact assessments for, 69; health-promoting strategies in, 6; hypertension and, 101; mental health and, 120; obesity, 103; respiratory diseases and, 94–95; vector-borne diseases and, 164–65
composite indices, 60, 62b
conceptual frameworks, 20, 21f, 42, 46–49, 47–48f, 65, 205, 269
conduct disorder, 115, 118, 118t
confidentiality. *See* privacy issues
construction. *See* design, construction, and operations
construction administration phase, 22f, 74, 209

276 INDEX

construction documents phase, 22f, 74, 206, 209
contract structures. See project delivery models
cooling centers, 51, 51f, 63, 87, 103, 128, 139, 216
COPD. See chronic obstructive pulmonary disease
core competencies: for ArchEPI assessments, 46, 54, 66, 68, 70, 77; for contract and financing structures, 264; professions covered by, 6, 7t; for project delivery process, 220; relevant to ArchEPI, 40
correlation vs. causation, 42–43
cost to build estimates, 225, 226
COVID-19 pandemic: co-impact pathways linking building design with, 80f; disasters/storms during, 153; geographic disparities and, 2; hierarchy of controls and, 27, 28f; infection control standards during, 155; lessons learned from, 24, 270; mortality rate during, 81, 89; respiratory diseases and, 89, 94, 96; risk factors for poor outcomes, 24; vaccination rates in, 34
crosswalk diagram, 167, 168–72f
CSOs. See combined sewer overflows

data: accessibility of, 53, 269; aggregated, 44, 63; aligning indicator definitions with, 54–55; buffering, 63–64, 65f; comparing indicators with, 55–56, 60; meta-analyses, 67–68; privacy issues, 39, 44, 52, 54, 63, 216; spatial analysis, 60, 63–65, 202–3; statistical analysis, 52, 60, 203; visualization, 63–64, 64–65f, 64b, 203. See also health data
Dell Children's Hospital (Austin), 254, 256–58b
dementia, 115, 118t, 119–21
dengue virus, 111, 132–33, 137, 153, 160–67, 161t, 163t
depression: air pollution and, 119; cancer diagnosis and, 107, 112–13; cardiovascular diseases and, 88; disasters/storms and, 153, 156; prevalence of, 81, 114; respiratory diseases and, 96; symptoms of, 115
design, construction, and operations: competing priorities in, 43; core competencies, 6, 7t, 40, 46, 54, 66, 68, 70, 77, 220, 264; environmental health and, 9b; health data for, 28–33, 39; health impact pyramid and, 26, 27f; hierarchy of controls and, 27, 28f; mediating factors, 51–52; population health and, 2, 9b, 29; social determinants of health and, 26, 27. See also project delivery process
Design-Bid-Build project delivery model, 174, 222, 223t
Design-Build project delivery model, 223t, 224–25
design development phase: ArchEPI during, 74, 202, 206; building code compliance in, 205; building information modeling in, 202–5, 203–4b, 203–4f; community engagement during, 206; Geographic Information Systems in, 202–3, 205; for green and healthy buildings, 22f, 202–4
developmental delays in children, 118t, 119
development teams: Aerotropolis Atlanta and, 200b; Bond University School of Sustainable Development and, 242b; Bon Pastor redevelopment and, 190b; Buckingham County Primary and Elementary Schools and, 227b; Chai Wan campus and, 212b; Dell Children's Hospital and, 257b; design strategies prioritized by, 34; Family Health Center on Virginia and, 196b; Floth Headquarters and, 252b; 425 Park Avenue and, 232b; Genentech Employee Center and, 248b; Gillett Square and, 184b; Harvard University Science and Engineering Complex and, 236b; Health and Wellness District at Frisco Station and, 246b; Heerema Marine Contractors B.V. Headquarters and, 238b; High Point redevelopment and, 187b; Jack London Gateway project and, 198b; JLL Shanghai Office and, 250b; New Karolinska Solna University Hospital and, 259b; St. Antony's School and, 207b; Santa Monica City Hall East and, 234b; sources of value creation for, 36; South Bronx Neighborhood and, 181b; Uberlândia housing development and, 219b; Vancouver Convention Centre West, 240b; Via Verde housing complex and, 210b
diabetes: air quality and, 102; built environment and, 82, 82t, 102; cardiovascular diseases and, 87; categorization of, 100; climate change and, 101–2; Community Health Initiative and, 176b; community planning and, 103; complications of, 81; disasters/storms and, 102, 149, 156; extreme heat and, 52, 102, 124; infographic on, 98–99; mortality rate, 100; obesity and, 97; prevalence of, 97, 100, 179b; primary care services for, 196b; symptoms of, 101, 101t; vulnerability to, 82, 103–6
disasters/storms: built environment and, 155; cancer and, 110, 156; cardiovascular diseases and, 83–86, 149, 156; climate change and, 124, 148–49, 150–57; community planning and, 155; diabetes and, 102, 149, 156; economic cost of, 148; health effects of, 148–49, 152–54, 153t; hypertension and, 102, 149, 156; infographic on, 150–51; mental health and, 120, 153, 156; respiratory diseases and, 93–94, 149, 153; vector-borne diseases and, 153; vulnerability to, 155–57. See also flooding
diseases. See chronic diseases; infectious diseases; specific diseases
displaced populations, 94, 120, 140, 141, 156–57
drought, 133, 137, 146, 148, 164, 177b, 234b, 252b

Edgewood Court Apartments (Atlanta), 31
elderly populations: air pollution and, 147; cancer and, 112; cardiovascular diseases and, 87; dementia and, 121; diabetes and, 101–2; disasters/storms and, 155–56; extreme heat and, 128; flooding and, 140; hypertension and, 103–4; obesity among, 103–4; respiratory diseases and, 95–96; vector-borne diseases and, 165
energy modeling, 203b, 203f, 204, 206, 215
Enterprise Green Communities, 6, 195, 206
environment, defined, 19, 273. See also built environment
environmental determinants of health: defined, 20, 273; natural, 49, 50b, 61t; in neighborhoods, 31. See also built environment determinants of health
environmental epidemiology, 19–20, 20t, 21f, 273
environmental exposures: ArchEPI and, 19, 20; cancer and, 111–12; categorization of, 49; chronic diseases and, 81, 82; health outcomes and, 42–43, 46; health situation analyses and, 36; infectious diseases and, 81; mental health and, 121; shifting among neighborhoods, 175b; social determinants of health and, 20; vulnerability to climate change and, 57t
environmental health: built environment and, 24; construction projects and, 9b; data sets for, 54, 195, 209; defining problems, 43–45; programming/visioning phase and, 194; schematic design phase and, 195

Environmental Protection Agency (EPA), 119, 129, 132
environmental public health hazards, 49, 51, 52, 273
environmental public health indicators (EPHIs): defined, 48, 273; development of, 49, 51–52; health mission statements and, 191; health situation analyses and, 175, 195; prioritization of, 65–66; spatial analysis and, 60; tracking, 73, 202, 205, 231; vulnerability to climate change by, 57–59*t*
environmental stewardship, 24, 176*b*, 191
epidemiology: core competencies, 6, 7*t*, 40, 46, 54, 66, 68, 70, 77, 220, 264; defined, 19, 273; environmental, 19–20, 20*t*, 21*f*, 273; roots in built environment, 23–24; social, 20, 20*t*, 21*f*, 274. *See also* architectural epidemiology
equity: climate, 267; health, 6, 8, 69, 80*f*, 178, 195, 206; social, 2, 43, 49, 52, 69, 128, 264
erosion, 137, 217*b*, 217*f*
ethnicity. *See* minorities and Indigenous populations
extreme heat: built environment and, 125–28; cardiovascular diseases and, 83, 87, 124; climate change and, 123, 124–29; community planning and, 128; COVID-19 pandemic and, 24; defining, 45, 49, 50*b*; diabetes and, 52, 102, 124; environmental determinants of health for, 50*b*, 61*t*; health effects of, 124–25; hypertension and, 102; infographic on, 126–27; mediating factors, 51; mental health and, 52, 119, 124, 128; mitigation strategies, 62*b*, 177*b*, 217*b*; mortality rate, 123, 124; obesity and, 102; regional priority credits and risk of, 4, 5*f*; resilience to, 182*b*; respiratory diseases and, 52, 93, 124; risk perceptions, 70, 71–72*t*; Uberlândia housing development and, 217*b*; vulnerability to, 128–29, 175*b*, 217*b*

facilities management, 216
Family Health Center on Virginia (McKinney, Texas), 196–97*b*, 196*f*
Federal Emergency Management Agency (FEMA), 31, 134, 139
Field Epidemiology Manual (CDC), 70–73, 71–72*t*
financing structures. *See* real estate investment models
Fitwel certification: building information modeling and, 205; establishment of, 33; net promoter scores and, 30; as real estate portfolio goal, 191; Viral Response Module, 2
flooding: access to outdoor activities and, 137; built environment and, 134, 136–37; cancer and, 110; climate change and, 123, 129, 130–41; combined sewer overflows due to, 177*b*, 217*b*; design strategies to protect against, 137–40; exposure to flood waters, 134; food insecurity and, 137; health effects of, 129, 132–33, 133*t*; infographic on, 130–31; mental health and, 120, 133; multimodal evacuation routes for, 138; North Houston Highway Improvement Project and, 47*f*; on-site food production and, 140; on-site renewable energy and microgrids and, 139; on-site water capture and treatment and, 139–40; regional priority credits and risk of, 4, 5*f*; resilience of utilities and infrastructure to, 136; respiratory diseases and, 93–94, 132; safety features for mitigation of, 236*b*, 246*b*; stress on plant and animal life from, 137; structural and moisture damage from, 136; SUDS installation for, 188*b*, 188*f*, 190*f*; Uberlândia housing development and, 217*b*; vector-borne diseases and, 136–37; vulnerability to, 140–41, 217*b*, 234*b*; water quantity and quality, 136

Floth Headquarters (Brisbane), 245, 252–53*b*
food insecurity, 50*b*, 104, 128, 133, 137, 152, 155, 227*b*
forest preservation, 9*b*, 10–11*t*, 12–13*f*
for-profit development projects, 230, 232–33*b*, 238–39*b*
425 Park Avenue (New York), 232–33*b*
Frieden, Thomas, 26
Frumkin, Howard, 2

Genentech Employee Center (South San Francisco), 245, 248–49*b*
gentrification, 69, 178, 182*b*, 184*b*, 236*b*, 273
Geographic Information Systems (GIS), 202–3, 205
geographic scales, 52, 53*f*
GHGs. *See* greenhouse gases
Gillett Square (London), 182–84*b*, 182*f*
Global Health Observatory (WHO), 44, 45
global warming. *See* climate change
government: data set availability from, 53; tax-credit and loan programs, 31. *See also* local government
Green Alley Program (Chicago), 177*b*
green and healthy buildings: affordable housing projects as, 31, 32; ArchEPI framework for, 21–22, 22*f*; building information modeling for, 202–4; community planning for, 21; construction documents for, 206; environmental stewardship and, 176*b*, 191; expansion of definition of, 268; health promotion through design, 28; indoor air quality of, 179*b*, 216*b*; mainstreaming of, 267; occupant health benefits, 30; project delivery process for, 21–22, 22*f*; tax-credit and loan programs for, 31
Green Guide for Health Care, 3, 191
greenhouse gases (GHGs), 9*b*, 23, 123, 125, 146, 154, 268
green space, 86, 120–23, 128, 137–38
grey literature, 273. *See also Technical Appendix online, p. 34*
Griffintown District (Montreal), 215*b*
ground-level ozone, 86, 119, 124, 141, 144–45
Guyer Problem-Solving Framework, 41–43, 66–67, 69, 77

Harvard University: Climate Action Plan, 8, 9–15*b*, 10–11*t*, 12–15*f*; Science and Engineering Complex, 236–37*b*
HEAL (Healthy Eating and Active Living) strategies, 254
health: built environment and, 5–6, 24–29, 25*f*, 39; computer software programs for promotion of, 202–5; sustainability and, 3, 191, 192–94*t*. *See also* community health; environmental health; mental health; population health; public health
health, safety, and welfare (HSW), 24, 33, 270
Health and Wellness District at Frisco Station (Texas), 245, 246–47*b*
health data: aggregated, 44; on cardiovascular diseases, 50*b*; for design and operations, 28–33, 39; facilities management and, 216; project delivery process objections to, 39; public health definitions, 45
health equity, 6, 8, 69, 80*f*, 178, 195, 206
health equity impact assessments (HEIAs), 69, 178
health impact assessments (HIAs): Aerotropolis Atlanta, 200*b*; Bruce Elementary School, 25, 26*f*, 61–62*b*, 61*t*; Cincinnati bridge demolition, 215*b*; communicating results of, 73; defined, 69, 273; Jack London Gateway project,

198*b*; North Houston Highway Improvement Project, 47–48*f*; in schematic design phase, 195; South Lincoln redevelopment, 32; time needed for completion of, 33
health impact pyramid, 26–28, 27*f*, 34
Health in All Policies (HiAP) approach, 69
health mission statements, 191–94, 192–94*t*, 196*b*, 273
health outcomes: air quality and, 61*t*; ArchEPI and, 20, 21; assessment of, 31, 32, 44–45; built environment and, 49–52, 50*b*; chronic diseases and, 30; disparities in, 20; environmental exposures and, 42–43, 46; from extreme heat, 50*b*, 52, 61*t*; health data on, 39; legal position on, 38; vulnerability to climate change and, 57*t*; wrong pocket syndrome and, 35
health situation analyses (HSAs): Aerotropolis Atlanta, 201*b*; Bond University School of Sustainable Development, 243*b*; Bon Pastor redevelopment, 189*b*; Buckingham County Primary and Elementary Schools, 228*b*; Chai Wan campus, 214*b*; communicating results of, 73; defined, 43, 174, 273; Dell Children's Hospital, 258*b*; of environmental conditions, 44–45, 175*b*; EPHIs and, 175, 195; Family Health Center on Virginia, 197*b*; Floth Headquarters, 253*b*; 425 Park Avenue, 233*b*; Genentech Employee Center, 249*b*; Gillett Square, 183*b*; Harvard University Science and Engineering Complex, 237*b*; Health and Wellness District at Frisco Station, 247*b*; Heerema Marine Contractors B.V. Headquarters, 239*b*; High Point redevelopment, 186*b*; Jack London Gateway project, 199*b*; JLL Shanghai Office, 251*b*; mapping technology for, 176*b*; New Karolinska Solna University Hospital, 260*b*; in programming/visioning phase, 174–78, 175–77*b*, 194–95; St. Antony's School, 208*b*; Santa Monica City Hall East, 235*b*; scale of development, 255; South Bronx Neighborhood, 180*b*; Texas Woman's University Master Plan, 261*b*, 262–63*f*; time needed for completion of, 33; Uberlândia housing development, 218*b*; value generation and, 36; Vancouver Convention Centre West, 241*b*; Via Verde housing complex, 211*b*
healthy buildings. *See* green and healthy buildings
Healthy Eating and Active Living (HEAL) strategies, 254
Healthy Housing Rewards program, 31
Healthy Neighborhoods Equity Fund (HNEF), 31, 255
Healthy People 2030 (US Health and Human Services Department), 6, 44, 55–56, 265, 266
heart attacks, 50*b*, 83, 86, 101
heart disease. *See* cardiovascular diseases
heat. *See* extreme heat; urban heat islands
Heerema Marine Contractors B.V. Headquarters (Leiden), 238–39*b*
HEIAs (health equity impact assessments), 69, 178
HiAP (Health in All Policies) approach, 69
HIAs. *See* health impact assessments
hierarchy of controls (HOC), 27, 28*f*, 34
high blood pressure. *See* hypertension
High Point redevelopment (Seattle), 185–87*b*, 185*f*, 187*f*
HNEF (Healthy Neighborhoods Equity Fund), 31, 255
homelessness, 94, 119, 128, 129, 141, 157, 166
housing: affordable, 31, 32, 179*b*, 206, 254, 256–57*b*; primitive and substandard, 97, 148, 166–67
HSAs. *See* health situation analyses

HSW (health, safety, and welfare), 24, 33, 270
hurricanes. *See* disasters/storms
hypertension: air quality and, 102; built environment and, 82, 82*t*, 102; cardiovascular diseases and, 88; climate change and, 101–2; Community Health Initiative and, 176*b*; community planning and, 103; diagnosis of, 101; disasters/storms and, 102, 149, 156; extreme heat and, 102; infographic on, 98–99; mortality rate, 100; obesity and, 97; prevalence of, 100; symptoms of, 101, 101*t*; vulnerability to, 82, 103–6

IgCC (International Green Construction Code), 24
immunocompromised persons, 96, 110–11, 147, 156, 165
Indigenous populations. *See* minorities and Indigenous populations
indoor air quality: cardiovascular diseases and, 86; extreme heat and, 50*b*; of green and healthy buildings, 179*b*, 216*b*; health care costs and, 31; LEED standards for, 204*b*, 204*f*, 216*b*; respiratory diseases and, 94; St. Antony's School and, 207*b*; Uberlândia housing development and, 217*b*
industrial pollution, 94, 120, 176*b*
infectious diseases: airborne, 16, 81, 270; environmental exposures and, 81; waterborne, 81, 132, 153, 175, 177*b*, 205, 217*b*, 270. *See also* vector-borne diseases; *specific diseases*
infographics: air quality, 142–43; cancer, 108–9; cardiovascular diseases, 84–85; diabetes, 98–99; disasters/storms, 150–51; extreme heat, 126–27; flooding, 130–31; hypertension, 98–99; mental health, 116–17; obesity, 98–99; respiratory diseases, 90–91; vector-borne diseases, 158–59
Integrated Project Delivery model, 224*t*, 226, 230
Intergovernmental Panel on Climate Change (IPCC), 125, 133, 146
International Green Construction Code (IgCC), 24
investment models. *See* real estate investment models

Jack London Gateway project (West Oakland), 198–99*b*, 198*f*
JLL Shanghai Office, 245, 250–51*b*
Joint Call to Action to Promote Healthy Communities (2017), 6, 38

Kaiser Permanente: Community Health Initiative, 176*b*; health mission statement for, 191
Kentucky Climate Center, 133–34, 135*f*

last mile problem, 34–35, 38
LEED (Leadership in Energy and Environmental Design) certification: building information modeling and, 205; Gold Certification, 30–31, 210*b*, 259*b*, 265; Healthcare rating system, 191; health impact assessment credits and, 6; indoor air quality and, 204*b*, 204*f*, 216*b*; operational revenue and, 30–31; Platinum Certification, 179*b*, 216*b*, 236*b*, 256*b*; regional priority credits and, 4, 5*f*; schematic design phase and, 195; Silver Certification, 179*b*
life expectancy, 20–21, 31, 81, 94, 96
literature and literature reviews, 29, 42, 62*b*, 66–69, 73, 124, 273, 274
Living Building Challenge, 139–40, 195, 205, 206, 234*b*, 236*b*

local government: Aerotropolis Atlanta and, 200*b*; Bon Pastor redevelopment and, 190*b*; Buckingham County Primary and Elementary Schools and, 227*b*; Chai Wan campus and, 212*b*; climate change commitments by, 23, 268; Dell Children's Hospital and, 257*b*; Family Health Center on Virginia and, 196*b*; Floth Headquarters and, 252*b*; Gillett Square and, 184*b*; Harvard University Science and Engineering Complex and, 236*b*; Health and Wellness District at Frisco Station and, 246*b*; Heerema Marine Contractors B.V. Headquarters and, 238*b*; High Point redevelopment and, 187*b*; Jack London Gateway project and, 198*b*; JLL Shanghai Office and, 250*b*; New Karolinska Solna University Hospital and, 259*b*; St. Antony's School and, 207*b*; Santa Monica City Hall East and, 234*b*; South Bronx Neighborhood and, 181*b*; Uberlândia housing development and, 219*b*; value streams for, 28, 35–38, 37*t*; Vancouver Convention Centre West, 240*b*; Via Verde housing complex and, 210*b*
lung cancer: air quality and, 94, 110; mortality rate, 89, 92, 106; smoking and, 96, 112; symptoms of, 93, 93*t*, 107, 110*t*; vulnerability to, 97, 112–14
Lyme disease, 124, 157, 160–61, 161*t*, 163–67, 163*t*

malaria, 89, 97, 153, 160–67, 161*t*, 163*t*
measurement and verification (M&V) programs, 215–16, 219
mental health: air pollution and, 119–22, 147; ArchEPI and, 23; built environment and, 120; cancer diagnosis and, 107, 112–13; cardiovascular diseases and, 88; chronic diseases and, 121–22, 147; climate change and, 119–20; cognitive ability and, 114–15, 118*t*, 119–21; community planning and, 120; cross-departmental collaboration and, 250*b*; daylighting and, 207*b*, 232*b*, 234*b*, 236*b*, 238*b*, 242*b*, 246*b*, 248*b*, 259*b*; diabetes and, 105; disasters/storms and, 120, 153, 156; extreme heat and, 52, 119, 124, 128; flooding and, 120, 133; hypertension and, 105; impact on physical health, 81; infographic on, 116–17; obesity and, 104–5; respiratory diseases and, 96; Sustainable Development Goals on, 268; vulnerability to issues with, 120–23. *See also* behavioral disorders; mood disorders
methane gas-to-electricity plants, 9*b*, 10–11*t*, 12–13*f*
minorities and Indigenous populations: air pollution and, 148; cancer and, 113; cardiovascular diseases and, 88; diabetes and, 105; disasters/storms and, 156; extreme heat and, 128–29; flooding and, 140; hypertension and, 105; mental health and, 122; obesity and, 105; respiratory diseases and, 96–97; vector-borne diseases and, 166
Montrose Whole Foods Market (Houston), 51, 51*f*
mood disorders: prevalence of, 115; PTSD, 115, 118, 118*t*, 120, 153, 156; symptoms of, 115, 118, 118*t*. *See also* anxiety
mosquito-borne diseases, 89, 97, 111, 124, 132–33, 137, 153, 157, 160–67, 161*t*, 163*t*. *See also specific diseases*
mouth cancer, 107, 110*t*

narrative literature reviews, 66–68
NASA Sustainability Base project (Ames Research Center), 203*b*, 203*f*
National Environmental Public Health Tracking System, 50*b*, 64*b*, 64*f*, 269

National Health Service (NHS), 191, 192–94*t*
National Institute of Building Sciences, 202
natural disasters. *See* disasters/storms
natural environment determinants of health, 49, 50*b*, 61*t*
New Karolinska Solna University Hospital (Solna, Sweden), 254, 259–60*b*
Nightingale, Florence, 29
noise pollution, 24, 212*b*
non-communicable diseases. *See* chronic diseases; *specific diseases*
non-profit development projects, 230–31, 236–37*b*, 242–43*b*
North Houston Highway Improvement Project (NHHIP), 47–48*f*

obesity: air quality and, 102; built environment and, 82, 82*t*, 102; cancer and, 112; cardiovascular diseases and, 87; climate change and, 101–2; community planning, 103; diabetes and, 97; extreme heat and, 102; hypertension and, 97; infographic on, 98–99; measurement of, 100; mortality rate, 100; musculoskeletal pain and, 81; prevalence of, 23, 97, 179*b*, 227*b*; prevention strategies, 234*b*, 236*b*, 240*b*, 242*b*, 246*b*, 248*b*, 250*b*, 257*b*, 259*b*; symptoms of, 101, 101*t*; vulnerability to, 82, 103–6
occupancy phase, 22*f*, 215–16, 219
occupational exposure and cancer, 106, 114
older adults. *See* elderly populations
operations. *See* design, construction, and operations
oppositional defiant disorder (ODD), 115, 118, 118*t*
overnutrition, 87, 104, 112
owner-occupied development projects, 244–45, 248–49*b*, 252–53*b*
ozone, ground-level, 86, 119, 124, 141, 144–45

Paris Climate Agreement (2015), 6, 23, 265, 267–68
participatory action research, 44, 55, 219*b*, 274
particulate matter (PM): air quality and, 141, 144, 144*t*; cancer and, 110; cardiovascular diseases and, 86, 87; construction sector and, 215*b*; distance-decay gradients, 145, 145*f*; health effects of, 145; mental health and, 119–21; mitigation strategies, 9*b*, 25, 266; monitoring programs, 215*b*; respiratory diseases and, 94; traffic-related air pollution and, 176*b*
payback period, 230, 232*b*, 234*b*
PDMs. *See* project delivery models
peer-reviewed literature, 274. *See also Technical Appendix online, p. 34*
philanthropy, core competencies for, 6, 7*t*, 40, 46, 54, 66, 70, 77, 220, 264
physical environment. *See* built environment
PLACES data portal (CDC), 50*b*, 56, 269
PM. *See* particulate matter
POEs. *See* post-occupancy evaluations
pollution: industrial, 94, 120, 176*b*; noise, 24, 212*b*; soil, 236*b*, 240*b*; water, 240*b*. *See also* air pollution
population, defined, 19, 274
population health: built environment and, 24; call to action for promotion of, 6; carbon offset projects and, 9*b*, 13*f*; data sets for, 32, 52, 178; design, construction, operations

and, 2, 9*b*, 29; location-based interventions, 176*b*; profit generation and, 29–32; vulnerability data and, 33

post-occupancy evaluations (POEs): in ArchEPI assessments, 70, 74; Bond University School of Sustainable Development, 242*b*; Buckingham County Primary and Elementary Schools, 227*b*; Dell Children's Hospital, 257*b*; Genentech Employee Center, 248*b*; health data integrated into, 219; High Point redevelopment, 185*b*; in occupany phase, 215–16; Raleigh elementary schools, 75–76*t*, 75*b*; Uberlândia housing development, 217*b*

post-traumatic stress disorder (PTSD), 115, 118, 118t, 120, 153, 156

poverty: air pollution and, 147–48; cancer and, 113–14; cardiovascular diseases and, 89; diabetes and, 105–6; disasters/storms and, 156; extreme heat and, 129; flooding and, 140–41; hypertension and, 105–6; mental health and, 122; obesity and, 105–6; respiratory diseases and, 97; vector-borne diseases and, 165–66

PPPs (public-private partnerships), 182*b*, 254–55, 256–60*b*

pregnancy: extreme heat and, 128; flooding and, 140; vector-borne diseases and, 162, 165

privacy issues, 39, 44, 52, 54, 63, 216

professional codes of conduct, 33

programming/visioning phase: ArchEPI during, 74, 191, 194–95; for green and healthy buildings, 22*f*; health mission statements in, 191–94, 192–94*t*, 196*b*; health situation analyses in, 174–78, 175–77*b*, 194–95; physical context and, 175; regulatory context and, 178; social context and, 178

programs, defined, 174, 274

project delivery, defined, 173, 274

project delivery models (PDMs), 221–26; CM-at-Risk, 224*t*, 225–26; defined, 221, 274; Design-Bid-Build, 174, 222, 223*t*; Design-Build, 223*t*, 224–25; Integrated Project Delivery, 224*t*, 226, 230

project delivery process, 173–220; case examples, 179–90*b*, 196–201*b*, 207–8*b*, 210–14*b*; construction administration phase, 22*f*, 74, 209; construction documents phase, 22*f*, 74, 206, 209; core competencies for, 220; design development phase, 22*f*, 74, 202–6, 203–4*b*; for green and healthy buildings, 21–22, 22*f*; health-promoting strategies in, 6; integration of ArchEPI into, 74, 174; objections to health data for, 39; occupancy phase, 22*f*, 215–16, 219; programming/visioning phase, 22*f*, 74, 174–78, 175–77*b*, 191–95, 192–94*t*; schematic design phase, 22*f*, 74, 195; variation among projects, 173, 174

PTSD. *See* post-traumatic stress disorder

publication bias, 68

public health: built environment and, 5–6, 24, 25*f*, 39; collaboration in, 5–6, 270–71; data definitions, 45; digital revolution in, 202; Geographic Information Systems in, 203; integrative design process and, 227*b*; problem-solving in, 41–42; real estate development and, 270–71; as social contract, 24

public-private partnerships (PPPs), 182*b*, 254–55, 256–60*b*

public-sector development projects, 230–31, 234–35*b*, 240–41*b*

quality control and improvement, 209, 225

race. *See* minorities and Indigenous populations

real estate, defined, 2, 274

real estate development: collaboration in, 5–6, 270–71; core competencies, 6, 7*t*, 40, 46, 54, 66, 70, 77, 220, 264; digital revolution in, 202; economic interests in, 35; external forces impacting, 267–68; for-profit, 230, 232–33*b*, 238–39*b*; futureproofing in, 31–32, 178, 236*b*; health impact pyramid and, 26, 27*f*; last mile problem and, 34–35, 38; non-profit, 230–31, 236–37*b*, 242–43*b*; payback period in, 230, 232*b*, 234*b*; profit generation in, 29–32; project-specific interests in, 35; public health and, 270–71; public sector, 230–31, 234–35*b*, 240–41*b*; regional priority credits for, 4, 5*f*; scale of development, 255; site analyses, 32, 43–44, 174–75, 178; site selection process, 21, 141, 146, 174–75; value streams for, 28, 30, 35–38, 37*t*; wrong pocket syndrome and, 35, 38. *See also* development teams; project delivery models; project delivery process; real estate investment models

real estate investment models, 230–60; for-profit developments, 230, 232–33*b*, 238–39*b*; non-profit developments, 230–31, 236–37*b*, 242–43*b*; owner-occupied development projects and, 244–45, 248–49*b*, 252–53*b*; public-private partnerships, 182*b*, 254–55, 256–60*b*; public-sector developments, 230–31, 234–35*b*, 240–41*b*; speculative development projects and, 244, 245, 246–47*b*, 250–51*b*

recovery and remediation workers, 141, 157

redlining, 36, 148

regional priority credits (RPCs), 4, 5*f*

resilience: of built environment, 32; to climate change, 191; community, 23, 175, 217*b*; enhancement of, 31–32, 42; to environmental hazards, 51; to extreme heat, 182*b*; of utilities and infrastructure to flooding, 136

respiratory diseases: acute lower respiratory infections, 89, 92, 93, 93*t*, 95–97; air quality and, 94, 178; built environment and, 82, 82*t*, 94; climate change and, 93–94; community planning and, 94–95; COPD, 89, 92–97, 93*t*, 144–45, 147; disasters/storms and, 93–94, 149, 153; extreme heat and, 52, 93, 124; flooding and, 93–94, 132; infographic on, 90–91; lung cancer, 89, 92–94, 93*t*, 96–97, 106; symptoms of, 92–93, 93*t*; TRAP exposure and, 176*b*, 178; tuberculosis, 89, 92, 93, 93*t*, 96–97, 149; vulnerability to, 82, 95–97. *See also* asthma

return on investment (ROI), 30, 221, 230

risk factors. *See* vulnerability

RPCs (regional priority credits), 4, 5*f*

rural areas, 97, 113, 121, 123, 133, 137

St. Antony's School (Gudalur, India), 207–8*b*, 207*f*

sanitation movement, 23–24, 81, 269

Sanitation Options for Sustainable Housing (SOSH) tool, 177*b*

Santa Monica City Hall East, 231, 234–35*b*

scale of development, 255

schematic design phase, 22*f*, 74, 195

SDGs. *See* Sustainable Development Goals

sedentary lifestyle, 82, 87, 97, 103, 104, 107, 112, 270

Single Overriding Health Communication Objectives (SOHCOs), 73–74

site analyses, 32, 43–44, 174–75, 178
site selection process, 21, 141, 146, 174–75
smoking: cancer and, 112; cardiovascular diseases and, 88; diabetes and, 104; hypertension and, 104; obesity and, 104; respiratory diseases and, 96
Snow, John, 24, 29
social determinants of health: defined, 20, 274; design and operations in relation to, 26, 27; environmental exposures and, 20; health disparities and, 20–21, 69; in neighborhoods, 31; POEs and, 75–76t, 75b; role of building sector in addressing, 268; site analyses and, 178; WHO on, 28
social epidemiology, 20, 20t, 21f, 274
social equity, 2, 43, 49, 52, 69, 128, 264
SOHCOs (Single Overriding Health Communication Objectives), 73–74
soil pollution, 236b, 240b
solar arrays: buffering and, 63; Bullitt Center and, 205; flooding and, 139; Gillett Square and, 182b; Harvard University Climate Action Plan and, 8, 9b, 10–11t, 12–13f; Santa Monica City Hall East and, 234b; South Bronx Neighborhood and, 180b; Via Verde housing complex and, 210b
Soman, Dilip, 34
SOSH (Sanitation Options for Sustainable Housing) tool, 177b
South Bronx Neighborhood (New York), 179–81b, 179f, 181f
South Lincoln redevelopment (Denver), 32
speculative development projects, 244, 245, 246–47b, 250–51b
stakeholders: prioritization of health concerns for, 44; trust and credibility established with, 72–73. See also community groups; development teams; local government
storms. See disasters/storms
stroke, 82–88, 83t, 101, 115, 145, 200b
sustainability: ArchEPI assessments and, 52; building information modeling and, 204; core competencies, 6, 7t, 40, 46, 54, 66, 68, 70, 77, 220, 264; health and, 3, 191, 192–94t; project-specific interests and, 35
Sustainable Development Goals (SDGs), 6, 44–45, 50b, 56, 60, 132, 137, 268
sustainable urban drainage systems (SUDS), 188b, 188f, 190f
systematic literature reviews, 67–68

Technological and Higher Education Institute Chai Wan campus (Hong Kong), 212–13f, 212–14b
Texas Woman's University Master Plan (Denton), 261–62b, 262–63f
throat cancer, 107, 110t
tick-borne disease. See Lyme disease
traffic-related air pollution (TRAP): built environment and, 146; cardiovascular diseases and, 86, 178; diabetes and, 102; mitigation strategies, 9b, 25, 62b, 147, 266; obesity and, 102; project-specific interests and, 35; proximity to busy roads and, 24, 64b, 234b, 256b; respiratory diseases and, 94, 178; street canyons and, 176b
tropical cyclones. See disasters/storms
tuberculosis (TB), 89, 92, 93, 93t, 96–97, 149

Uberlândia housing development (Minas Gerais, Brazil), 217–19b, 217f
unconscious bias, 68

United Nations: country-level data sets, 53; Sustainable Development Goals, 6, 44–45, 50b, 56, 60, 132, 137, 268
Upstream Thinking program, 137
urban heat islands: air pollution and, 146; car-centric land use and, 86, 102, 120; climate change vulnerability and, 60; extreme heat and, 50b, 125; measurement of, 53; mitigation strategies, 33, 51, 62b, 128, 188b, 236b, 257b; project-specific interests and, 35
US Green Building Council, 4, 33
US National Climate Assessment, 125, 134

value engineering (VE), 206, 209, 210b
Vancouver Convention Centre West, 231, 240–41b
vector-borne diseases: built environment and, 164; cancer and, 110–11; climate change and, 124, 157, 158–60; community planning and, 164–65; dengue virus, 111, 132–33, 137, 153, 160–67, 161t, 163t; disasters/storms and, 153; flooding and, 136–37; health effects of, 160–62, 163t; infographic on, 158–59; Lyme disease, 124, 157, 160–61, 161t, 163–67, 163t; malaria, 89, 97, 153, 160–67, 161t, 163t; mitigation strategies, 270; prevalence of, 157, 161t; vulnerability to, 165, 167t; West Nile virus, 157, 160–65, 161t, 163t, 167; Zika virus, 111, 124, 137, 160–67, 161t, 163t
Via Verde housing complex (New York), 210–11b, 210f
visioning. See programming/visioning phase
vulnerability: to air pollution, 147–48; to cancer, 97, 111–14; to cardiovascular diseases, 87–89; to climate change, 56b, 57–59t, 60; data on, 29, 31–33, 205; to diabetes, 82, 103–6; to disasters/storms, 155–57; EPHIs and, 51; to extreme heat, 128–29, 175b, 217b; to flooding, 140–41, 217b, 234b; to heat, 175b, 256b; to hypertension, 82, 103–6; to mental health conditions, 120–23; to obesity, 82, 103–6; to respiratory diseases, 82, 95–97; social, 234b; to vector-borne diseases, 165–67

waterborne diseases, 81, 132, 153, 175, 177b, 205, 217b, 270
water pollution, 240b
WELL certification: building information modeling and, 205; health impact assessment credits and, 6; Health-Safety Rating, 2; operational revenue and, 30; as real estate portfolio goal, 191; schematic design phase and, 195
West Nile virus (WNV), 157, 160–65, 161t, 163t, 167
wicked problems, 3, 123, 124
World Bank, 53, 137
World Health Organization (WHO): on cancer deaths, 106, 110; on cholesterol, 87; on chronic diseases, 81; country-level data sets, 53; on COVID-19 deaths, 81; on determinants of health, 28; on flooding, 129; Global Health Observatory, 44, 45; health data portal, 50b; on hypertension, 100; on mental health conditions, 114; on particulate matter, 86, 141, 144, 144t, 145; on respiratory diseases, 94; on smoking deaths, 96; on vector-borne diseases, 157, 160, 162, 165
wrong pocket syndrome, 35, 38

Zika virus, 111, 124, 137, 160–67, 161t, 163t
zoning codes, 35, 178, 266

Explore other books from HOPKINS PRESS

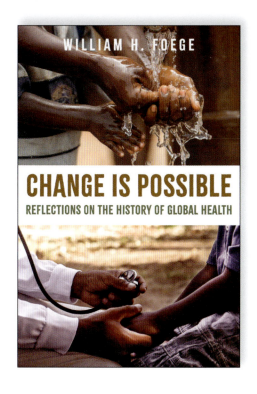
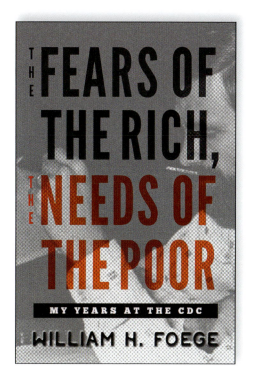
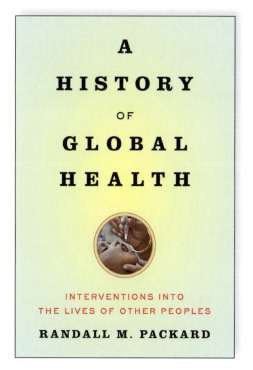